Atlas of
Surgery
of the
Facial Nerve

An Otolaryngologist's Perspective

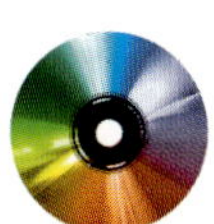

System requirement:
- **Windows XP or above**
- **Power DVD player (Software)**
- **Windows media player 11.0 version or above (Software)**

Accompanying DVD ROM is playable only in Computer and not in DVD player.

Kindly wait for few seconds for DVD ROM to autorun. If it does not autorun then please do the following:
- Click on my computer
- Click the **CD/DVD drive** and after opening the drive, kindly double click the file **Jaypee**

DVD Contents

Atlas of Surgery of the Facial Nerve

An Otolaryngologist's Perspective

SECOND EDITION

DS Grewal
MS DLO FACS FIAO
Former Professor and Head
Department of ENT and Head and Neck Surgery
TN Medical College and BYL Nair Charitable Hospital, Mumbai, Maharashtra, India
President, Association of Otolaryngologists of India (AOI)–2005
E-mail: *drdsgrewal@rediffmail.com*

Foreword
O Nuri Özgirgin

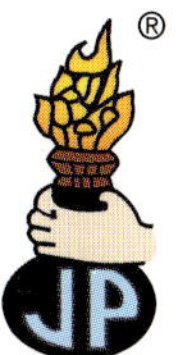

JAYPEE BROTHERSS MEDICAL PUBLISHERS (P) LTD
New Delhi • Panama City • London

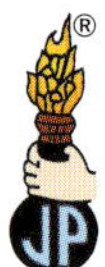

Jaypee Brothers Medical Publishers (P) Ltd

Headquarter

Jaypee Brothers Medical Publishers (P) Ltd
4838/24, Ansari Road, Daryaganj
New Delhi 110 002, India
Phone: +91-11-43574357
Fax: +91-11-43574314
Email: jaypee@jaypeebrothers.com

Overseas Offices

JP Medical Ltd
83 Victoria Street, London
SW1H 0HW (UK)
Phone: +44-2031708910
Fax: +02-03-0086180
Email: info@jpmedpub.com

Jaypee-Highlights Medical Publishers Inc
City of Knowledge, Bld. 237, Clayton
Panama City, Panama
Phone: 507-301-0496
Fax: +50-73-010499
Email: cservice@jphmedical.com

Website: www.jaypeebrothers.com
Website: www.jaypeedigital.com

Atlas of Surgery of the Facial Nerve

First Edition: 2006
Second Edition: **2012**

ISBN: 978-93-5025-789-0

Printed at: Ajanta Offset & Packagings Ltd., New Delhi

Dedicated to

My father, Prof Dr GS Grewal, an ENT Surgeon par excellence
My mother, Daljit Grewal
Robule, my wife
Dr Amrit Sandhu, Dr Jasbir Grewal, my sisters
Dr Milan Sangha
and all my students

Contributors

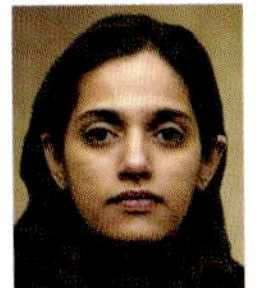

Aditi N Modi
Specialist Registrar, Anesthesia
James Paget University Hospital
East of England Deanery
Norfolk, UK

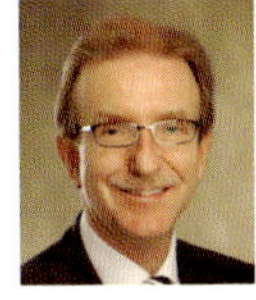

David Moffat
Consultant
Otoneurological and
Skull Base Surgery, Box 48
Addenbrooke's, Cambridge University
Teaching Hospitals NHS Trust
Hills Road, Cambridge CB2 2QQ, UK

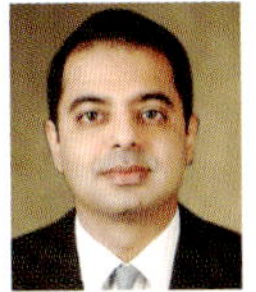

Alok Mohorikar
ENT Registrar
Royal Darwin Hospital
Northern Territory, Australia

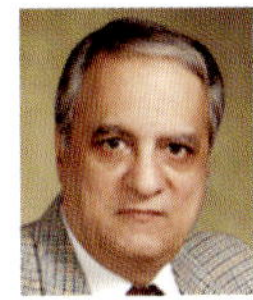

DS Grewal
Former Professor and Head
Department of ENT and
Head and Neck Surgery
TN Medical College and
BYL Nair Charitable Hospital
Mumbai, Maharashtra, India
President, Association of
Otolaryngologists of India (AOI)–2005

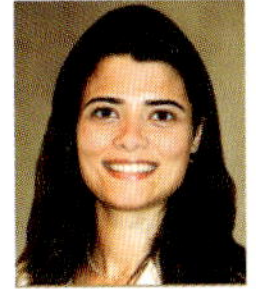

Anna Carolina O Fonseca
Fellow in Otology and Skull Base Surgery
Department of Otorhinolaryngology
Faculty of Medicine
University of Sao Paulo, Brazil

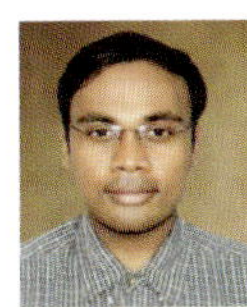

Ganeshan
Post MS Resident
Department of ENT
Head and Neck Surgery
Grant Medical College and
Sir JJ Group of Hospitals
Mumbai, Maharashtra, India

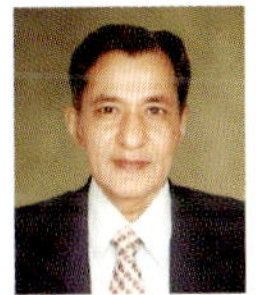

Ashok Shah
Hon Professor and Head
Department of Plastic Surgery
Grant Medical College and
Sir JJ Group of Hospitals
Consultant Plastic Surgeon
Harkisandas Hospital Breach Candy Hospital
Mumbai, Maharashtra, India

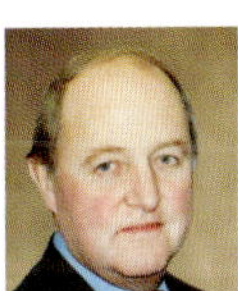

Guy Kenyon
Senior Consultant
Wipps Cross University Hospital, London
Former Editor and now Emeritus Editor
Journal of Laryngology and Otology, UK

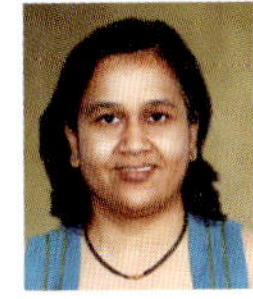

CM Deshpande
Professor
Department of Anesthesiology
TN Medical College and
BYL Nair Charitable Hospital
Mumbai, Maharashtra, India

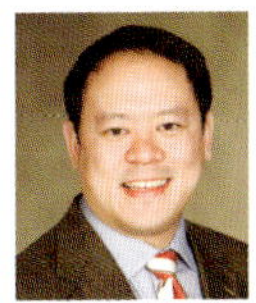

James Lin
Assistant Professor
Otology and Neurotology
Louisiana State University
Health Sciences Center
Department of Otolaryngology
Head and Neck Surgery
New Orleans, Louisiana 70112, USA

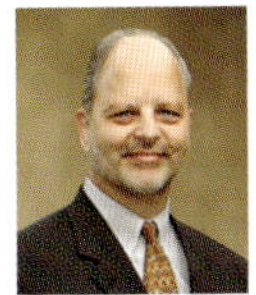

Daniel W Nuss
George D Lyons Professor and Chairman
Head Neck Surgical Oncology and
Skull Base Surgery
Louisiana State University
Health Sciences Center
Department of Otolaryngology
Head and Neck Surgery
New Orleans, Louisiana 70112, USA

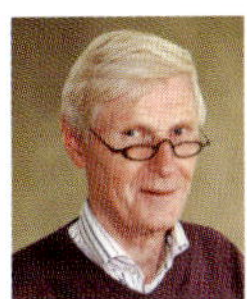

JJ Manni
Professor
Department of Otolaryngology
Head and Neck Surgery
University of Maastricht
Maastricht, The Netherlands

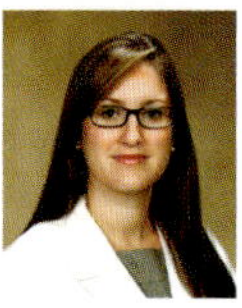

Laura Hetzler
Assistant Professor
Facial Plastics and Reconstructive Surgery
Louisiana State University
Health Sciences Center
Department of Otolaryngology
Head and Neck Surgery
New Orleans, Louisiana 70112, USA

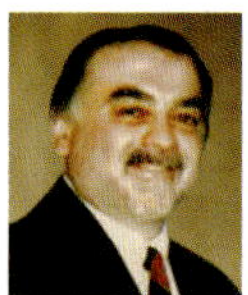

Mohan Jagade
Professor and Head
Department of ENT
Head and Neck Surgery
Grant Medical College and
Sir JJ Group of Hospitals
Mumbai, Maharashtra, India

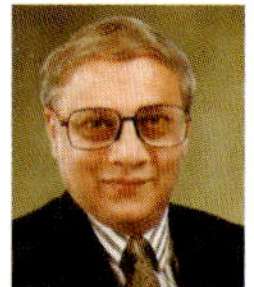

Narendra Pandya
Honorary Surgeon Commodore
Diplomate, American Board of Plastic Surgery
Hon Cosmetic Surgeon, Jaslok Hospital
Breach Candy Hospital
Ex Hon Professor of Plastic Surgery
TN Medical College and
BYL Nair Charitable Hospital
Mumbai, Maharashtra, India

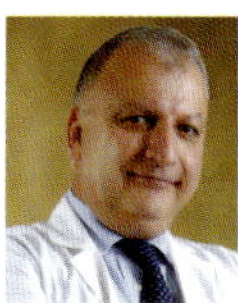

O Nuri Özgirgin
Department of ENT
Bayindir Hospital, Ankara, Turkey
Editor, The Journal of International
Advanced Otology
President, Politzer Society

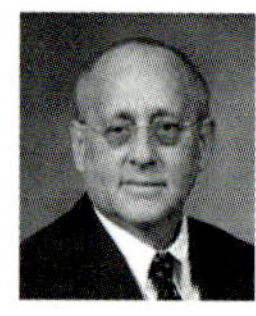

Peter D Oliver
Louisiana State University
Department of Cell Biology and Anatomy
New Orleans, Louisiana 70112, USA

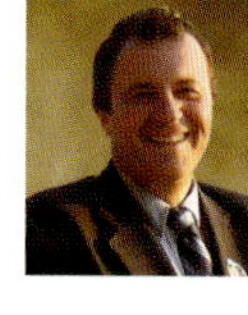

Ricardo F Bento
Professor and Chairman
Department of Otorhinolaryngology
Faculty of Medicine
University of Sao Paulo, Brazil

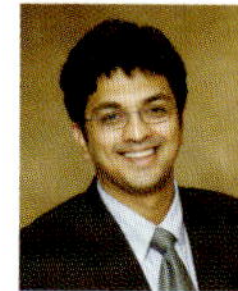

Rohan R Walvekar
Assistant Professor
Head Neck Surgical Oncology
Skull Base Surgery and Sialendoscopy
Louisiana State University
Health Sciences Center
Department of Otolaryngology
Head and Neck Surgery
New Orleans, Louisiana 70112, USA

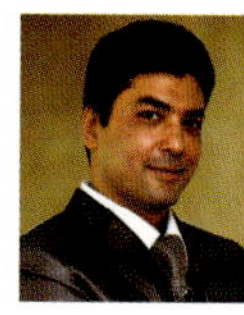

Syed Mohammad Hashmi
Consultant
BCJ Hospital and Asha
Parekh Research Centre
Teaching Faculty
Tibia Medical College and Kalsekar Hospital
Mumbai, Maharashtra, India

Foreword

The facial nerve as it functions, the mimics of the face is very important in expressing the feelings, emotions and social behavior. The face, the beauty, mimics, smile are the expressions that we build-up our individual relations on. Fear, anger, surprise, contempt, disgust, happiness, and sadness, are all expressed in the same manner regardless of culture. Charles Darwin noted in his book "The Expression of the Emotions in Man and Animals" ... the young and the old of widely different races, both with man and animals, express the same state of mind by the same movements.

The course of the facial nerve that contributes these functions is mainly in the ear, and this makes the temporal bone unique only for ear surgeons. Evolution of ear surgery in regard to allowing patients better quality of life has focused the attention on the facial nerve. One of the primary tasks for a resident before starting for the ear surgery is to learn the anatomy of the facial nerve and explore it in temporal bones.

The book which is dedicated to the facial nerve and its abnormalities will reserve its place in the bookshelves of the ear surgeons and physicians to be the primary reference tool for their professional life.

I appreciate the work done by Dr Grewal and congratulate for publishing such an important guide for understanding and treating the facial nerve diseases.

O Nuri Özgirgin
Department of ENT
Bayindir Hospital, Ankara, Turkey
Editor, The Journal of International Advanced Otology
President, Politzer Society

Preface to the Second Edition

I am very happy to bring out the second edition of *Atlas of Surgery of the Facial Nerve*. Whilst preparing this, many thoughts came to my mind, I believe in Sir William Osler saying—a person deep versed in books may not be able to use his knowledge to practical effect, or more likely his failures are not because he has studied books much, but because he has not studied men more. Keeping this in mind, I prepared the second edition of Atlas as a balance between books and practical knowledge required to diagnose and treat the patients of facial nerve disorders, so that the book becomes a simulator like tool and thereby gives the reader the experience to gain practical knowledge.

To achieve this:

1. I added two DVDs which cover various aspects of surgery of facial nerve thereby providing insight into surgical techniques commonly used in a simple and straightforward manner. I feel this has an advantage as they can be seen at leisure and also repeatedly if required.
2. I requested more of my colleagues to contribute to the Atlas and/or DVD. I am grateful to all of them as they have enthusiasm, deep love and full knowledge of the subject and a desire to teach. They have a sense of obligation, a feeling that compels a teacher to be a contributor.
3. Revised and updated the existing chapters.

I would like to thank Dr Syed Mohammad Hashmi for drawing sketches for the book for chapters written by myself, Dr Mohan Jagade, Dr Narendra Pandya and Dr Ashok Shah. I would also like to thank Dr Rohan Walvekar, Dr Alok Mohorikar, Sanjay Chabria, Kaushal Sheth, Rajiv Manudhane for their help, and Dinaz Irani and Brandon Hitchcock for contributing photographs of the Surgery of the Parotid Gland.

I am grateful to all the Deans and staff of the ENT Department, TN Medical College and BYL Nair Charitable Hospital, Mumbai, Maharashtra, India, during my tenure where I worked for nearly 32 years. Professor Ninad Gaikward has been always extremely helpful to me.

I am also grateful to Dr O Nuri Özgirgin for writing the foreword and my teacher Dr LH Hiranandani, who was my constant source of inspiration.

It is well said that we are not here to get all we can out of life for ourselves but try to make lives of others happier.

DS Grewal

Preface to the First Edition

The facial nerve has fascinated and interested almost all Otologists since several decades leading to extensive studies being carried out on the nerve and its functions. In spite of this, a comprehensive atlas featuring various intraoperative photographs of the facial nerve and its pathologies is conspicuous by its absence.

My fascination with the facial nerve goes back several decades when I operated more and more cases of carcinoma of the cheek. Earlier, the trend was to functionally reconstruct the face postoperatively and this was achieved by reconstructing the outer and inner lining of the cheek. However, invariably, this was followed by sagging of the face. According to my experience, there was a failure to realize that, with the inner and outer lining of the cheek, there is a middle layer, which includes the facial nerve and hence, is most important from the functional and cosmetic viewpoint. This concept got me interested in facial nerve surgery, and slowly and steadily prompted me to study facial nerve in the middle ear.

The conception of the "Atlas" however, was not only because of my keen interest in the facial nerve but also in the art of photography for which I received professional training from the Indo-American Society, Bombay in 1976. The magic of photography is that it allows you to capture a moment before it is gone. I personally believe that a photograph should be such that once the audience sees it, they should be able to visualize the mind of the photographer, and actually feel the pulse of the subject. Pondering over a photograph later may also help a surgeon to observe something new that was previously unnoticed and give him ideas to improvise on his technique.

In my experience, the facial nerve can be considered as the most photogenic structure in the middle ear due to its long and tortuous course. It is best captured on a photograph as it does not reflect light but absorbs it. Its exact intraoperative color is best seen in the light of the operating microscope, photographed without the use of a flash. All these features of facial nerve along with a good surgical exposure make the facial nerve an interesting subject for an atlas. The constant use of Zeiss operating microscopes have significantly contributed to the quality and precision of my photography.

Also, I would like to emphasize that the facial nerve should be considered very much as a part of mainstream ENT surgical practice and should be dealt with confidence by trainee and budding otologists, rather than being scared of it and avoiding it. The purpose of this atlas is to achieve this through exhaustive photographic depiction of the nerve and its various features (anatomical and pathological), which will allow the young otologist to visualize and indeed understand this so-called complex structure as a thing of beauty, and fall in love with the facial nerve. Surgery of facial nerve has proven to increase the chance of cure and hence the perspective towards surgical treatment needs to be changed.

I would like to thank our **Dean, Dr Sanjay Oak** and our **ex-Dean, Dr GV Koppikar** for giving me all the facilities for facial nerve surgery. I would also like to thank **Dr LH Hiranandani,** my constant source of inspiration as well as **Dr NL Hiranandani** my colleague and friend; **Prof William House,** a legend in Otoneurosurgery for writing the foreword; **Prof John Ballantyne** one of our senior colleagues and a renowned otologist who has always guided me; **Dr David Moffat,** Cambridge; **Dr Johannes J Manni,** Netherlands; and **Dr Narendra Pandya, Dr Ashok Shah, Dr CM Deshpande,** and **Dr AN Modi,** India; for their contribution. I am thankful to **Dr Mohammed Hashmi** for drawing the diagrams for the Atlas. I also would like to thank my lecturer, **Dr Nilam Sathe** and my past and present residents—Dr Manoj Bhaskaran, Dr Trupti Manjrekar, Dr Neha Shah, Dr Paresh Tankwal, Dr Rahul Mehta, Dr Ashwin Dwivedi, Dr Shobhit Srivastava, Dr Ritu Agarwal, Dr Lovneesh Kumar, Dr Santhosh Davis, Dr Minal Shroff, Dr Rajeev T, Dr Mukesh Kumar, Dr Vijay Prakash, Dr Palak Shroff, Dr Prashant Sharma and Dr Mitul Chamadia, as they were associated during various stages of preparation of the Atlas. My special thanks to **Dr Alok Mohorikar** and **Dr Vicky Khattar** who have not only contributed a chapter, but have worked tirelessly with us throughout the making of this Atlas. **Dr Sonal Saraiya** was a great help in the proofreading of the Atlas. I would also like to thank **Dr Rohan Walvekar** and **Dr Kaushal Sheth,** my past residents for all their help in the basic stages of the Atlas.

I sincerely hope that this Atlas serves its purpose of enlightening the readers about the various aspects of the facial nerve and the photographs capture the essence of facial nerve surgery, which is important for maintaining the normalcy of the face—truly the index of man.

The facial nerve is considered as a "friend of the otologist" and through our experience, we feel that the facial nerve sheath is a boon to the otologist as it is not only a barrier in limiting the spread of disease to the facial nerve but also prevents iatrogenic trauma to the nerve. This firm belief of mine forms the principle of unhesitant atraumatic facial nerve surgery.

I am indeed grateful to my colleague and co-author of this Atlas, **Dr Bachi T Hathiram** for making this belief a reality.

Jointly through this Atlas, we have made an effort to familiarize you with our concepts of facial nerve surgery.

DS Grewal

Acknowledgments

I wish to thank sincerely:

- All contributors.

- Shri Jitendar P Vij (CMD), Mr Tarun Duneja (Director-Publishing), Mr Tarun Vij (Director-Pharma), Mrs Chetna Malhotra Vohra (Sr Manager-Business Development), Mr Ramesh Krishnamachari (Commissioning Editor, Mumbai Branch) and all staff members of M/s Jaypee Brothers Medical Publishers (P) Ltd, New Delhi, India.

- Mr Raju Shinde for making the Video.

Contents

1

Anatomy of the Facial Nerve

DS Grewal

The facial nerve is the nerve of the second branchial arch. It is a mixed nerve. Its course can be broadly classified into (Fig. 1.1):
1. Intracranial
2. Intratemporal
3. Extratemporal.

SUPRANUCLEAR PATHWAY

The facial nucleus is represented in the precentral gyrus of the cerebral cortex. The facial nerve fibers run downwards from the precentral gyrus through the genu of the internal capsule and then through the pons, where majority of the fibers cross over to reach the opposite facial nerve nucleus. Some fibers continue on the same side to terminate in the ipsilateral nucleus. The facial nerve nucleus is located in the pons; ventrolateral to the abducens nucleus. The fibers of the facial nerve emerging from the facial nucleus curve around the abducens nucleus and later pass ventrolaterally and downwards to lie between the facial nucleus and the spinal nucleus of the trigeminal nerve. They emerge from the lower border of the pons between the olive and the restiform body as a motor root and a sensory root (nerve of Wrisberg) and it is from here that the infranuclear pathway starts.

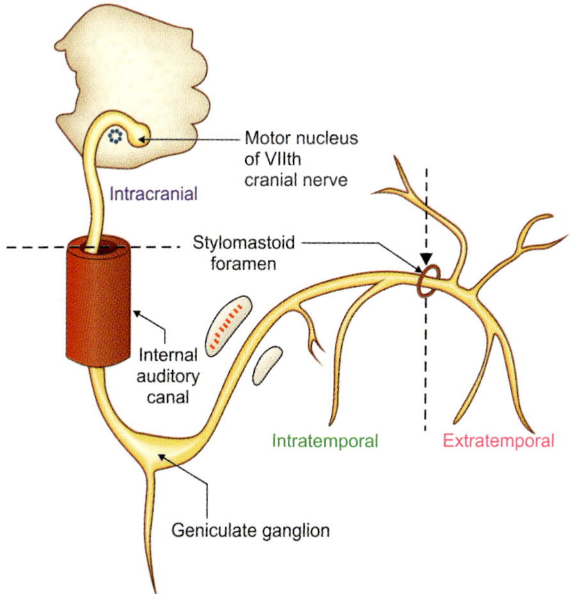

Fig. 1.1: Diagrammatic representation of the course of the facial nerve

INFRANUCLEAR PATHWAY

The facial nerve after leaving its nucleus travels along with the eighth cranial nerve in the cerebellopontine angle to enter the internal auditory canal (IAC). The facial nerve consists of a motor root, carrying fibers to the muscles of the second pharyngeal arch (muscles of facial expression, scalp, auricle, stylohyoid, stapedieus and the posterior belly of the digastric). While the sensory root consists of:

- *Special visceral afferent (SVA)*: Taste to anterior 2/3rd of the tongue via the chorda tympani
- *General visceral efferent (GVE)*: Salivary glands via the petrosal nerves
- *Special visceral efferent (SVE)*: To the facial muscles.

Upon entering the porus (IAC), the seventh cranial nerve and the nervus intermedius join to form a common trunk, which lies slightly above and anterior to the eighth cranial nerve. A dural prolongation containing a narrow subarachnoid space and spinal fluids surrounds the seventh and the eighth cranial nerves to the lateral end of the internal auditory canal (fundus) (Fig. 1.2). After leaving the internal auditory canal, the facial nerve enters a separate bony canal, the fallopian canal (Fig. 1.3) in the temporal bone.

The facial nerve has a unique course through the long, narrow and tortuous bony fallopian canal in its intratemporal segment. This renders it more susceptible to damage following trauma or disease pathology and the symptoms depend on which portion of the nerve is involved.

The total length of the facial nerve in the temporal bone is 22–33 mm and its course can be broadly subdivided into the following segments:

- The first horizontal segment, from the fundus of the internal acoustic meatus to the geniculate ganglion, is 3–5 mm in length and is known as the labyrinthine segment
- The nerve then takes an acute angled turn to enter the tympanic cavity. This is the first genu.
- It then runs posteriorly on the medial wall of the middle ear above the promontory, forwards to backwards. This is the tympanic segment and is 10–12 mm in length
- It then curves down at the pyramid and oval window at an angle. This is the second genu
- The mastoid segment or the vertical segment runs from the second genu to the stylomastoid foramen and is 9–16 mm in length.

As the nerve enters the facial (fallopian) canal, three morphologic peculiarities are noted as described by Gerrier (1977):

1. Individual sheath of pia mater curves up and continues with arachnoid.
2. Slight constriction of nerve is seen just prior to its labyrinthine segment about 0.68 mm (Fisch, 1981) in diameter, which is a normal constriction of the nerve.
3. Change in the direction of the nerve that produces an angle of 132°, open anteriorly and medially.

Labyrinthine Segment

It contains the seventh nerve and nerve of Wrisberg, inclined slightly from above to below and from behind to forwards. It is 3–5 mm in length and extends from the fundus of the internal acoustic meatus to the geniculate ganglion.

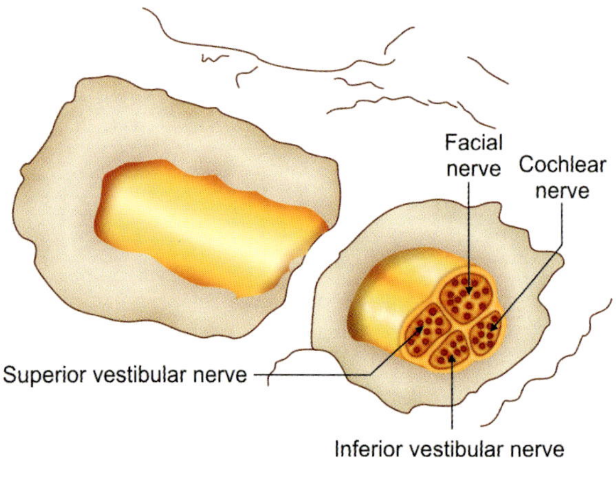

Fig. 1.2: Diagrammatic representation of course of facial nerve through the internal auditory canal

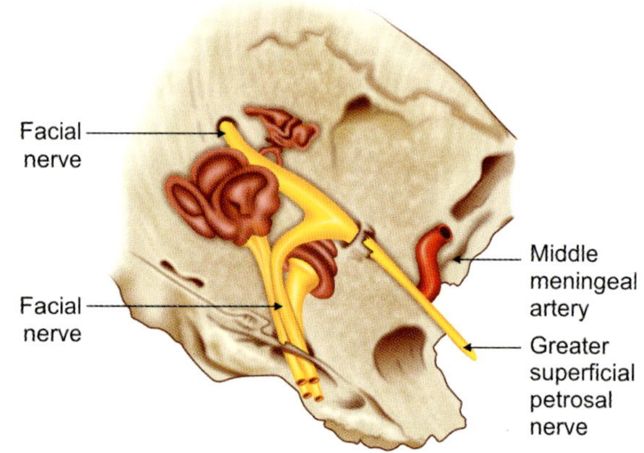

Fig. 1.3: Diagrammatic representation of labyrinthine and tympanic segment of the facial nerve

First turn of the facial nerve and the geniculate fossa; which is the crossroad of four-nerve canals, as follows:

- Central and peripheral extremities of the facial canal
- Conduit for the greater superficial petrosal nerve
- Conduit for the lesser superficial petrosal nerve.

The fossa is quadrangular in shape measuring 2–3 mm. It is completely enclosed in a bone but it is occasionally only covered with dura. The geniculate fossa contains the geniculate ganglion—the bulbous enlargement of the facial canal. The nerve of Wrisberg terminates in the ganglion but emerges as the greater superficial petrosal nerve passing through the facial hiatus.

Second Part or Tympanic Segment (Fig. 1.3)

The facial canal is horizontal and 10–12 mm in length. It extends from the geniculate fossa to the posterior wall of the tympanum. It is inclined slightly inferiorly and forms an angle of less than 10° with the plane of the horizontal canal. It does not give any branches in this segment.

Second Turn of the Facial Canal or Second Genu

It is a curvature with a wide radius which starts in the horizontal plane and then becomes almost vertical. The angle formed varies from 95°–125°.

Vertical/mastoid Segment

It extends from the second genu to the stylomastoid foramen measuring 9–16 mm in length. It forms an angle of 95°–125° with the tympanic portion of the facial canal (second genu). It runs through the mastoid process. The vertical portion tends to swing laterally and at the level of the stylomastoid foramen the nerve is found more superficial than at the level of the second genu.

The second genu lies beneath the posterior portion of the horizontal semicircular canal. The facial canal is separate from the posterior fossa by a distance of 4–5 mm; this retrofacial space is usually occupied by retrofacial air cells. The mastoid portion of the facial canal deviates posteriorly from the vertical by 5°–35°.

We have observed that in the mastoid portion just prior to entering the stylomastoid foramen, the nerve takes a distinct obtuse angled turn forward towards the foramen deviating from its vertical course. This is an important landmark for the stylomastoid foramen. We term this as the third genu (Figs 1.4A and B).

Stylomastoid Foramen

It opens at the base of the petrosa between the mastoid and styloid groove, facing forward towards the base of the styloid process. In the newborn, the stylomastoid foramen is at a higher level with the facial nerve emerging at the level of the mastoid antrum.

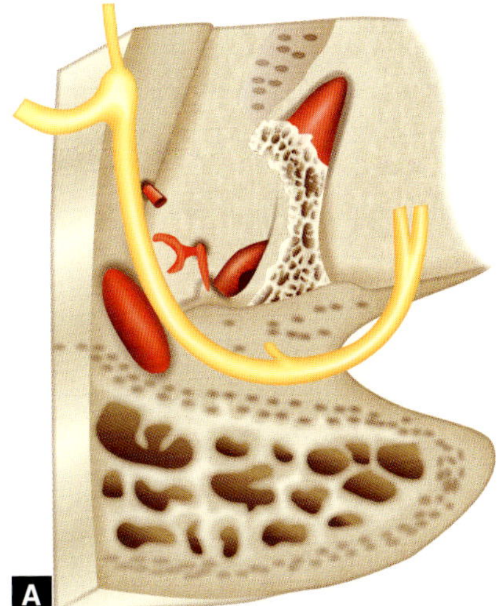
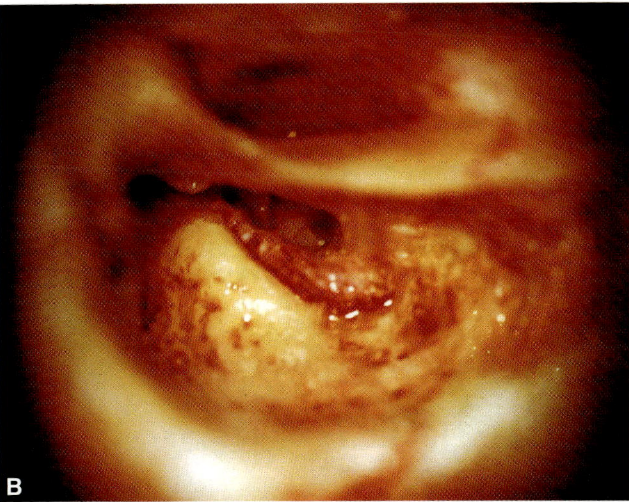

Figs 1.4A and B: (A) Diagrammatic representation showing the angulation of the facial nerve anteriorly prior to entering the stylomastoid foramen (third genu); (B) Intraoperative photograph showing the third genu

Extratemporal Facial Nerve

After it emerges from the stylomastoid foramen, the nerve turns anteriorly in the substance of the parotid gland and divides at the posterior border of the ramus of the mandible into two primary branches:

1. Superior (temporofacial) branch which is larger and horizontally directed.
2. Inferior (cervicofacial) branch which is smaller and longer and vertically directed.

From this, a plexiform arrangement of nerves arises called the parotid plexus or the Pes Anserinus (as it resembles goose feet). These nerves are distributed over the head, face and upper part of the neck. In the parotid gland, the facial nerve presents a curvilinear course and then as it emerges from the parotid, it rapidly becomes superficial and is related to the external wall of the parotid space; which is a thin glandular bed.

BRANCHES OF THE FACIAL NERVE (FIG. 1.5)

INTRACRANIAL

Greater superficial petrosal nerve: It is the first branch, which arises from the geniculate ganglion and carries secretomotor fibers to the lacrimal gland.

INTRATEMPORAL BRANCHES

They arise from the mastoid segment:

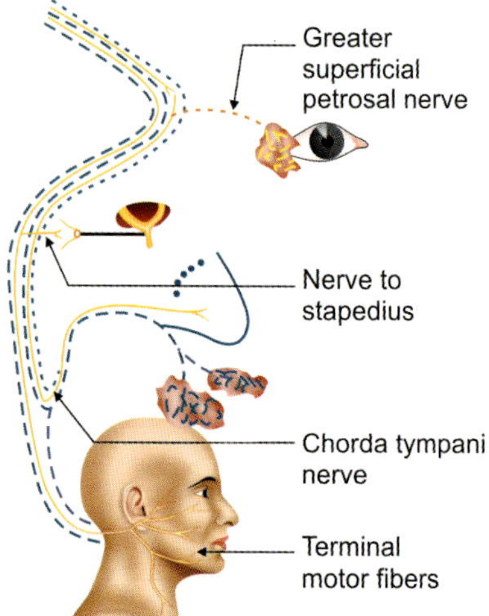

Fig. 1.5: Diagrammatic representation of the branches of the facial nerve for topodiagnostic tests

- *Nerve to the stapedius muscle*: Arises from the mastoid segment and supplies the stapedius muscle.
- *Chorda tympani nerve*: Arises from the mastoid segment, slightly more distal to the nerve to the stapedius, courses anteriorly across the middle ear space between the incus and malleus, to join the lingual nerve and supplies the anterior 2/3rd of the tongue. It also supplies secretomotor fibers to the submandibular gland.
- The *sensory fibers* of the nerve which join the auricular branch of the vagus and supply the skin of the external auditory canal.

BRANCHES OF FACIAL NERVE IN THE NECK AND FACE

1. The *Ansa Haller* (inconstant) which arises immediately below the stylomastoid foramen and anastomosis with the glossopharyngeal nerve, while passing lateral to the jugular vein.
2. *Posterior auricular branch* arises 1–2 mm below the stylomastoid foramen, winds around the digastric muscle and extends posteriorly upon the anterior surface of the mastoid. There it is joined by a filament from the auricular branch of the vagus and communicates with the posterior branches of the greater auricular nerve and with the lesser occipital nerve. Between the external auditory canal and the mastoid process, it divides into auricular and occipital branches.
3. *Stylohyoid branch* frequently arises in conjunction with the digastric branch and enters the stylohyoid muscle in its mid-portion.
4. *Branch to the posterior belly of digastric muscle*
5. The *lingual branch*, which follows the styloglossus muscle and replaces the Ansa Haller.

Branches Forming Parotid Plexus

- Temporal branches of facial expression
- Zygomatic branches of facial expression
- Buccal branches of facial expression
- Marginal mandibular branch, which supplies orbicularis oris and muscles of lips and chin
- Cervical branch which supplies the platysma.

SURGICAL LANDMARKS OF THE FACIAL NERVE

Anatomical landmarks provide the surgeon with various ways to locate the facial nerve, which is distorted by trauma, tumor or infection.

Landmarks for Extratemporal Part

The pinna is important since the incision for all facial nerve surgeries is decided on its position. Parotidectomy is the most common procedure, in which the extra-temporal facial nerve is dissected. Different methods to locate the nerve during surgery are:

- *Tragal pointer (of Conley):* The nerve is located medial and about 1 cm inferior to the tragal cartilage
- *Tympanomastoid suture (TMS):* This is located at the apex of the vagino-mastoid angle or valley of the nerve. It is the angle where the vaginal process of the tympanic portion of the temporal bone meets the mastoid process. The facial nerve runs just deep to this suture.
- *Styloid process:* The nerve passes lateral to the styloid process at the skull base
- By tracing the terminal branches of the facial nerve backwards:
  - The ramus frontalis is located by a line from the tragus to lateral canthus
  - The ramus buccalis is located by a line from the tragus towards the alae of the nose parallel to the zygoma but 1 cm below
  - Ramus mandibularis is near the angle of the mandible at a point 4–4.5 cm from the attachment of the lobule of the pinna
- Tendon of the posterior belly of digastric muscle
- Posterior auricular vein or the retromandibular vein.

During submandibular gland excision, to save the marginal mandibular branch, dissection should be carried out in the plane deep to the fascia overlying the submandibular gland.

Landmarks in the Mastoid and the Middle Ear

- The cog, which is a bony ridge, hangs from the tegmen, anterior to the head of the malleus, is useful in identifying the first genu
- Cochleariform process is immediately inferior to the anterior portion of the tympanic segment of the facial nerve. When the cochleariform process is inapparent, it may be located by identifying the Jacobson's nerve on the promontory and tracing it superiorly
- The oval window is a useful guide to the posterior portion of the horizontal segment of the nerve. The nerve lies above the oval window

- The lateral semicircular canal lies postero-superior to the second genu. This is a very constant landmark
- Retrofacial air cells help in delineating the medial aspect of the vertical segment of the facial nerve
- The chorda tympani is used as a landmark when performing a Combined Approach Tympano-plasty
- The upper portion of the vertical segment lies in the base of the bony ridge that separates the sinus tympani from the facial recess. The processus pyramidalis attaches to the superior aspect of this ridge
- Digastric ridge points to the lateral and inferior aspect of the vertical segment of the facial nerve
- The nerve is located medial to the inferior portion of the tympanic annulus
- In our experience, while decompressing the facial nerve in case of trauma and palsy due to injury/tumor/disease, most of these anatomical land-marks are destroyed; but we have observed a constant relation of the facial nerve in the angle formed by the posterior canal wall and the floor of the mastoid. The posterior canal wall meets the floor of the mastoid below the lateral semicircular canal with an inclination and forms an angle with it. The facial nerve lies within the apex of this angle (Fig. 1.6). Using a 2–3 mm diamond burr, to drill the mastoid bone, the facial nerve can be easily exposed in this angle. By further thinning the posterior meatal wall anteriorly, the facial recess is opened.

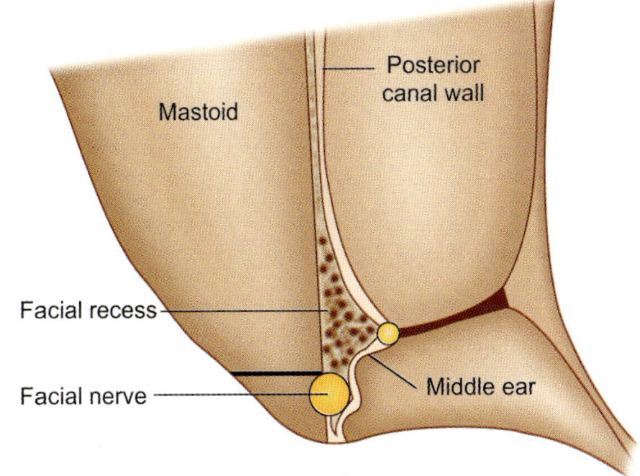

Fig. 1.6: Diagrammatic representation of the relation of facial nerve to the posterior canal wall and floor of the mastoid

Landmarks in the Middle Cranial Fossa

As the middle cranial fossa approach is a neurosurgical approach, most of the otologists are not familiar with it. The standard landmarks are different from the ones used in the mastoid, middle ear and the parotid. These include the greater superficial petrosal nerve, which is the most common landmark. The greater superficial petrosal nerve is identified and followed backwards to the geniculate ganglion and the facial nerve is identified. Another landmark is the identification of the internal auditory canal. The external auditory canal and the internal auditory canal lie in the same coronal plane. Drilling begins in the same plane as the external auditory canal; then the internal auditory canal is identified followed subsequently by the geniculate ganglion and the facial nerve. Also, the bulge of the superior semicircular canal can be identified and subsequently the internal auditory canal is identified.

ANATOMICAL VARIATIONS AND ANOMALIES INVOLVING THE FACIAL NERVE AND ITS CANAL

All components of the temporal bone are subject to variation. The facial canal may display:
- Congenital bony dehiscence
- Variations and anomalies of its usual course
- Rarely, a persisting embryonic artery or vein may also be seen.

Congenital Bony Dehiscence

A gap in the continuity of the bony fallopian canal may be observed in any portion. It is more commonly seen in the tympanic portion (Figs 1.7 A and B) and it may involve the medial, inferior or lateral walls. Most frequent site is above and posterior to the oval window. Occasionally, the dehiscence may be near the cochleariform process or over the superior aspect and medial to the geniculate ganglion. Occasionally, there may be more than one site of dehiscence. Baxter (1971) has derived more accurate information concerning the site and incidence of dehiscence from histological examination of temporal bones at Massachusetts Eye and Ear Infirmary. In a series of 535 temporal bones, dehiscence was detected in 55% cases out of which 91% were intratympanic and 9% were in the mastoid segment. Of all the dehiscences in the tympanic segment, 83% were located adjacent to the oval window involving the lateral, medial and inferior portion with the facial nerve protruding from its bony canal in 26% (Figs 1.8 A to C). In less than 1%, the dehiscence involved the entire tympanic segment.

Variation of the Course of the Facial Nerve

Fowler (1961) collected the most pertinent forms of literature and his observations were as follows:
- Variations involving the mastoid segment may be found in a normally developing temporal bone
- A variation involving the tympanic segment frequently is associated with a lack of differentiation or agenesis of the oval window
- Severe dysplasias of the middle ear or inner ear are regularly accompanied by an aberrant course of the nerve.

Aberrant course of the nerve is classified according to the site at which it occurs:
- *Canalicular segment (Intracranial segment)*: The canalicular segment may enter the petrous pyramid instead of going through the internal acoustic meatus, through the subarcuate fossa and may run through the center of the superior semicircular canal to the stylomastoid foramen bypassing the middle ear cavity as described by Dworacek (1960). Bifurcation of the nerve may be seen.
- *Labyrinthine segment*: Bifurcation of the labyrinthine segment may be seen rarely as described by Altmann (1933) and Miehlke and Partsch (1963).
- *Tympanic segment*:
  - Facial nerve crossing along the superior aspect of the lateral semicircular canal has been documented by House as described by Nager and Proctor (1991)
  - Bifurcation of the nerve anterior or proximal to the oval window has been noticed by Nager and Proctor (1991), Baxter (1971), Dietzel (1961) and Fowler (1961) (Figs 1.9 and 1.15)
  - Facial nerve crossing horizontally over the oval window (Figs 1.10 A and B)
  - Facial nerve crossing through the stapedial arch as documented by Butler (1968), Caparosa and Kalassen (1966) and Ombredanne (1960)
  - Nerve crossing posteriorly between the oval and round windows as described by Durcan et al. (1967) (Fig. 1.11)
  - Facial nerve crossing postero-inferiorly to the round window

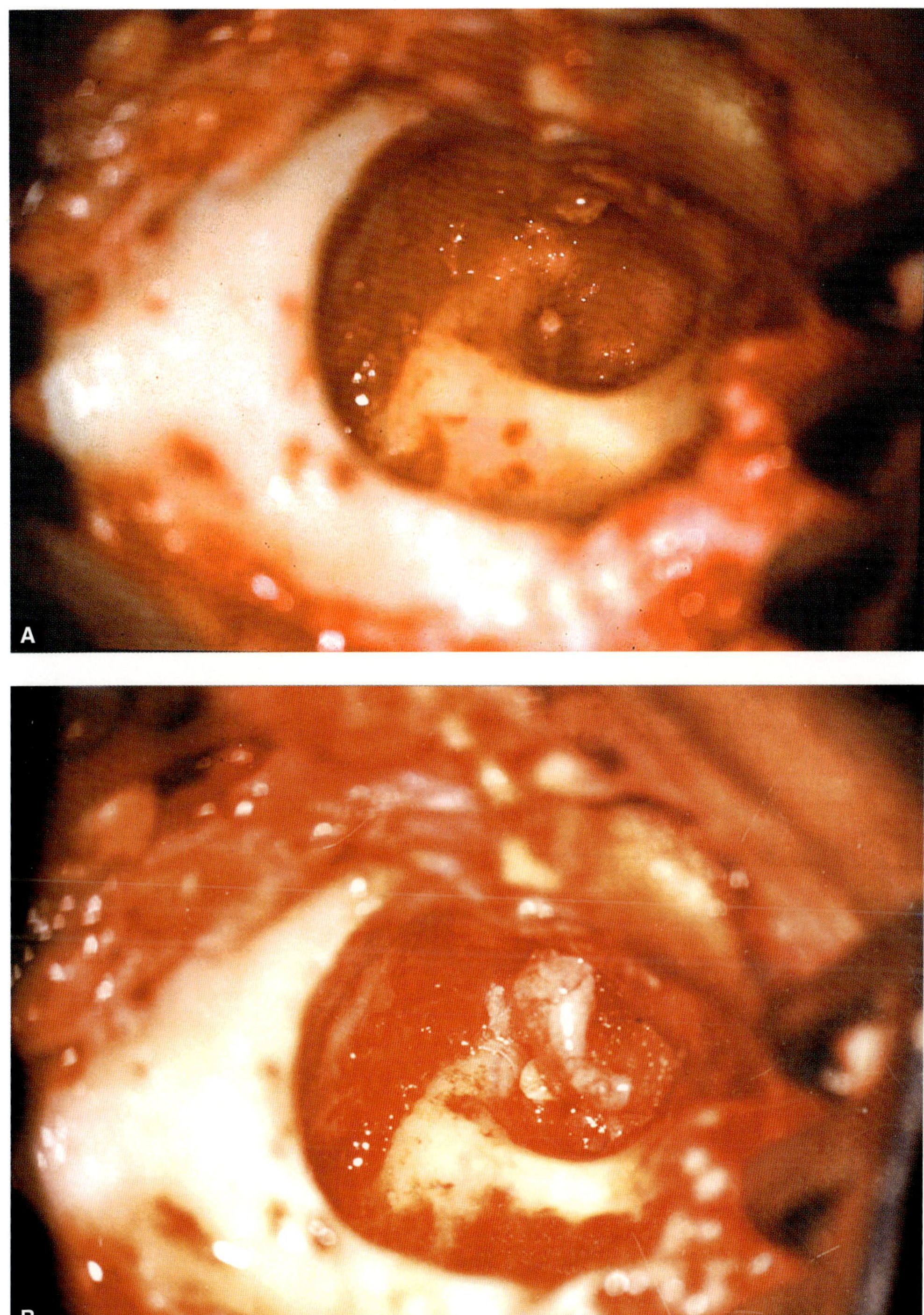

Figs 1.7A and B: Intraoperative photograph showing a dehiscence of the bony fallopian canal in the tympanic segment

– Facial nerve passing from the geniculate ganglion straight downwards over the promontory anterior to both oval and round windows and exiting through the hypotympanum as reported by Dickinson et al. (1968) (Fig. 1.12)
– Hypoplasia of the facial nerve as seen by Kodama et al. (1982).

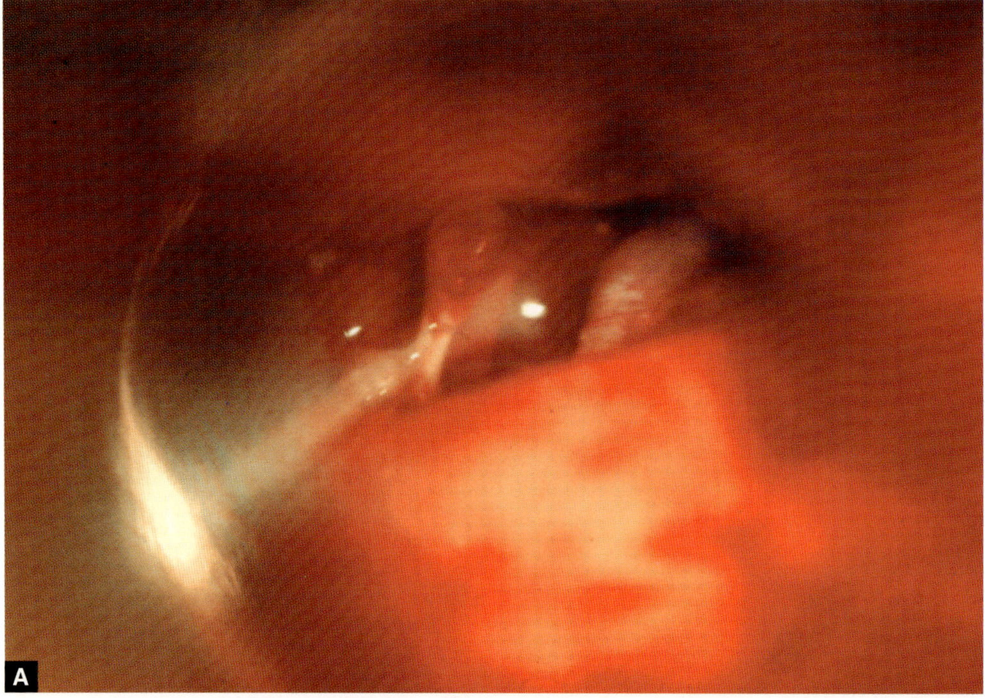

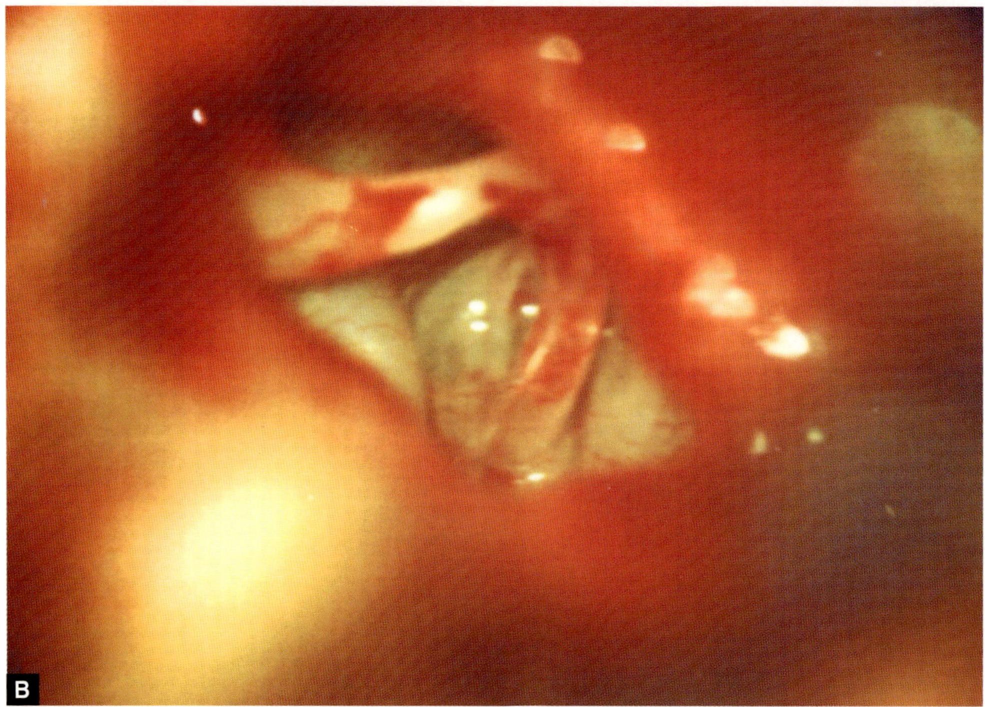

Figs 1.8A and B: Intraoperative photograph showing facial nerve overhang

- *Anomalies of the mastoid segment:*
  - Most frequent is a posterior and lateral bulge (dorsal hump) of the canal beneath the prominence of the lateral semicircular canal as described by Fowler (1961) and Kettel (1946) (Fig. 1.13)
  - The nerve may follow an abnormal posterior, lateral or anterior course as seen by Kettel (1963) (Fig. 1.14)

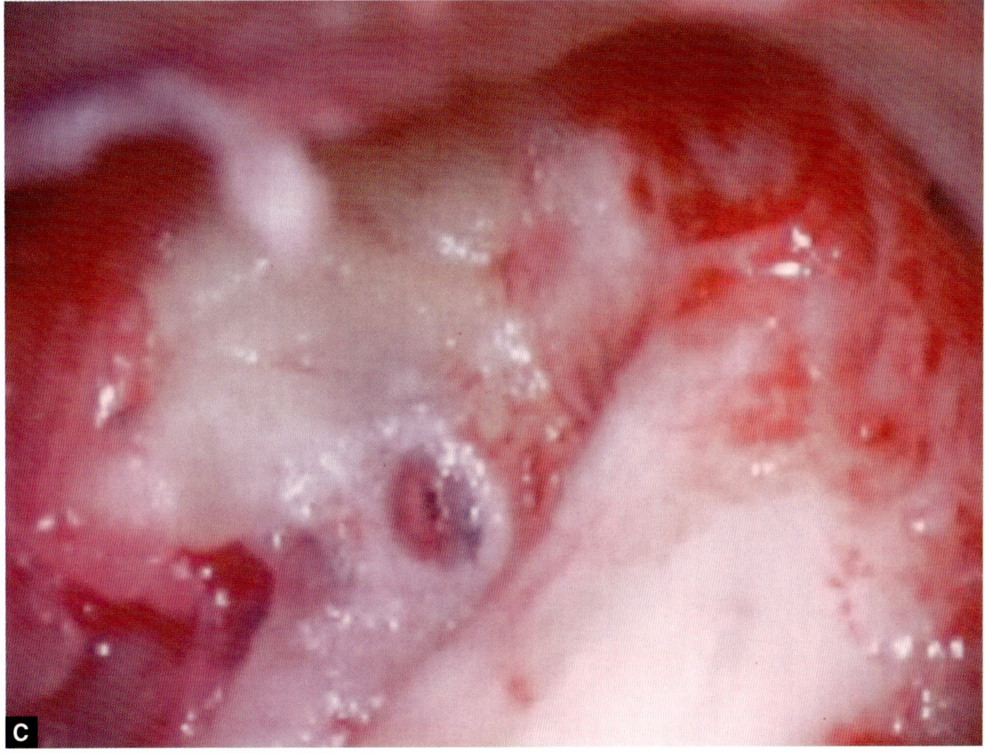

Fig. 1.8C: Facial nerve overhang with promonterial fistulae

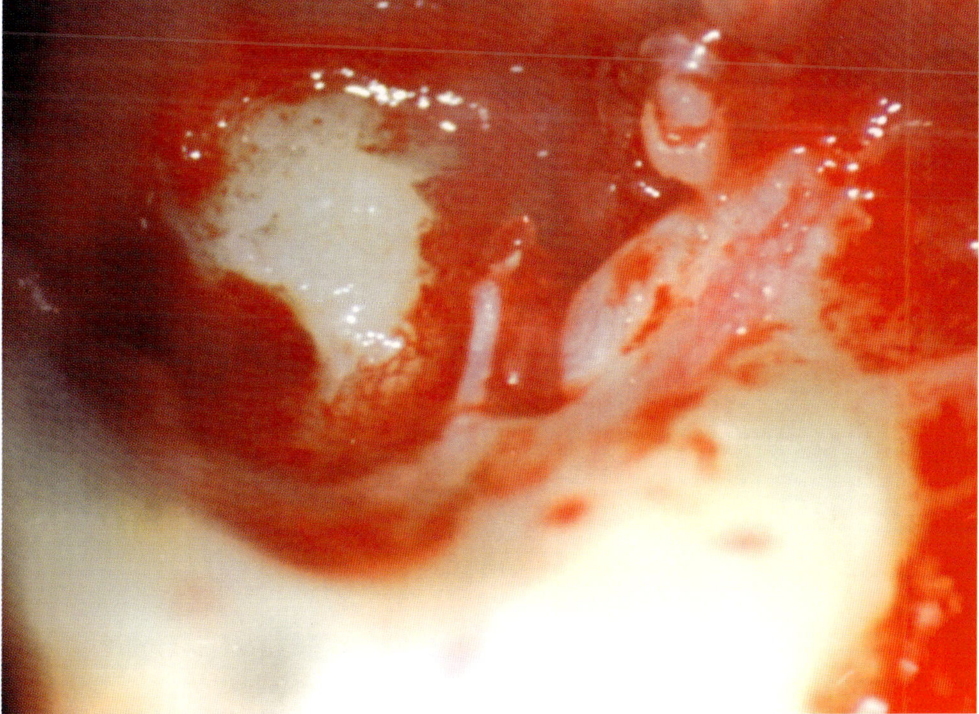

Fig. 1.9: Intraoperative photograph of a bifid facial nerve in the tympanic segment (proximal to the oval window)

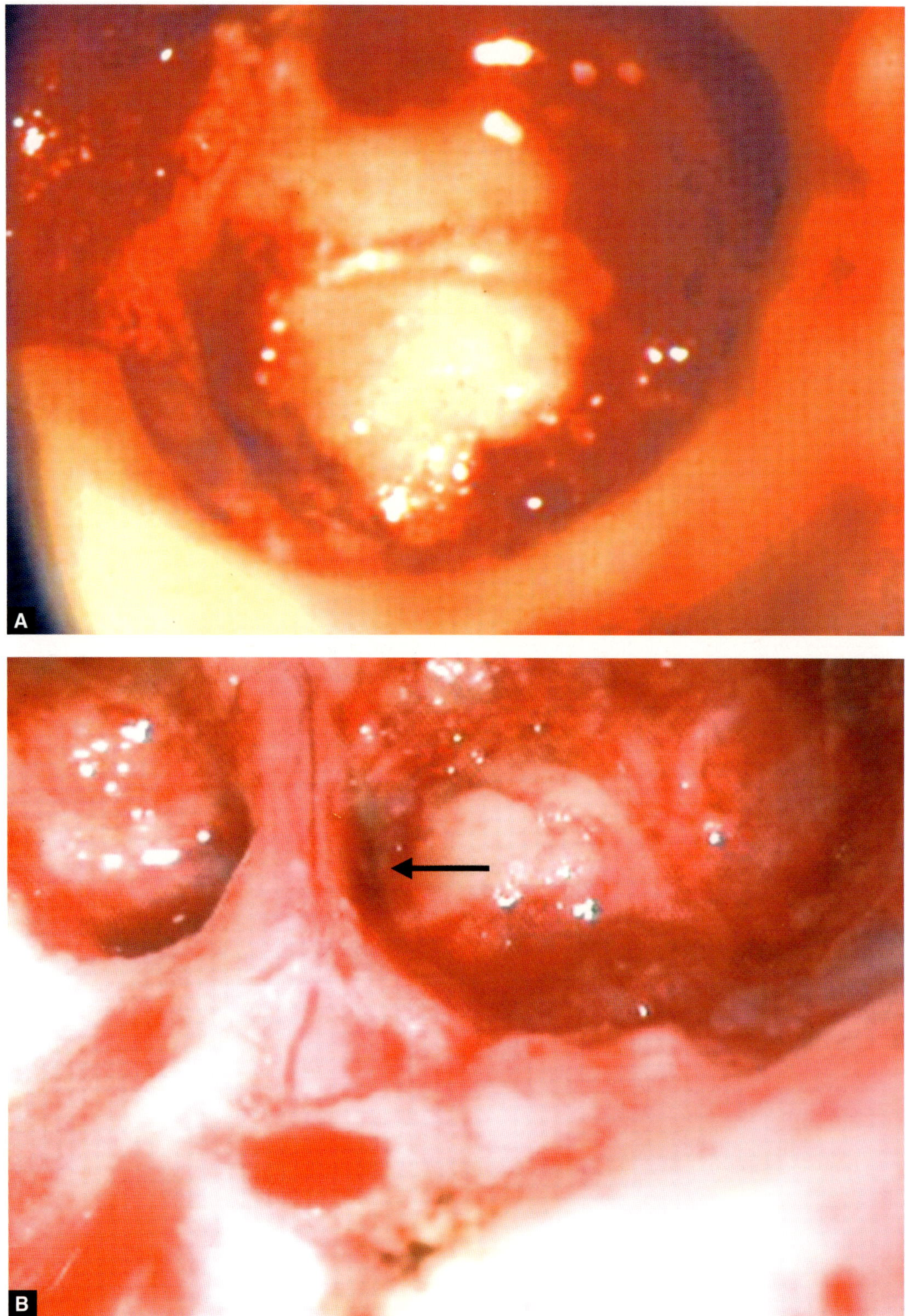

Figs 1.10A and B: (A) Intraoperative photograph of tympanomastoidectomy showing the seventh nerve running over the stapes footplate; (B) Intraoperative photograph showing the facial nerve running over the stapes footplate with only the small inferior portion of the footplate being seen (arrow)

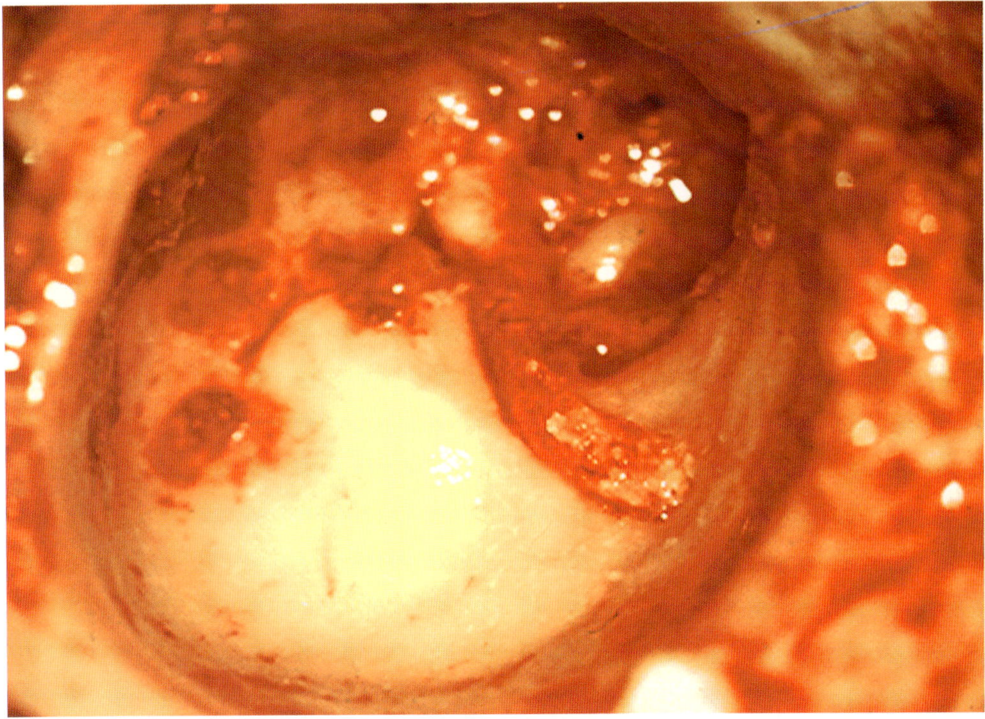

Fig. 1.11: Intraoperative photograph of the anomalous facial nerve which is anteriorly displaced and running between the round window and the stapes footplate over the promontory

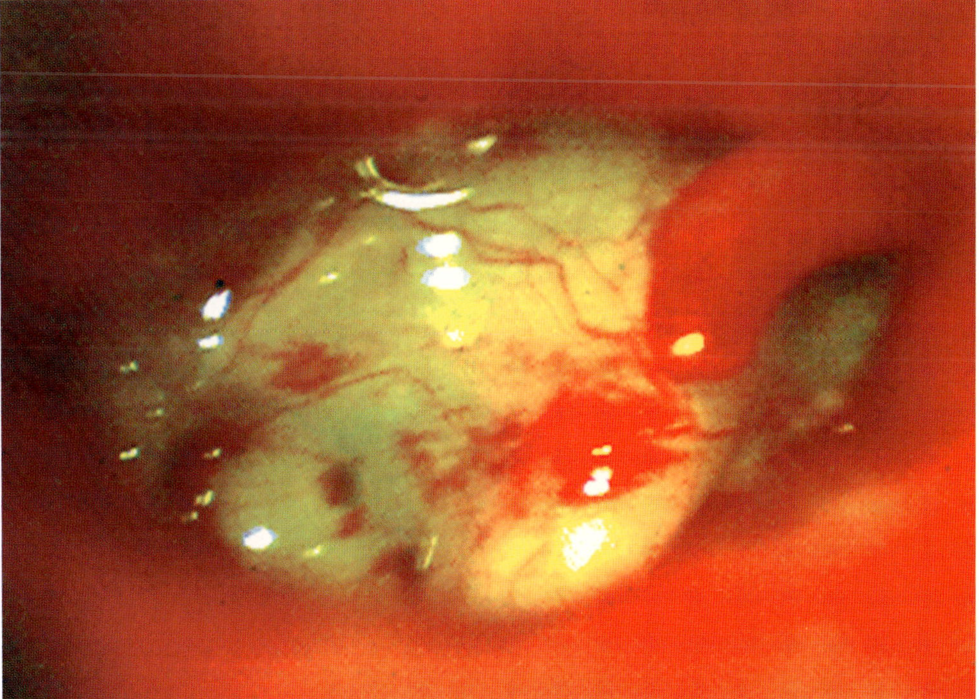

Fig. 1.12: Intraoperative photograph of exploratory tympanotomy showing facial nerve running over the promontory. The round window is covered by bone

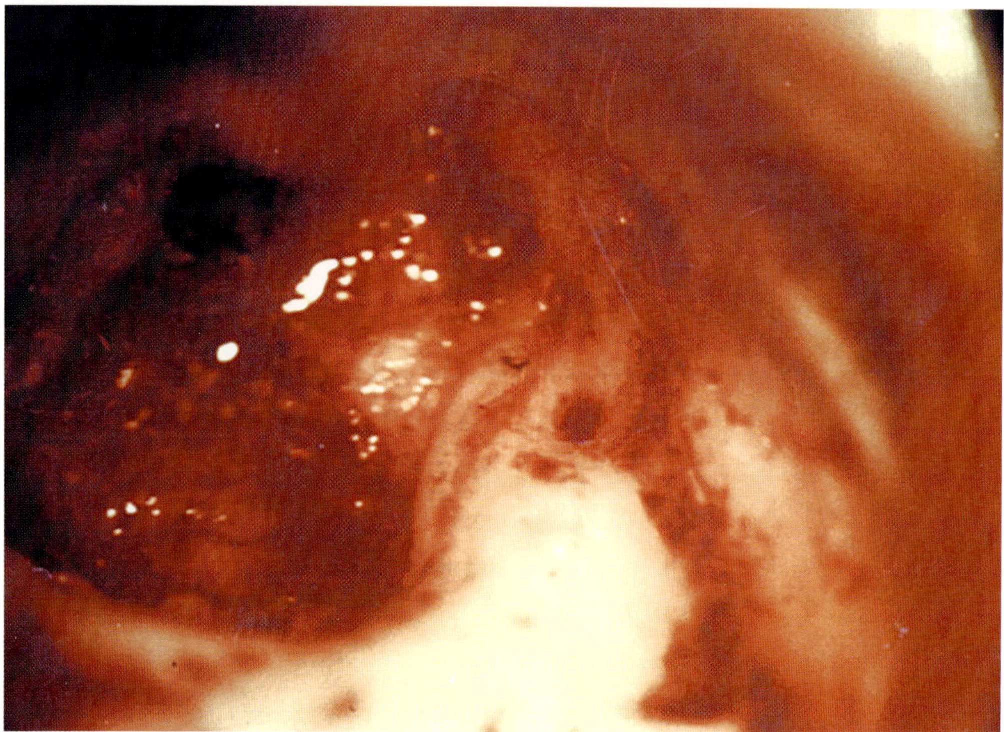

Fig. 1.13: Tympanomastoid surgery showing an anteriorly placed facial nerve in relation to the lateral semicircular canal

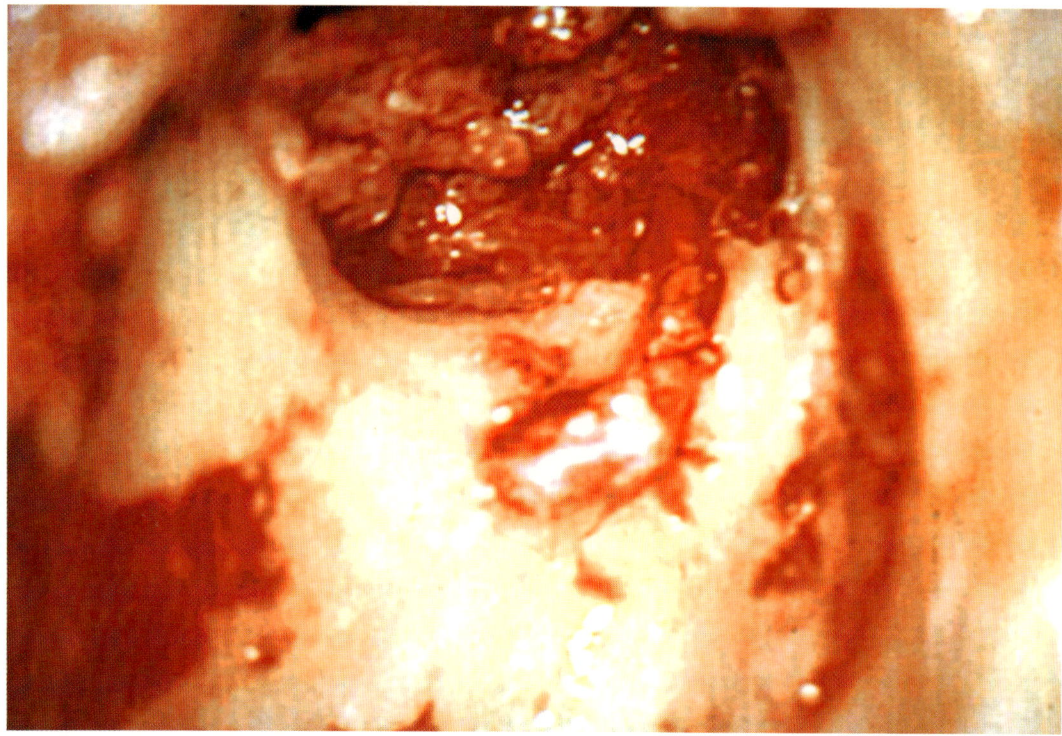

Fig. 1.14: Intraoperative photograph of a dehiscent facial nerve entering the middle ear through aditus ad antrum and running posterior to its normal course in the mastoid segment

– Bifurcation of the facial nerve posterior or distal to the oval window with the two branches continuing in separate canals and the mastoid process through separate foraminae has been mentioned by Arndt (1967), Hahlbrock (1960) and Mielhke (1973). The separate branches may join on their way into a single trunk before passing through the stylomastoid foramen or just outside it as seen by Arndt (1967) and Wright (1991) (Figs 1.15 and 1.16). Occasionally, the nerve is trifurcated.
– Hypoplasia of the nerve
– Anomalous branches arising in the mastoid segment (Fig. 1.17).

ANATOMIC VARIATION IN THE EXTRATEMPORAL COURSE OF THE FACIAL NERVE

Though the facial nerve terminates into its terminal branches within the parotid gland the branching pattern is extremely variable. Various researchers have studied this. However, the most recent study is by Katz and Catalano (1987) where they have classified this branching pattern into five types (Figs 11.4A to D):
1. *Type I (25%)*
   • Splitting and reunion of the zygomatic branch
   • Splitting and reunion of the mandibular branch.
2. *Type II (14%)*: Buccal branch fuses distally with the zygomatic branch.
3. *Type III (44%)*: Major communication between the buccal branch and the other branches.
4. *Type IV (14%)*: Complex anastomotic branching patterns between the major divisions.
5. *Type V (3%)*: Facial nerve leaves the skull as more than 1 trunk.

Anatomic Variations of Chorda Tympani

The origin varies from 1 mm distal to 11 mm proximal to the stylomastoid foramen as described by Nager

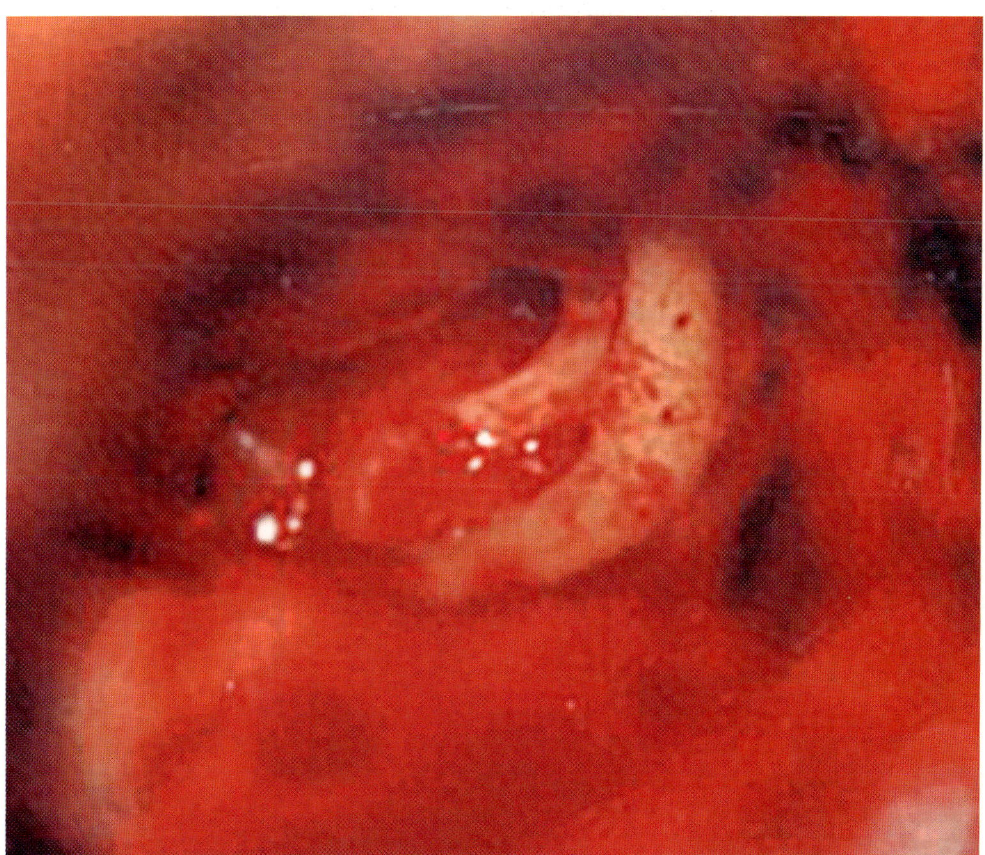

Fig. 1.15: Exploratory tympanotomy showing a bifid facial nerve over the promontory

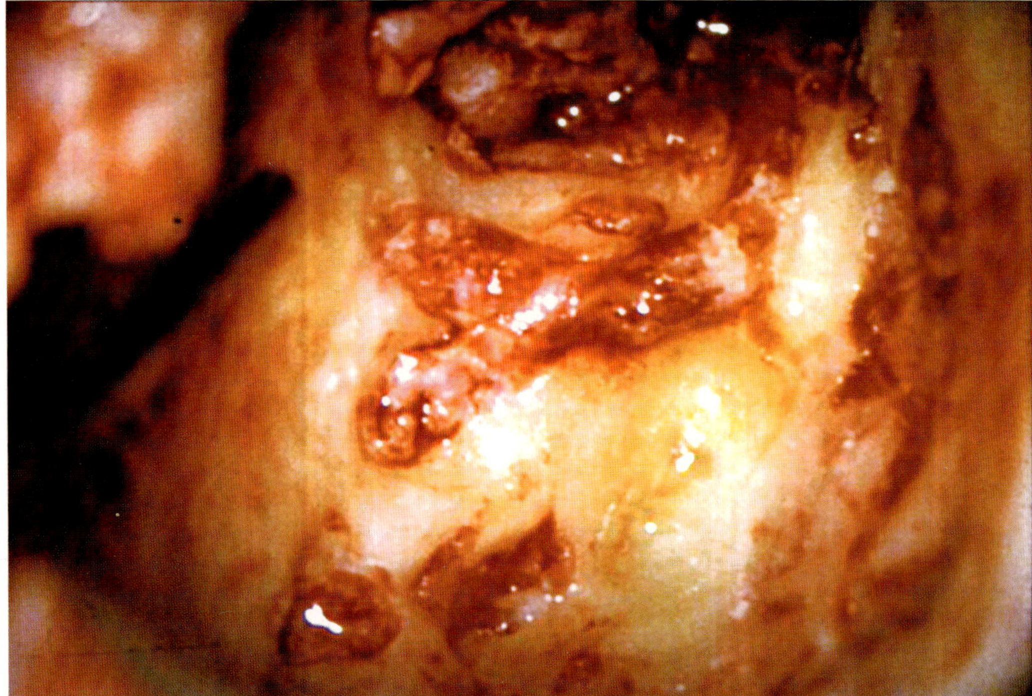

Fig. 1.16: Tympanomastoid surgery showing a bifid facial nerve in the mastoid segment

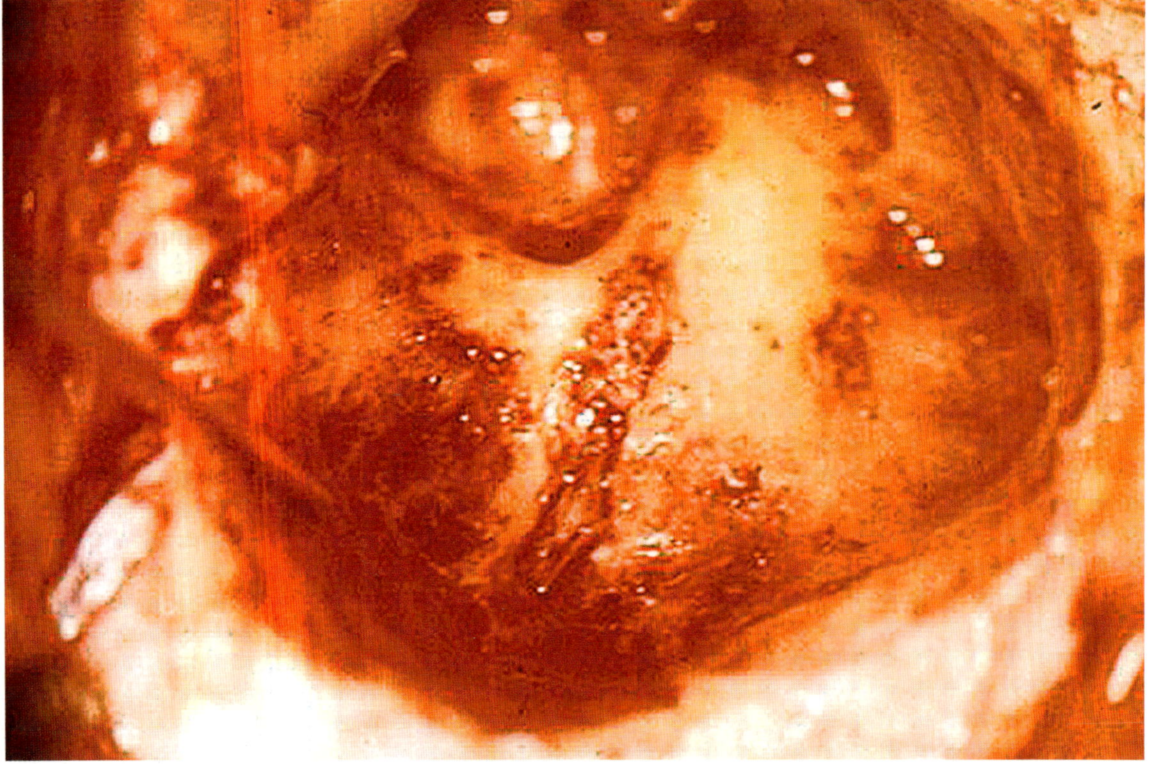

Fig. 1.17: Intraoperative photograph of tympanomastoid surgery showing a branch of facial nerve to the occipitofrontalis muscle abnormally arising from the mastoid segment and running across the mastoid cavity

and Proctor (1991). Rarely, bifurcation may occur as reported by Durcan et al. (1967).

Abnormal Veins and Arteries Along the Facial Nerve

A persistent stapedial artery may be encountered in the tympanic segment of the facial nerve through the stapedial arch. In a rare instance, a large vein of equal size or larger than the nerve may be observed joining the nerve in the facial canal near the geniculate ganglion, accompanying it to the stylomastoid foramen. The vein represents a persistent lateral capital vein.

FACIAL NERVE SHEATH

Throughout the fallopian canal, the nerve (and its two infrageniculate branches) is enclosed in a fibrous sheath. As exposed during surgical procedures, this sheath consists from without inwards of:
- A tough, shiny, grey periosteal layer
- A vascular plane of arteries and venous plexus embedded in loose connective tissue
- A firm fibrous layer perforated by the vessels and on its deep surface in contact with the perineural connective tissue.

Although a clear plane of dissection is found between the sheath and the nerve, this plane is crossed by innumerable connective tissue strands, which require careful division and separation if a length of the nerve is to be decompressed.

At the internal auditory meatus the sheath blends with the dural coverings of the nerve, while at the stylomastoid foramen it fuses with the periosteum and with the adjacent facial layers covering the diagastric muscle, the parotid gland and carotid vessels. The sheath is easily recognized under the operating microscope and it is a valuable barrier against mechanical injury and infection. It should be incised only if there are proper surgical indications for doing so.

BLOOD SUPPLY OF THE FACIAL NERVE

Within the confined space of the fallopian canal, special attention to the blood supply of the nerve is necessary. A detailed account is given by Blunt (1954). The stylomastoid artery, a branch of the occipital artery, enters the stylomastoid foramen and runs upwards anterior and slightly medial to the nerve, sending short branches at intervals around and into

it. At the geniculate ganglion, the petrosal branch of the middle meningeal artery enters the canal and runs distally to anastomose with the stylomastoid artery. Within the internal auditory meatus, the nerve is supplied by the internal auditory artery and in the posterior cranial fossa by the anterior inferior cerebellar artery. The veins form a plexus around the nerve, from which efferent vessels run obliquely, first between the sheath and the nerve and then through the sheath to lie on its outer surface. Apart from small veins accompanying the chorda tympani, the venous drainage leaves the canal mainly at the stylomastoid foramen and at the second genu.

The anterior inferior cerebellar artery, petrosal branch of middle meningeal artery and stylomastoid branch of posterior auricular artery anastomose proximal to the geniculate ganglion. Facial nerve is vulnerable to ischemia in the labyrinthine segment. Sympathetic nervous control of vasomotor tonus is presumed to be effective through the cervical sympathetic fibers distributed around the branches of the external carotid artery.

BIBLIOGRAPHY

1. Altmann F. Zur anatomie und formalen genese der atresia auris Congenita. Monatasschr Ohrenheilkd Laryngorhino. 1933;67:765-71.
2. Arndt HJ. Zweiteilung des nervus facialis zwischen ganglion geniculi und foramen stylomastoideum; HNO (Berlin). 1967;15:116-8.
3. Baxter A. Dehiscence of the fallopian canal. J Laryngol Otol. 1971;85:587-94.
4. Blunt M.J. The blood supply of the Facial nerve Journal of Anatomy 1954;88:520-6.
5. Butler GE. Transtapedial congenital malposition of the facial nerve. Arch Otolaryngol. 1968;88:268.
6. Caparosa RJ, Klassen D. Congenital anomalies of the stapes and facial nerve. Arch Otolaryngol. 1966; 83:420-1.
7. Dickinson JT, Srisomboon P, Kamerer DB. Congenital anomaly of the facial nerve. Arch Otolaryngol. 1968;88:357-9.
8. Dietzel K. Ueber die Dehiszenzen des Facialis Kanals; Z Laryngol Rhinol Otol. 1961;40:366-76.
9. Durcan DJ, Shea JJ, Sleeckx JP. Bifurcation of the Facial nerve. Arch Otolaryngol. 1967;86:619-31.
10. Dworacek H. Die anatomischen Verhaltnisse des Mittelohres unter operations microscopischer Betrachtung; Acta Otolaryngologica (Stockholm). 1961;51:31-45.

11. Fisch U. Surgery for Bell's palsy. Arch Otolaryngol. 1981;107:1-11.
12. Fowler EP Jr. Variations in the temporal bone course of the facial nerve. Laryngoscope. 1961;71:937-44.
13. Gerrier Y. Surgical anatomy particularly vascular supply of the facial nerve. In: Fisch U (Ed): Facial Nerve Surgery. Birmingham AL:Aesculapius;1977.
14. Hahlbrock KH. Zweiteilung des N facialis im warzenfortsatz; Arch Ohren Nasen Kehlkopfheilkd. 1960;174:465-70.
15. Katz AD, Catalano P. The clinical significance of the various anastomotic branches of the facial nerve. Report of 100 patients; Arch Otolaryngol Head Neck Surg. 1987;113(9):959-62.
16. Kettel K. Abnormal course of the facial nerve in the fallopian canal. Arch Otolaryngol. 1946;44:406-8.
17. Kettel K. Surgery of the facial nerve. Archiv Otolaryngol. 1963;77:327-41.
18. Kodama A, Sando I, Meyers EN, et al. Severe middle ear anomaly with underdeveloped facial nerve. Arch Otolaryngol. 1982;108:93-8.
19. Miehlke A. Surgery of the facial nerve Munchen, Urban and Schwarzenberg Verlag; Philadelphia:WB Saunders;1973.
20. Miehlke A, Partsch CJ. Ohrmissbildung Facialis and Abducenslahmung als Syndromder Thalidomidsc-hadigung. Arch Ohren Heilk Z Hals Heilk. 1963;181:154-74.
21. Nagher GT, Proctor B. Anatomic variations and anomalies involving the facial canal; Otolaryngol Clin North America. 1991;24(3):531-53.
22. Ombredanne M. Chirurgie des surdites congenitales par malformation ossicularre. Annals Otolaryngol. 1960;77:423.
23. Wright JW Polytomography and congenital external and middle ear anomalies, Laryngoscope. 1991;91:1806-1911.

2

Neurophysiology of the Facial Nerve and Nerve Regeneration

DS Grewal

INTRODUCTION

Facial expression depends on 7000 motor fibers of the facial nerve firing in unison to bring about muscular contraction. Each of the nerve fibers consists of a central protoplasmic process of parent neuron—the axon which is surrounded by an insulating layer of myelin and by the thin protoplasmic cytoplasm of Schwann cells that constitute the neurilemmal sheath. Around each nerve fiber is a connective tissue tubule, the endoneurium. Many tubules are held together by the perineurium and these bundles are bound together by epineurium (Fig. 2.1).

The facial nerve is highly organized at the CNS level; the degree of topographic organization of the peripheral nerve is controversial. Although clinical observation suggests such a spatial orientation, laboratory investigations demonstrate progressive diffusion and fiber mixing as the nerve courses peripherally.

DEGREES OF NERVE INJURY

Seddon in 1943 described three types of nerve injuries:

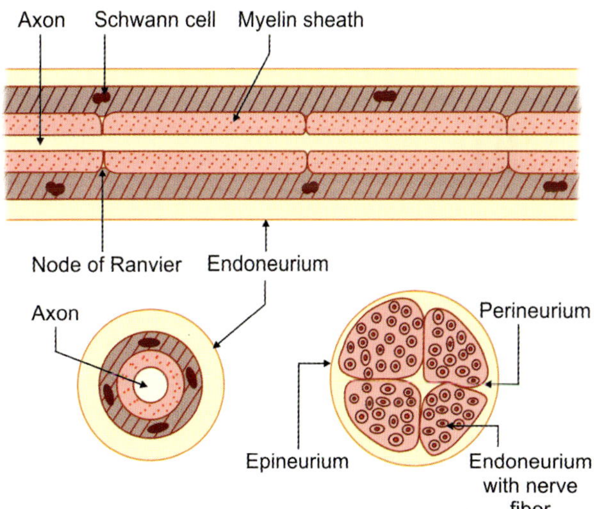

Fig. 2.1: Diagrammatic representation of a nerve fiber

1. Neurapraxia
2. Axonotemesis
3. Neurotmesis.

Neurapraxia: Pressure on a peripheral nerve can block the transmission of the impulses without death and degeneration of the axon beyond the site of pressure and may be associated with the loss of myelin at the site of pressure. Release of pressure results in rapid and complete recovery of function, without residual deficit. This is a reversible conduction block.

Axonotmesis: Sectioning of an axon or sufficient pressure to block off axoplasm in the distal segment completely results in the death of the distal segment not at once but after several days.

Neurotmesis: Sectioning or disruption of the entire nerve trunk.

After the classification by Seddon, it was Sunderland in 1978 who described five degrees of nerve injury:
1. *First degree*: Indicates compression of the nerve that is reversible and the recovery is complete. This is similar to neuropraxic damage to the nerve.
2. *Second degree*: There is interruption of the axoplasm and the myelin. This occurs when the compression persists. It results in loss of axons but the endoneurium remains intact. Recovery may take more than 1-2 months but is usually complete. This correlates well with the axonotmesis type of nerve injury.
3. *Third degree*: In the third degree of nerve injury, there is loss of myelin tubes due to an increased intraneural pressure. In this case recovery may take as long as 2-4 months, there may not be a complete recovery or the recovery though complete may be accompanied by complications of faulty regeneration. The third degree nerve injury correlates with the neurotmesis type of damage.
4. *Fourth degree*: Fourth degree of nerve injury implies a partial transection of the nerve and recovery is poor.
5. *Fifth degree*: In the fifth degree of nerve damage, there is a complete transection of the nerve and there is absolutely no recovery.

Thus, by knowing the type of nerve injury it may be possible to assess the prognosis of recovery of the facial nerve function in various disorders. It was found that in Bell's palsy and herpes zoster cephalicus, the first three types of nerve injury were seen. Since, the pathological process in these disorders does not progress beyond the first or the second degree, the patients usually recover satisfactorily. Partial or complete transection of the nerve is seen more commonly with trauma, tumor or cholesteatoma. In these conditions, it is seen how recovery even under ideal conditions is never as good as with the first three degrees of nerve injury.

NERVE REGENERATION

Nerve regeneration can be defined as a complex interaction of neurons, Schwann cells, extracellular matrix and neurotrophic substances (Selzer, 1987). Regeneration is influenced by various factors and processes. These can be studied by *in vivo* and *in vitro* studies. Of the various factors and processes all do not have a clinical application, as they are not very practical. Regeneration follows degeneration, which is usually of the Wallerian type. During regeneration, there is sprouting at the axonal end. This is an early process during regeneration and one regenerating axon may produce as many as 20 sprouts. These sprouting ends usually restore the nerve continuity, which is accompanied by reformation of myelin.

Regeneration of the nerve may cause three major changes in the axon:
1. The distance between the node of Ranvier is altered.
2. The myelin covering the axons is much thinner than normal.
3. There is a splitting and crossing of axons that re-innervate the denervated muscle groups, without necessarily corresponding to the cell-body unit arrangement that was present prior to degeneration.

This may result in the various complications of regeneration such as synkinesis, crocodile tears, facial myokimias, hemifacial spasms and stapedius muscle contraction (Schaitkin and May, 1997).

Factors Affecting Regeneration

- *Site of lesion*: Higher the site of the lesion poorer is the prognosis. Closer the lesion to the neuron, poorer is the quality of regeneration.
- *Duration of the injury*: Longer the duration of the injury, poorer is the prognosis and quality of regeneration.
- *Age*: Regeneration is better in children than in adults due to a better neural plasticity seen in children.

- *Nutrition*: A good nutrition is essential for a better functional recovery. Malnourishment deters the process of regeneration.
- *Blood supply*: Better the blood supply to the injured segment faster is the recovery. Poor blood supply or a compromised blood supply will hamper the chances of regeneration.
- *Associated injury or infection*: Other associated injuries or infections will produce poorer functional results. The chances of regeneration are poor or nil in an infective bed. Hence, a clean field free from infection is very important for regeneration.

Along with the above mentioned factors, there are certain other biochemical and pharmacological adjuvants that help in the process of regeneration. Though all of them cannot be used *in vivo*, they provide a promising approach to the regeneration process and may find some use in the future.

- *Gangliosides*: These agents can be used *in vivo* for aiding the process of regeneration. Biochemically, gangliosides are complex glycosphingolipids, while functionally they have two properties:
  1. Neuronotrophic: Aiding in survival and maintenance of the neurons.
  2. Neuritogenic: Increasing the number and size of branching processes.

Gangliosides of bovine origin are commercially available and can be used in peripheral neuropathies.

- *Immunomodulators*: A nerve injury causes the release of nerve proteins in the blood, which may act as a "foreign antigen." This leads to neuritis and thus hampers regeneration. A similar process may be seen in diseases like amyotrophic lateral sclerosis and Guillain-Barré syndrome.

Also, immunomodulators in the form of imm-unosuppressive agents decrease the non-specific inflammation and subsequently cause fibrosis by limiting the response of macrophages and histiocytes. MacKinnon et al. (1987) have found that the immunosuppresssive agents like Azathioprine and Hydrocortisone aid in nerve regeneration.

Growth Factors

The growth factors important for nerve regeneration include nerve growth factor (NGF) and neurite promoting factor (NPF).

Nerve growth factor (NGF) was first described by Levi-Montalcini (Levi-Montalcini and Hamburger, 1953). The peripheral nerve injuries lead to the increased production of NGF.

NGF promotes:
- Increased axonal branching
- Increased dendritic branching
- Prevention of death of neurons.

Neurite promoting factor (NPF) has not proven to be of great importance consistently in the process of regeneration. However, it can be considered as a mixture of different growth factors and can be used in certain cases.

Hormones

ACTH (Strand & Smith, 1980); T3 (Stelmack & Kiernan, 1977); T4 (Danielsen et al. 1986) and testosterone (Kujawa et al. 1989) have been implicated to increase the rate of regeneration.

FACIAL NERVE GRADING SYSTEM

House and Brackmann's Grading System for Recovery of Facial Nerve Function

Approved by 1984 Facial Nerve Disorder Committee of the American Academy of Otolaryngology.

Grade 1 : Normal

Grade 2 : Mild dysfunction

Grossly there is a slight weakness noticeable on close inspection, at rest there is normal symmetry and tone. Motion as observed in the forehead, is moderate to good. Eye closure is complete with slight asymmetry of the mouth.

Grade 3 : Moderate dysfunction

Grossly there is obvious but no disfiguring difference between two sides and at rest there is normal symmetry and tone. Motion as seen in the forehead is slight to moderate, there is weakness of the angle of the mouth on maximal effort and eye closure is complete with effort.

Grade 4 : Moderately severe dysfunction

Grossly, there is obvious asymmetry or disfigurement or both. At rest, there may be normal symmetry and tone. There is no motion in the forehead, the eye closure is incomplete even with maximal effort and there is mouth movement with asymmetry on maximal effort.

Grade 5 : Severe dysfunction

Grossly there is only barely perceptible motion at rest. Forehead motion is none and eye closure is incomplete with maximal effort and there is very slight mouth movement.

Grade 6 : Total paralysis, i.e. no movement.

BIBLIOGRAPHY

1. Danielsen N, Dahlin LB, Ericson LE, et al. Experimental hyperthyroidism stimulates axonal growth in mesothelial chambers. Experimental Neurology. 1986;94(1):54-65.
2. House JW, Brackmann DE. Facial nerve grading system. Otolaryngol Head Neck Surgery. 1985;93:146-7.
3. Kujawa KA, Kinderman NB, Jones KJ. Testosterone induced acceleration from facial paralysis following crush axotomy of the facial nerve in male hamsters. Experiment Neurol. 1989;105:80-5.
4. Levi Montalcini R, Hamburger V. A diffusible agent of mouse sarcoma producing hypoplasia of lymphatic ganglia and hyperneurotization of viscera in chick embryos. J Experiment Zool. 1953;123:233-388.
5. MacKinnon SE, Hudson AR, Bain JR, et al. The peripheral nerve allograft: An assessment of regeneration in an immunocompromised host. Plast Reconstruct Surg. 1987;79:436-44.
6. Schaitkin B, May M. Disorders of the Facial Nerve. (6th edn). Scott-Brown's Otolaryngology. 1997;3: 24/1-38.
7. Seddon HJ. Three types of nerve injury. Brain. 1943;66:237-88.
8. Selzer ME. Nerve regeneration. Seminars in Neurology. 1987;7:88-96.
9. Strand FL, Smith CM. LPH, ACTH, MSH and motor systems. Pharmacol Therapeut. 1980;11:509-33.
10. Stelmack BM, Kiernan JA. Effects of Triiodothyronine on the normal and regenerating facial nerve of the rat. Acta Neuropathologica (Berlin). 1977;40:151-5.
11. Sunderland S. Nerve and nerve injuries (2nd edn). London: Churchill Livingstone. 1978:88-9:96-7;133.

3

Causes of Facial Palsy

DS Grewal

BIRTH

1. Forceps delivery
2. Moebius syndrome
3. Dystrophia myotonica

TRAUMA

A. Accidental
1. Skull base fractures
2. Penetrating injury to middle ear
3. Barotrauma
4. Scuba diving
B. Iatrogenic
1. Mastoid surgery
2. Parotid surgery
3. Postaural local anesthesia
4. Anti-tetanus serum
5. Rabies vaccine
6. Embolization

INFECTIONS

A. Bacterial
1. Malignant otitis externa
2. Otitis media—acute and chronic with/without cholesteatoma
3. Tuberculosis
4. Botulism
5. Lyme disease
6. Mastoiditis
B. Viral
1. Herpes zoster cephalicus (Ramsay Hunt syndrome)
2 Poliomyelitis
3. Encephalitis
C. Fungal—mucormycosis.

NEOPLASTIC

A. Cerebellopontine angle tumors
1. Vestibular schwannoma

2. Facial nerve tumors
3. Cochlear neuromas
4. Meningioma
5. Ependymoma
6. Arachnoid cyst
B. Temporal bone tumors
1. Primary
    i. Glomus jugulare
    ii. von Recklinghausen's disease
    iii. Hans-Schüller-Christian disease
2. Secondary
    i. Teratoma
    ii. Leukemia
    iii. Sarcoma
C. Parotid tumors
1. Benign
    i. Pleomorphic adenoma
    ii. Adenolymphoma
    iii. Oxyphil adenoma

2. Malignant
    i. Mucoepidermoid carcinoma
    ii. Acinic cell carcinoma
    iii. Adenocarcinoma
    iv. Epidermoid carcinoma

NEUROLOGICAL

1. Opercular syndrome
2. Millard-Gubler syndrome
3. Encephalitis
4. Multiple sclerosis
5. Myasthenia gravis
6. Charcot-Marie-Tooth disease.

MISCELLANEOUS

1. Toxic
    i. Tetanus
    ii. Diphtheria
2. Metabolic—diabetes.

4

Testing of the Facial Nerve

Alok Mohorikar

INTRODUCTION

Basic knowledge of the testing of the facial nerve needs to be a part of the armamentarium of a neurotologist in this day and age. One needs to know not only how to evaluate facial palsy but also to treat it at the right time. It is recognized that 90% of facial nerve disorders originate in the temporal bone (Shambaugh and Clemis, 1973). Facial nerve testing includes not only topognostic tests and prognostic tests but also intra-operative facial nerve monitoring. Intra-operative monitoring is almost imperative nowadays and facial nerve monitors are common-place in the operating theaters.

There are various tests, subjective or objective and tests that may or may not use electrical stimulation of the nerve. Facial nerve or the VII cranial nerve is a mixed nerve and even though the motor component of the nerve is relatively more important and more commonly used for testing, the sensory component can also be used less reliably for its testing.

The intratemporal location of most facial nerve injuries precludes direct assessment of the damaged segment, so facial nerve testing depends upon:

- Determining the degree of axonal degeneration (electrodiagnosis)
- The function of accessory branches (topognosis).

FACIAL NERVE TESTING

Topognostic Tests

- Lacrimation test (Schirmer's test)
- Stapedial reflex
- Salivary flow test
- Test for the sensation of taste on anterior two-thirds of the tongue.

Prognostic Tests

- Electromyography (EMG)
- Nerve excitibility test (NET)
- Nerve conduction time
- Maximal stimulation test (MST)
- Electroneuronography (ENoG).

Intraoperative Monitoring

- Electrically evoked potential
- Mechanically evoked potential

Imaging

- Computed tomography
- Magnetic Resonance Imaging.

Topognostic tests should form a part of the clinical assessment of the patient. However, electrodiagnosis of the nerve palsy is more reliable. Imaging and intraoperative monitoring are relevant in specific settings and should be used if required.

ELECTRODIAGNOSTIC TESTS

These tests are most reliable prognostic indicators of facial nerve recovery. The tests can be of two types depending upon the direction of the stimulated impulses traveling along the nerve:

1. Orthodromic conduction tests: Where the nerve is stimulated proximally and muscle response is recorded distally.
2. Antidromic conduction tests: Where the nerve is stimulated in a retrograde manner. Antidromic tests can detect the nerve injury earlier than Orthodromic tests but have a disadvantage of having multiple artifacts and the responses are difficult to detect.

Correct method of performing the tests and its interpretation is of vital importance.

Principle

All the nerve conduction studies assess the strength and speed of the action potential that is generated when a peripheral nerve is stimulated by using a skin electrode. As the stimulus is increased in intensity, more and more number of axons are stimulated. The stimulus at which all the axons are stimulated is the maximal stimulus. A supramaximal stimulus is used (just above the level needed to stimulate all axons) and the summated waveform is recorded. This can be used for sensory as well as motor nerves. The time lag between the nerve stimulation and recording of the waveform is nerve latency (in milliseconds) and this can be used to calculate the nerve conduction velocity. The amplitude of the waveform and the nerve conduction velocity both are used to point to the status of the nerve. Amplitude of the waveform indicates the integrity and the latency or velocity indicates the myelination.

ELECTROMYOGRAPHY (EMG)

First used by Weddell and colleagues (1944) for facial paralysis. It measures electric responses during needle insertion, at rest and during volitional movement (Crumley, 1982).

There are five criteria of measurement. They are insertional activity, spontaneous activity, motor unit action potential, recruitment pattern and interference pattern.

Insertional activity: Increased activity is the characteristic of a denervated muscle.

Spontaneous activity: Active denervation usually due to injury.

Motor unit action potential: When the motor unit APs appear increasingly complex, larger and of a higher duration, it indicates a chronic axonal injury. These APs are called neurogenic APs and appear due to collateral innervation. Collateral innervation is the re-innervation of the denervated muscle fibers from the uninjured axons of the same nerve. The process usually takes many months and is seen in partial injuries to the nerve.

Recruitment pattern: This is characterized by rapid firing of motor APs. However, there are no extra motor units added and this pattern is also a feature of a denervated muscle.

Interference pattern: An incomplete interference pattern is when the axons do not transmit their APs to the motor units. This produces gaps in the overlapping AP waveforms.

Possible responses include:
- *Silent resting potential*: Indicates normal innervated muscle in a state of rest or severe muscle wasting caused by fibrosis
- *Voluntary motor unit potential*: Characterized by triphasic or biphasic morphology with amplitude of 50-1500 microvolts
- *Fibrillation potential*: Has smaller amplitude and represents involuntary, invisible contraction of a single denervated muscle fiber—indicating degeneration of the muscle nerve supply
- *Polyphasic re-innervation potential*: Precedes recovery of denervated muscle fibers and is seen during nerve regeneration.

NERVE CONDUCTION VELOCITY (LATENCY)

This test is similar to evoked EMG in technique. It is used to test the latency response of a muscle (innervated by facial nerve) on electrical stimulation. EMG equipment is used to stimulate the nerve at the stylomastoid foramen and record over one of the facial muscle group such as frontalis (Rogers, 1978), midface (Esselen, 1977) or mentalis (Brown et al. 1970) is obtained. The latency for each compound action potential is defined as the time between onset of stimulus and onset of response.

Esselen (1977) and May et al. (1974) found this to be the least reliable prognostic test. We have found that nerve conduction velocity is less reliable as well. This is possibly due to the fact that there is a variable transmission of stimulus across the neuromuscular junction.

As mentioned in the earlier paragraph, conduction velocity correlates with the degree of myelination and hence low velocity or high latency indicates demyelination.

NERVE EXCITABILITY TEST (NET)

It is most commonly used because it is easy to perform, easily available and inexpensive.

It is performed by stimulating the nerve at the stylomastoid foramen and then determining subjectively the presence of a twitch response in the facial musculature. The lowest electric current (threshold) to elicit a facial twitch on the paralyzed side of the face is compared with the threshold value of the normal side. A difference of 3.5 milliampere (mA) between sides suggests a poor prognosis.

The main problem with this test is that only large myelinated fibers are stimulated because of their lower threshold, smaller fibers are not recruited until higher thresholds are used and 50% fibers have to be lost before the results are seen. However, it has been seen that despite a normal NET some patients of Bell's palsy had an incomplete recovery.

MAXIMAL STIMULATION TEST (MST)

It is best defined as a modified NET, in which maximal rather than minimal stimulation is given to peripheral branches of the facial nerve. The same stimulator is used as in NET with the current set initially at 5 mA and increased to the level of the patient's tolerance. The paralyzed side is compared subjectively to the normal side and is assigned a grade of equal, slightly decreased, markedly decreased or no movement. The latter two responses correlate to a poor prognosis.

ELECTRONEURONOGRAPHY (ENoG)

Described by Esselen (1977), popularized by Fisch (1981) as electroneuronography (ENoG) and May et al. (1981) called it as evoked electromyography (EEMG). It differs from EMG in that bipolar electrodes are used for stimulating as well as recording. Two techniques have been proposed for positioning of electrodes:
1. Hughes (1981 and 1983) recommends a standard lead placement (SLP)
2. Kartush and colleagues (1985) recommended optimized lead placement (OLP).

OLP has shown to be more reliable than SLP and has a better subject tolerance. We have found alae nasi to be an optimum site for lead placement.

After placing the electrodes, the stimulating intensity is gradually increased until smooth biphasic waveform of maximal amplitude is achieved. The response amplitude of the paralyzed side is compared with that of the normal side and the percentage reduction is calculated which correlates most commonly with the axonal degeneration. The rate of amplitude reduction is also correlated with prognosis. Impedance, stimulus amplitude and stimulus frequency affect the response in electroneuronography.

Electroneuronography has been shown to be the most accurate prognostic indicator of all electro-diagnostic tests.

MAGNETIC STIMULATION TEST

This test was first introduced by Barker in 1985 (Barker et al. 1985). Barker stimulated the motor cortex by time varying magnetic fields to induce electrical depolarization. Magnetic fields cause depolarization of the facial nerve at the root entry zone (REZ) by a transcranial penetration. The response can be recorded indirectly by surface electrodes on individual muscles. This test shows a longer latency than ENoG as it tests the nerve at a more proximal site, i.e. REZ.

This test helps to eliminate the delay in testing nerve function due to its ability to stimulate the intratemporal segment of the facial nerve. Another benefit of magnetic stimulation is the decreased pain in testing compared to electrical stimulation.

OTHER TESTS

Some of the other tests that can be performed include:

- *Trigeminofacial (Blink) reflex*: This test was first introduced by Overend (1896) by tapping the glabellar surface. Nowadays, it can be done electrically by stimulating the nerve at the supraorbital foramen and recording the EMG response of the orbicularis oculi. The reflex arc in this case uses trigeminal nerve as its afferent and facial nerve as its efferent. It can be considered as a test for the intracranial and the intratemporal portion of the facial nerve.
- *Strength duration curve*: This test can be considered as an extension of NET. In this the electrical intensities required for the stimulation of various muscles to evoke contraction is plotted graphically. Depending on their response the degree of axonal degeneration is determined.

Merits of Electrodiagnostic Testing

- Helps to detect subclinical evidence of early regeneration
- Helps to differentiate birth trauma from embryo-genic etiology (Harris et al. 1983)
- Helps in determining the completeness of neural blockade by testing for subclinical voluntary potentials.

Demerits of Electrodiagnostic Testing

- EMG is not of much use in evaluation of acute paralysis because 14–21 days are required for the development of fibrillation potentials from the time of onset of the facial nerve injury; hence EMG is use only after 14–21 days of nerve injury
- Slight electrodental positioning may produce variations in amplitude of response making accurate assessment impossible
- Temperature affects all electrodiagnostic studies. Although most of the modern EMG machines will have a temperature probe, optimum warmth and/or temperature correction options are used.
- Suboptimal stimulation can mimic demyelinations and conduction blocks. This can be caused by inadequate stimulation, improper electrode placement, sweat/dirt/electrode gel/dead skin causing a significant barrier or obesity.
- Excessive stimulation can result is spread of the stimulus in the surrounding areas and may result in a larger waveforms.

Clinical Application of Electrodiagnostic Tests in Facial Nerve Palsy

- Facial nerve testing provides data, which when combined with the history and physical examination of the patient facilitates adequate counseling and appropriate surgical intervention
- In patients with poor recovery following Bell's palsy it will help in deciding the exact time for intervention
- If ENG shows 90% or greater reduction amplitude within 21 days of onset, surgery is indicated
- ENoG can be used to document the degree of subclinical facial nerve involvement and prognosis prior to CP angle and skull base tumor surgery. It also plays a role in the diagnosis of occult tumor involving the facial nerve
- In managing patients with malignant otitis externa the progression or regression of an underlying neuritis can be monitored by serial ENoG
- In temporal bone fracture, these tests help in taking decisions about the time of surgery.

INTRAOPERATIVE FACIAL NERVE MONITORING

The use of nerve stimulator has become one of the commonplace practices in otology, neurotology and Head-Neck surgery. Most of the larger centers use it routinely and continuous monitoring intra-operatively is recommended. The common procedures where the monitors are used are facial nerve decompression, revision mastiodectomy, cochlear implant, parotidectomy, posterior and middle cranial fossa approach, thyroidectomy. It, however, is important to note that nerve monitor is not an alternative of any sort to knowledge of anatomy or surgical skills.

Goals of Intraoperative Monitoring

- Early identification of facial nerve by using electrical stimulation in the soft tissue, tumor or bone

- Warning the surgeon of an unexpected facial nerve in the temporal bone or tumor
- Mapping the course of the facial nerve in the temporal bone or tumor
- Reducing the mechanical trauma to the facial nerve during re-routing or tumor dissection
- Evaluation and prognosis of facial nerve function at the conclusion of surgery.

The reasons for use of intraoperative facial nerve monitoring routinely are:
- The surgeon can judge when it will be needed in a particular case
- The operating room personnel become familiar with the equipment
- The surgeon learns how to interpret the sounds produced by the monitor and how to correlate them with the surgical manipulation around the facial nerve.

Facial nerve monitors are of different types depending on the institutional preference and hence it is important for the surgical and the non-operative staff to be familiar with the instrument. Visual and acoustic inputs are important for the surgeon when he/she is working around the facial nerve.

Aspects to be Considered while Using Facial Nerve Monitors

1. *Local anesthetic agents (lignocaine, cocaine, bupivacaine, etc.):* Increase latency and decreased amplitude of APs.
2. *Inhalational agents (halothane, isoflurane):* Delay in wave V 0.5–1.0 m/S, prolonged I–V latency on ABRs.
3. *Neuromuscular blockade (succinylcholine, atracurium, vecuronium, etc.):* Spontaneous and triggered EMG blocked.
4. *Temperature:* Decreases the activity. Tissues need to be warm as also the body by warm blankets, Bair Huggers, etc.
5. Testing of the nerve monitor pre and intra-operatively for optimum functioning.

FACIAL NERVE IMAGING MODALITIES

MRI has supplemented CT as the imaging modality for evaluation of the brainstem, cisternal segment and the intracanalicular segment because:
- Of superior soft tissue contrast
- No change in the position with multiple planes
- Interpetrous streak artifacts seen in CT are avoided.

Intravenous administration of Gadolinium-DTPA when combined with T1 weighted imaging sequences increases the sensitivity of acoustic neuroma diagnosis.

Intratemporal Evaluation of the Facial Nerve

High resolution CT (HRCT) using bone algorithms is the main-stay for evaluating the intratemporal segment. Direct axial and coronal scanning with slice thickness of no more than 2 mm consistently will display the bony labyrinth, facial nerve canal and the tympanic cavity and its contents. High field strength magnets using standard lead coil and low field strength magnets using a specialized surface now are capable of imaging the facial nerve directly.

Extratemporal Evaluation of the Facial Nerve

Both MRI and CT scan can be used to demonstrate lesions affecting this segment of the facial nerve. Direct imaging of the facial nerve is possible with MRI. Both CT with contrast and MRI provide the same diagnostic information regarding parotid tumors, it's relationship to facial nerve and it's aggressiveness.

TOPOGNOSTIC TESTS

They help to determine the site of nerve injury. Not used frequently nowadays because of unreliable information.

Lacrimal Flow Assessment

It was popularized by Tschiassny (1953).

Schirmer's test: Lacrimation is studied objectively by Schirmer's test. A strip of filter paper of 5 cm × 0.5 cm is placed in the lower conjunctival fornix of each eye for 5 min and the (soakage) lacrimation of both the sides is compared with inhalation of ammonia to enhance lacrimation. A comparison between the amount of soaked filter paper on the normal and affected side establishes whether there is lessening of tear secretion. A reduction of lacrimation by 30% as compared to the normal side or bilateral reduction to less than 25 mm is considered significant.

Salivary Flow Test

It was introduced by Magielski and Blatt (1958). Techniques include introduction of a no. 50/60 polyethylene catheter in both Wharton's papillae for about 3 mm. The patient is given a few lemon drops to suck for 1 min and the number of drops of saliva over 1 or 5 min is monitored. (Huges, 1989). A 25% reduction between the sides is considered significant.

Stapedial Reflex

This test provides an advantage of easy and repeated assessment. It is an objective test and eliminates subjective variation and variation in interpretation. Hence, it is commonly called the "Otologist's electromyogram." Koike and colleagues (1977) found that restoration of the stapedial reflex within three weeks after onset of facial palsy indicates a functional recovery.

Taste Sensation (Anterior two-thirds of the Tongue)

This provides useful information in the diagnosis and management of facial palsy and is best assessed by electrogustometry. However, it has not proved to be a useful diagnostic tool.

FACIAL NERVE INJURY/RECOVERY CLASSIFICATION SYSTEM

Sunderland's classification of nerve injury describes five degrees of injury (1977):

1. Class I   : Neurapaxia
2. Class II   : Axonotmesis
3. Class III   : Disruption of endoneurium
4. Class IV   : Disruption of endoneurium and perineurium
5. Class V   : Neurotmesis.

Electrical testing can distinguish Class I from Class II through V but cannot make distinction between Classes II through V. The same test results may be obtained from a Class II injury with excellent chances of recovery as from Class V injury with no recovery potential (Sunderland, 1978).

Class	General	Symmetry at rest	Synkinesis	Movement	Eye closure
1	Normal	Yes	No	Normal	Yes
2	Slight Weakness	Yes	No	Weak	Yes
3	Can close eye	Yes	Yes	Weak	Yes
4	Cannot close eye	Yes	Yes	Weak	No
5	Slight movement	No	Yes	Slight	No
6	Paralyzed	No	N/A	No	No

Classification System for Reporting Results of Recovery from Facial Paralysis (House and Brackmann, 1985)

This system has been approved and adopted by the Facial Nerve Disorders Committee of the American Academy of Otolaryngology-Head and Neck Surgery, 1984.

House-Brackmann Facial Nerve Paralysis Classification

BIBLIOGRAPHY

1. Barker A, Jalinous R, Freeston I. Noninvasive magnetic stimulation of the human motor cortex. Lancet. 1985;1:1106-7.
2. Brown E, Arno S, Twedt DC. Bells Palsy. Nerve conduction and recovery time. Physical Therapy. 1970;50:799-806.
3. Crumley RL. Electromyography and muscle biopsy in facial paralysis. In: Graham MD, House WF (Eds). Disorders of the Facial Nerve. New York: Raven Press,1982.
4. Esslen E. Electromyography and electroneurography. In: Fisch U (Ed). Facial Nerve Surgery. Birmingham: AL Aesculapius Publishing. 1977.pp. 93–100.
5. Esslen E. Investigations on the localization and pathogenesis of meatolabyrinthine palsies. In: The Acute Facial Palsies New York: Springer-Verlag;1977.
6. Fisch U. Surgery for Bell's palsy. Archives of Otolaryngology. 1981;107:1-11.
7. Harris JP, Davidson TM, May M, et al. Evaluation and treatment of congenital facial paralysis. Archives of Otolaryngology. 1983;109:145.

8. House JW, Brackmann DE. Facial Nerve Grading System. Otolaryngology-Head and Neck Surgery. 1985;93:146-7.

9. Huges G, Nodar R, Williams G. Analysis of test-retest variability in facial electroneurography. Otolaryngology Head and Neck Surgery. 1953;91:290-3.

10. Huges G, Josey A, Glasscock M, et al. Clinical electroneurography Statistical analysis of controlled measurements in 22 normal subjects. Laryngoscope. 1981;91:1834-46.

11. Huges GB. Prognostic tests in acute facial palsy. American Journal of Otolaryngology. 1989;10:304-11.

12. Kartush J, Lilly D, Kermink J. Facial electroneurography: Clinical and experimental investigations. Otolaryngology Head and Neck Surgery. 1985;93:516-23.

13. Koike Y, Hojo K, Iwasaki E. Prognosis of facial palsy based on the stapedial reflex test. In: Fisch U (Ed): Facial nerve surgery. Birmingham:AL Aesculapius Publishing. 1977. p.159-64.

14. Magielski JE, Blatt IM. Submaxillary salivary flow-a test of chorda tympani nerve function as an aid in diagnosis and prognosis of facial nerve paralysis. Laryngoscope. 1958;68:1770-89.

15. May M, Blumenthal F, Klein SR. Acute Bell's palsy: Prognostic value of evoked electromyography, maximal stimulation and other electrical tests. American Journal of Otology. 1983;5:1-7.

16. May M, Blumenthal F, Taylor FH. Bell's palsy: Surgery based upon prognostic indicators and results. Laryngoscope. 1981;91:2092-103.

17. Overend W. Preliminary note on a new cranial reflex. Lancet. 1896;1:619.

18. Rogers RL. Nerve conduction time in Bell's palsy. Laryngoscope. 1978;88:314-26.

19. Shambaugh G, Clemis J. Facial nerve paralysis. In: Paparella M, Shumrick D (Eds) Otolaryngology. Philadelphia: W.B. Saunders. 1973. p.275.

20. Sunderland S. Nerve and Nerve Injuries. 2nd Ed. London:Churchill Livingstone. 1978. p. 88-9:96-7/133.

21. Tschiassny K. Eight syndromes of facial paralysis and their significance. Annals of Otology, Rhinology and Laryngology. 1953;62:677.

22. Weddell G, Feinstein B, Pattle RE. The electrical activity of the voluntary muscle in man under normal and pathologic conditions. Brain. 1944;67:178-257.

5

Bell's Palsy

DS Grewal

INTRODUCTION

Facial nerve is unique among motor nerves. It has a long course through a narrow bony canal called the fallopian canal. It is due to this that it is more prone to paralysis than any other nerve in the body. The most frequent type of facial palsy is Bell's palsy. Bell's palsy is described as an acute idiopathic lower motor neuron palsy of the facial nerve that is usually unilateral, self-limiting, non-progressive, non-life threatening and spontaneously remitting after 4-6 months and always by 1 year. The diagnosis of Bell's palsy is that of exclusion and theoretically it is considered to be accurate only when there is no evidence of any other cause for facial palsy. Nevertheless, there is evidence that a typical idiopathic palsy is mediated by a viral inflammatory immune reaction.

Today various modes of treatment have been documented for the management of this condition including medical line of therapy, surgery and physiotherapy as the understanding of this disease has improved. Thus, it is important for every physician to diagnose this condition and to refer such disease to the otologic surgeon at the earliest, remembering the dictum of the celebrated neurologist Gower—"A complete unilateral palsy of the face without other symptoms must mean disease of the nerve, as it passes through the temporal bone."

HISTORICAL ASPECTS

In 1829, Sir Charles Bell, an anatomist and a surgeon first described facial palsy and named it "Bell's palsy." He was subsequently knighted for his work. In 1919, Antoni using physical diagnostic techniques labeled the disease as "Acute infectious polyneuritis cerebral acousticofacialis," while in 1960, Dalton identified "Ramsay Hunt syndrome" as a florid form of Bell's palsy.

In 1904, Riek suggested that the cause may be a subclinical middle ear infection and proposed a combined medical and surgical treatment. However, Watermann in 1909 showed that the middle ear was normal in cases of Bell's palsy. There was a divergence of opinion regarding the treatment. In Pietersen's landmark article (Pietersen, 1982), 1101 patients were followed up for a period of one year. It showed that almost 80% of the patients had some return of facial function without any kind of intervention.

The concept of spasm of middle meningeal artery or the stylomastoid artery and paralysis due to ischemia gradually came in. 1950s saw many treatment regimens that included low dose Histamine (Skinner, 1950) to massive doses of Histamine (De Blasio, 1959) and Prednisolone (Taverner, 1954). Korkis (1961) classified patients into two groups:

1. The "vasospastic group" who showed good results with a cervical sympathetic block
2. The "organic thrombosis group" who did not benefit from the same.

Various adjuvants were used like galvanic stimulation, physical therapy-facial support, massage, exercises and splints. They have been recommended and condemned.

For a very long time, it was believed that decompression at the stylomastoid foramen was a sufficient treatment for Bell's palsy till Fisch (1977), recommended middle cranial fossa approach to decompress the facial nerve. However, Brackmann (1974) felt that decompression of the mastoid portion of the facial nerve was important as the pathology lies there. Transmastoid extralabyrinthine subtemporal approach was described by May in 1976. Thus, at present, we have a number of approaches for decompression of the nerve, however, its role is still debatable.

ETIOLOGY

There are three theories regarding the etiology of Bell's palsy:

1. The vascular ischemia theory
2. The viral theory
3. The hereditary theory.

Features of each theory support surgical decompression of the facial nerve in selected individuals.

Vascular Ischemia Theory

In the theory of vascular ischemia, the central feature of the pathophysiology is a decrease in the circulation to the facial nerve. Some investigators believe that a primary interruption of one of the major nutrient vessels to the facial nerve is responsible (primary ischemia), but most theorize that the ischemia is secondary to compression of the nerve within the rigid fallopian canal (secondary ischemia). The presence of a thickened fibrous sheath in certain cases causes

Tertiary ischemia (Grewal et al., 2002) and this theory is recently proposed and elaborated further.

Primary Ischemia

Vasospasm of the blood vessels leads to decrease in the blood supply to the facial nerve. Though epineurium has a rich vascular supply, the nerve is relatively avascular due to which primary ischemia will cause a palsy of the nerve.

However, the opponents of this theory cite that the nerve has an adequate blood supply with numerous anastomosis between the stylomastoid and the petrosal blood vessels. Drachmann (1969) has stated that primary ischemic neuropathy is rare occurring only in certain conditions like the Liereche's syndrome and possibly Diabetes mellitus.

Proponents of this theory have demonstrated lack of significant anastomosis between the stylomastoid and the petrosal vessels (Donath and Lengyel, 1957); decreased vascularity of the horizontal segment of the facial nerve (Blunt, 1954); acute onset facial paralysis following the embolization of the middle meningeal artery (Calcaterra, 1976).

Secondary Ischemia

Hilger (1949) proposed that the process of primary ischemia leads to secondary ischemia. Iilger described the mechanism of secondary ischemia as follows. The essential features are arteriolar constriction, followed by capillary dilatation with an increase in permeability and resultant transudation. The capillary dilatation may follow ischemic damage or may result reflexly from a fall in venous pressure. The pressure of fluid transudate is rapidly transmitted to the walls of the lymph capillaries and they may be closed by compression. Additional fluid then accumulates and compression of capillaries and venules within the fallopian canal creates further zonal ischemia so that a vicious cycle arises. In severe cases, this may lead to necrosis of the nerve, the continuity of which is accordingly interrupted.

This theory of secondary vascular ischemia was the most widely accepted theory for many years. Fundamental investigation of nerve injury has demonstrated that the damaging effect of pressure on nerves is related to blood vessel occlusion rather than to nerve compression alone. Investigators have induced facial paralysis in animals by cold and by constriction of the nerve with a suture and demonstrated histological changes similar to those seen in Bell's palsy. Sunderland (1945) has pointed out the delicate balance of pressures within the fallopian canal that are necessary for continued nutrition of the nerve. Slight swelling that leads to obstruction of venous outflow would then initiate the vicious cycle that results in interference to the arterial blood supply of the nerve.

The cause for the initial swelling within the fallopian canal is not explained. However, it has been theorized that autonomic dysfunction predisposes to vasospasm, but there is no proof for this theory. Mc Govern et al. (1966), on the basis of experimental studies, proposed that the triggering mechanism in Bell's palsy is an immunological process of mast cell degranulation, activated by complement or specific allergens. The pathophysiology of edema within the confines of the fallopian canal is the same. The initial vasospasm, increased capillary permeability and edema are due to the histamine release mechanism in immediate hypersensitivity reactions.

According to Fisch (1981), the fundus of the internal auditory meatus is the narrowest portion of the fallopian canal measuring approximately 0.61 mm in diameter while according to Proctor (1991), this narrow segment measures 0.68 mm. This explained why in the presence of edema, the facial nerve fibers (and their vessels) would most often be strangulated at the meatal foramen. The massive bulbous swelling of the meatal segment of the facial nerve occurring in severe cases of Bell's palsy is a typical demonstration of the engagement of the axonal flow, which according to Weiss (1969) is always proximal to the point of pathological constriction of mature nerve fibers.

Tertiary Ischemia

In certain longstanding cases of Bell's palsy, the process of secondary ischemia leads to what is called as tertiary ischemia (Grewal et al. 2002). This is because of the presence of a thickened unyielding facial nerve sheath, which has strangulating effect on the nerve and is responsible for residual facial paresis in cases of Bell's palsy (Grewal et al. 2002).

The nerve sheath has three distinct layers:
1. A tough shiny periosteal layer
2. A layer of loose connective tissue containing blood vessels
3. A firm layer of fibrous tissue that sends strands that connect the perineural connective tissue.

The nerve itself has perineurium, epineurium and endoneurium. The epineurium has a rich vascular supply that communicates freely with the larger vessels, however, the nerve itself is relatively avascular. With this basis of nerve sheath anatomy, the concept of tertiary ischemia can be explained.

In secondary ischemia, the vascular events that take place in the nerve sheath cause vasospasm of the arterioles in the layer of loose connective tissue. This is a temporary reversible event. In most of the cases, this temporary vasospasm resolves with complete return of function within 4-6 months. However, in certain cases, it may persist leading to the permanent event of endarteritis of the blood vessels of the nerve sheath. This phenomenon can be demonstrated histologically and is dealt with later in this chapter. Due to this, the nerve sheath becomes thickened, fibrous and cord-like. There may be formation of fibrous band in the nerve sheath near the stylomastoid foramen or second genu. There can be even more than one fibrous band in the course of facial nerve in the mastoid segment. A thicker nerve sheath and fibrous band or bands further enhances the compressive effects on the nerve and it persists even after the resolution of inciting factors. This leads to a permanent residual facial palsy and to prevent this early surgical intervention is required. There may be even associated subacute mastoiditis in a few cases.

Viral Theory

This theory proposes that Bell's palsy may be a part of polyneuropathy of viral origin. Adour et al. (1978) have found involvement of multiple cranial nerves in cases of Bell's palsy. Also, they have found a stationary titer to Herpes simplex virus or a rising titer to Herpes zoster and also an abnormality in spinal fluid in some patients. Thus, they have concluded that Bell's palsy is an acute benign cranial polyneuritis caused by reactivation of Herpes simplex virus. Djupesland et al. (1977) also proposed that Bell's palsy may be caused due to cranial polyneuropathy that may be viral in origin. This view is supported by May and Hardin (1977) and Tomita (1977) who have also concluded that Herpes simplex or Herpes zoster is a cause of infection. Murakami et al. (1996) also reported the involvement of the herpes simplex virus type 1 (HSV-1) in Bell's palsy as a causative agent.

It is proposed that the virus replicates in the ganglion cells causing local damage and hypofunction of the nerves. It then passes down to the axons causing radiculitis. It infects the Schwann cells causing inflammation and autoimmune response. Lymphocytic infiltration follows leading to fragmentation of myelin, demyelination and chromatolysis. When the inflammation and the autoimmune reaction resolve, remyelination follows. Minkowski in 1891, was the first to provide a careful histological description of the nerve in Bell's palsy. Eight weeks following onset of the palsy, the nerve appeared to be normal from the nucleus to the geniculate ganglion. Distally, within the fallopian canal there were pronounced degenerative Schwann cells, with no signs of inflammation.

Studies of the nerve sheath by Kettle (1963) and Sade et al. (1965) also failed to reveal inflammatory cells. These data would not support an inflammatory etiology for Bell's palsy.

Hereditary Theory

A familial anatomic variation in the facial canal may account for tendency towards a greater incidence of development of facial palsy later in life. The bony constriction of the fallopian canal leads to acute recurrent attacks of facial palsy. This is commonly seen in osteoporosis group of diseases in which the fallopian canal is of an abnormally small diameter. It also makes the nerve more prone for primary ischemic insult or viral infections. Kakar (1966) has concluded this trait of development of recurrent attacks of facial palsy to be a recessive trait. The anatomical variations in the middle ear cleft, can be of:

- Pneumatization pattern
- Size of mastoid antrum (Grewal et al. 2007)
- Fallopian canal: The fallopian canal may vary in its diameter and course, it may be even dehiscent.

These anatomical variations in the presence of cold or viral prodome may lead to primary and thereafter secondary ischemia leading to Bell's Palsy and ultimately tertiary ischemia leading to permanent facial palsy if not timely treated (Flow chart 5.1).

CLINICAL FEATURES

In our experience, the patient usually has a history of exposure to a cold draught of wind while traveling or a history of splashing cold water on the face followed by pain in the postauricular region which may begin as a deep seated ache and progresses to a severe catch in the upper part of the neck on the ipsilateral side. After a few days, the patient notices soap getting into the ipsilateral eye and inability to gargle while washing his/her face in the morning and realizes that there is a facial asymmetry with deviation of the face to the opposite side.

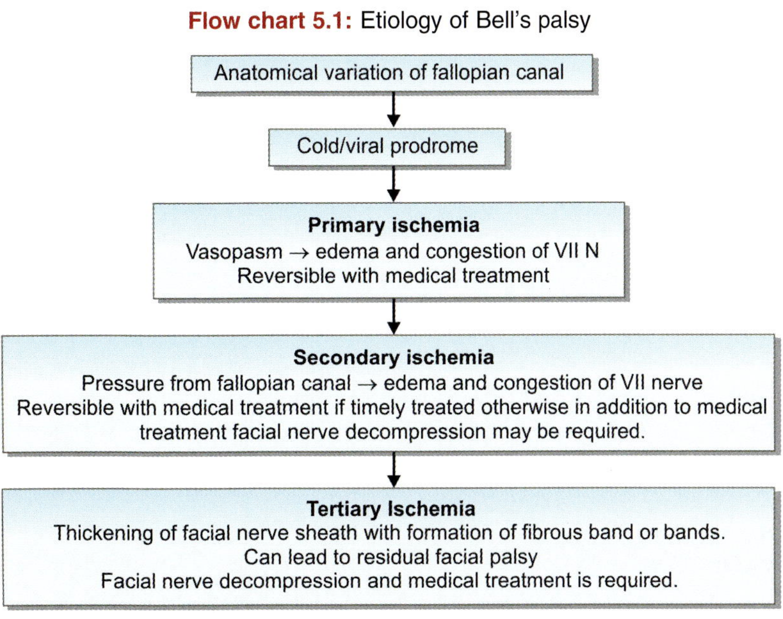

Flow chart 5.1: Etiology of Bell's palsy

The characteristic features of Bell's palsy are that the facial palsy is usually acute in onset and unilateral with an associated numbness and weakness of the side of the face involved. Some patients may give history suggestive of a viral prodrome or there may be a family history of facial palsy. There may be history of recurrent ipsilateral palsy as well as decreased lacrimation and salivation on the side of the lesion. All patients present with a facial asymmetry with deviation of the face to the opposite side. Almost 90% of the patients show an absent stapedial reflex on impedance audiometry and in some patients the chorda tympani nerve appears red on otoscopic examination within 10 days of onset of the palsy.

The features of presentation in this patient also include upward movement of the eyeball on attempting to close the eye (Bell's phenomenon), epiphora, deviation of the face and the angle of the mouth to the normal side of the face, dribbling of saliva and liquids on attempts to drink, collection of food in the cheek as a result of the paralysis of the buccinator muscle and an inability to blow or whistle. There may be a loss of taste sensation and hyperacusis due to the involvement of the chorda tympani nerve and the stapedius muscle respectively.

However, it is important to know that the classical features of Bell's palsy are that it is "self limiting, non progressive, non-life-threatening and spontaneously remitting usually within 4-6 months and always by 1 year".

HISTOLOGICAL ASPECTS

The biopsy of the nerve sheath in cases of Bell's palsy during its surgical decompression shows the presence of endarteritis of the nerve sheath. The microscopic features include the presence of vessels with thickened walls along with a few vessels showing features of obliterative endarteritis. These features are typically seen in cases that have a residual facial palsy.

Also, the other features that can be appreciated are the presence of edema in early cases. In some cases with residual palsy, marked amount of fibrosis can be seen in the nerve sheath and thus a thickened nerve sheath is seen microscopically. These typical features can be very well demonstrated by some special stains like the Masson's trichrome which stains the connective tissue green (Fig. 5.5).

MANAGEMENT OF BELL'S PALSY

The management of Bell's palsy can be divided into:
- Medical management
- Surgical management.

There exists controversies over what line of treatment should be adopted first and there are various studies, which show the benefit of one over the other. The palsy may be either complete or incomplete, when the patient presents to the otologist. It is seen that almost one-third of the patients with incomplete palsy show an evidence of recovery with medical management within three weeks and eventually progress to complete recovery. However, we prefer to start with the medical line of management as soon as the patient presents to us and monitor the progress of the palsy using serial EMG and Nerve Excitability Test repeated every week. Acoustic reflex monitoring is also performed weekly, since it is the first sign of return of nerve function.

Medical Management

This comprises of high dose steroids (starting with Prednisolone-1 mg/kg/day or 60 mg) given orally in tapering doses over a period of three weeks, antibiotics, vasodilators like Xanitol nicotinate, Ascorbic acid, multi-vitamins and vitamin B1, B6 and B12, eye care (eye pad, dark goggles, artificial tears, etc.) along with active and passive physiotherapy. Steroids help by providing a protection to the nerve tissue against degeneration of the nerve. Ascorbic acid is known to have antiviral properties. Adour (1991) advocates the use of Acyclovir orally in the dose of 200-400 mg five times per day.

The medical treatment forms the main stay of Bell's palsy and it results in improvement of most of the cases. However, if signs of recovery fail to appear within three weeks of medical management, we advocate surgical decompression of the nerve.

Surgical Treatment

This includes the decompression of the facial nerve that may be done by various approaches. They include middle cranial fossa approach; translabyrinthine approach; transmastoid extralabyrinthine subtemporal approach and total decompression that may be a combination of the approaches mentioned above.

It still remains controversial whether a case of Bell's palsy should be offered surgical treatment and at what point of time should it be offered. There are no strict criteria so as to when the facial nerve should be decompressed. Various researchers have debated on the role of surgical decompression. The Marsh and Coker criteria (1991) state the following indications:

- Complete denervation
- Paralysis for more than 4-6 weeks
- Incomplete return of function in 60 days
- Recurrent facial palsy
- Nerve excitability test shows a difference of 3.5 mA on both the sides.

Schirmer's test can be used to decide the mode of surgical decompression if the tear flow is reduced by more than 50% on the affected side then a total decompression or middle fossa approach is indicated.

We advocate facial nerve decompression in a case of Bell's palsy if there is no improvement of the palsy after three weeks of medical treatment or if the palsy appears to be progressively worsening inspite of the patient being on medical management. Facial nerve decompression can be carried out for a patient presenting up to two years, after onset of palsy. However, if a patient presents after 2 years of onset of palsy, regeneration usually does not occur and plastic surgical repair has to be considered.

It is known that in a case of Bell's palsy, the facial nerve shows "skip lesions", i.e. segments of normal nerve tissue in between areas of pathology. Keeping this in mind, we prefer to do decompression of the nerve during its course in the tympanic and mastoid segments, till the stylomastoid foramen and labyrinthine part is dealt with as much as possible without dislocating the incus.

We carry the decompression of the facial nerve through a transmastoid approach via a posterior tympanotomy. We consider posterior tympanotosmy is a very useful and versatile approach for facial nerve surgery because it is a relatively small opening through which one can expose and operate upon the longest structure in the middle ear and mastoid i.e. facial nerve. A standard postauricular incision is taken with an anteriorly based pedicled flap. A complete cortical mastoidectomy is done and a posterior tympanotomy is performed. The facial nerve is then decompressed and while decompressing it is important that more than half of its circumference is decompressed to achieve good results. (Figs 5.1 to 5.3).

During facial nerve decompression, we have seen that the nerve sheath in a case of Bell's palsy appears unusually thickened due to fibrosis (Figs 5.4A to D). This is an important factor in creating a vicious cycle of further compressing the edematous nerve resulting in tertiary ischemia due to the compressive

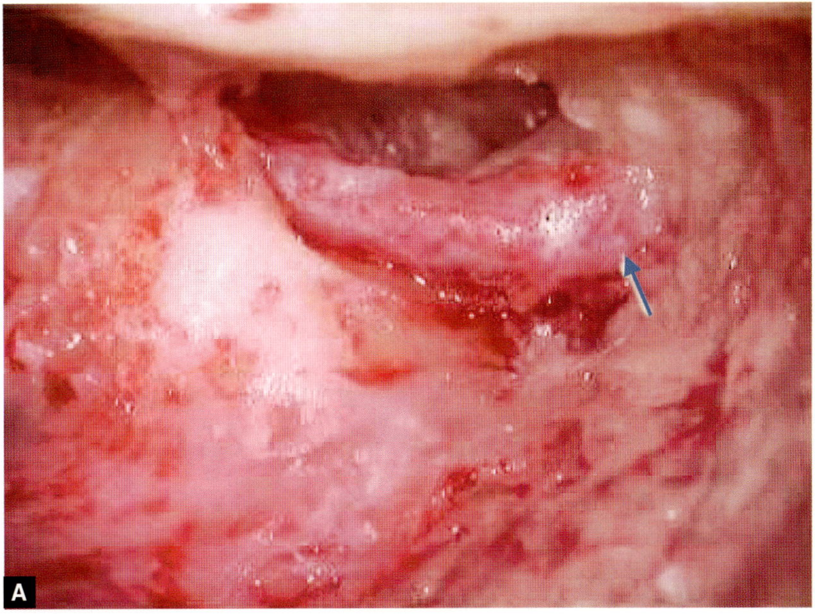

Fig. 5.1A

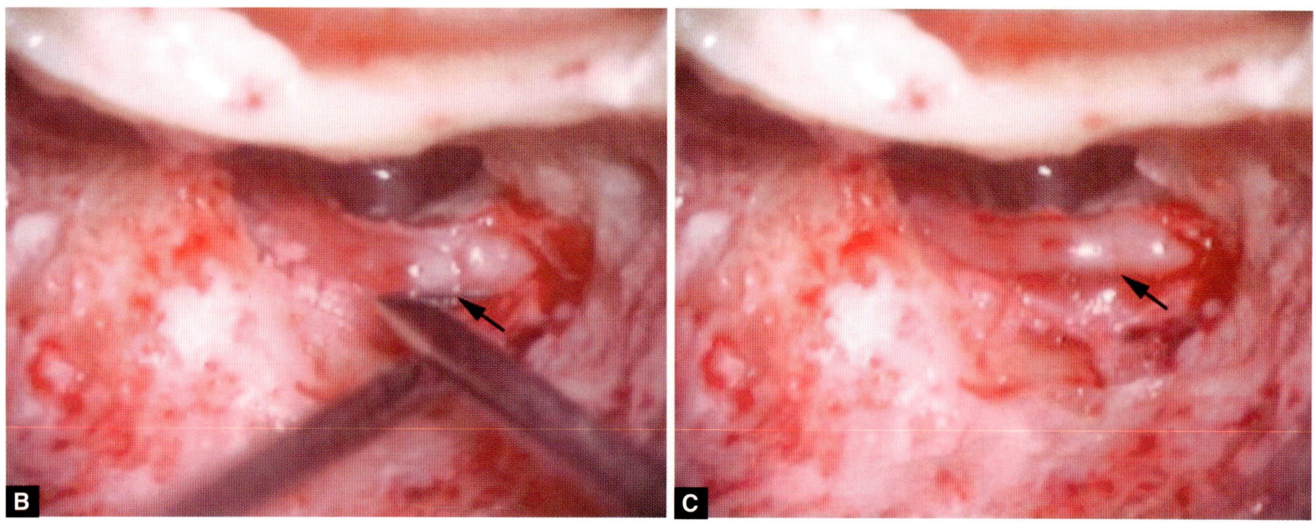

Figs 5.1B and C

Figs 5.1A to C: Facial nerve decompression done. Note the thickened facial nerve sheath and fibrous band compressing it in the mastoid segment. Fibrous band is cut. Note the effect of compression on the facial nerve by the fibrous band. The fibrous band near the stylomastoid foramen can lead to classical edema described of facial nerve in this region and perhaps the cause of catch like pain in the stenomastoid region.

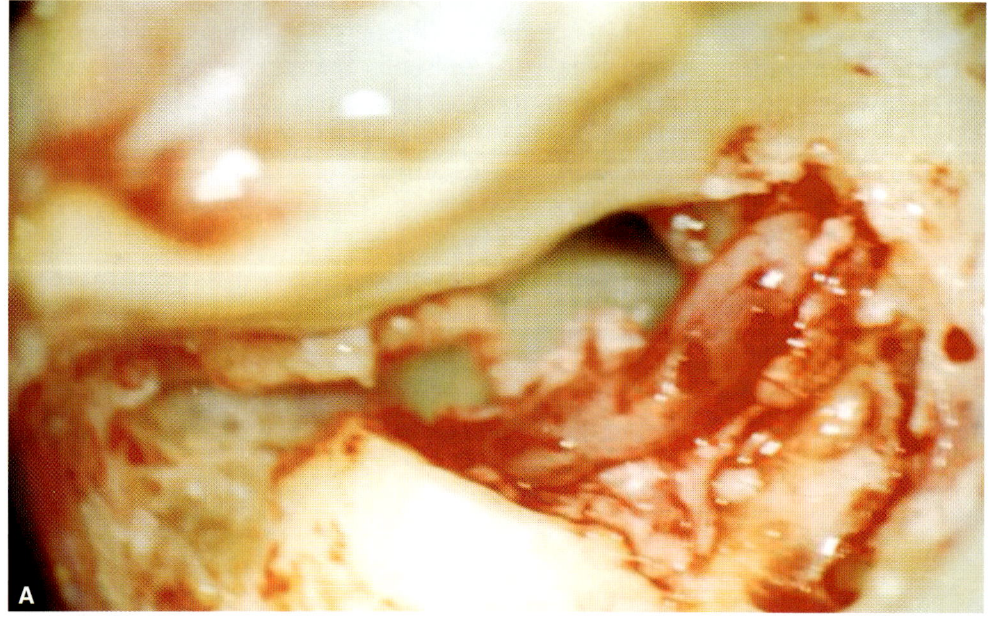

Fig. 5.2A: Intraoperative photograph of the facial nerve decompressed in a case of Bell's palsy with slitting of its thickened sheath.The nerve is edematous and congested

effects of the rigid thickened nerve sheath, even after removing the compression caused by the bony facial canal in addition to secondary ischemia due to a rigid bony fallopian canal and worsening of the edema. Hence, we prefer to slit the nerve sheath and cut the fibrous band or bands if present. The nerve is then gently separated from its thickened sheath thus relieving the nerve of the strangulating effects of the nerve sheath. Also, we have seen varying pictures of nerve pathology after the sheath is slit and depending

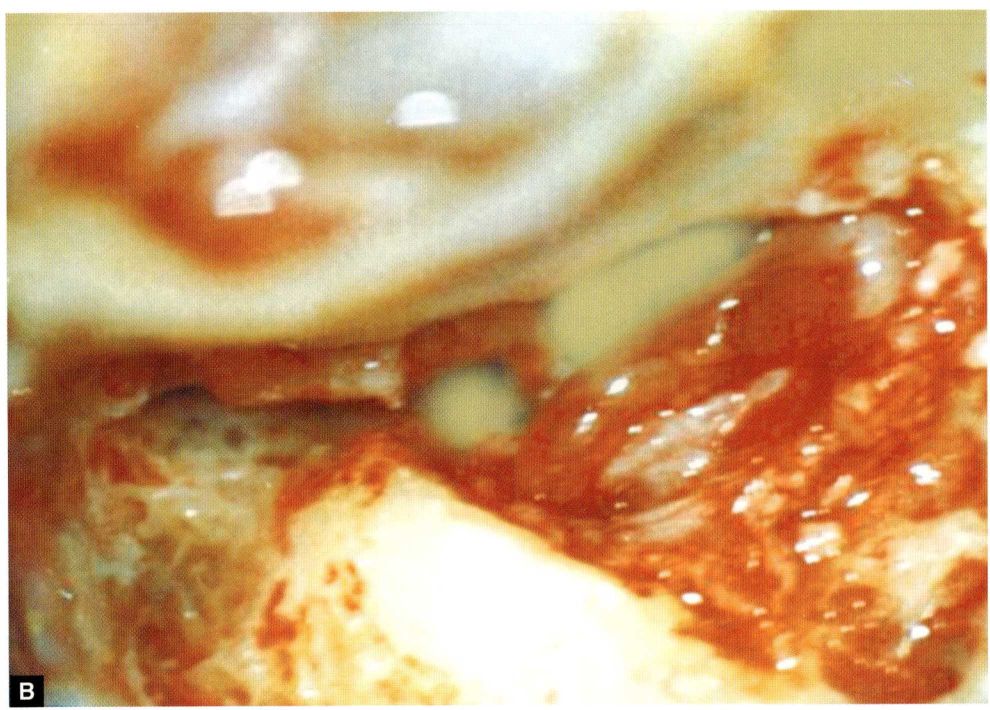

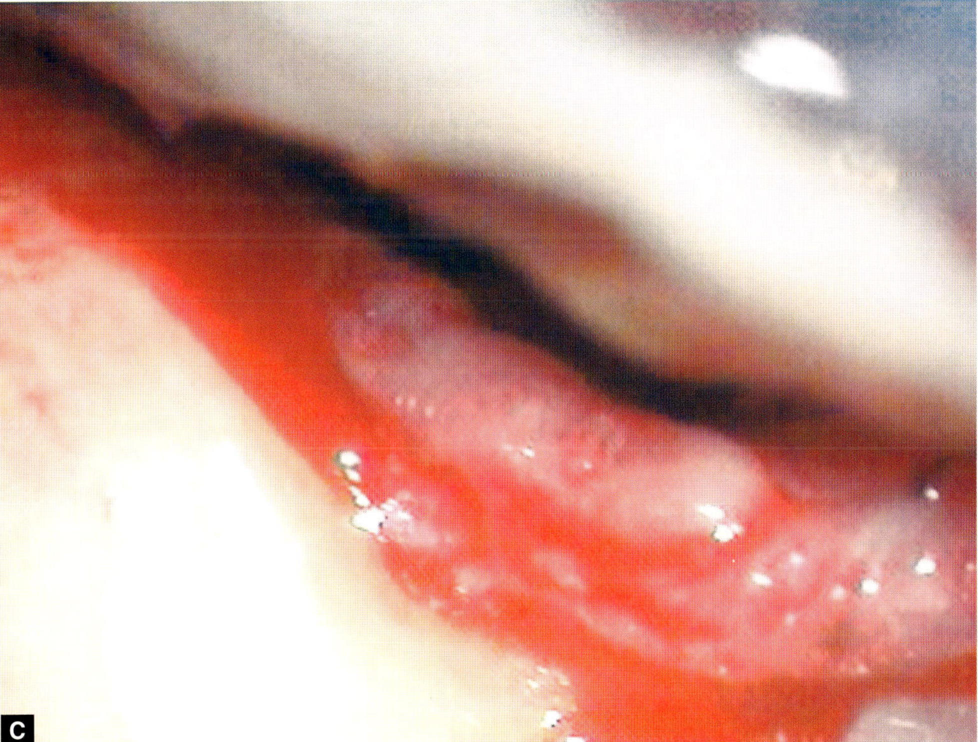

Figs 5.2B and C: (B) A case of long-standing Bell's palsy (18 weeks duration) where decompression of the nerve, with slitting of its sheath revealed multiple sites of nerve compression due to fibrous bands which were cut; (C) The decompressed nerve with severe edema and multiple indentations due to the compressive effect of the fibrous bands even after they were cut. The nerve is seen bulging out of the cut sheath

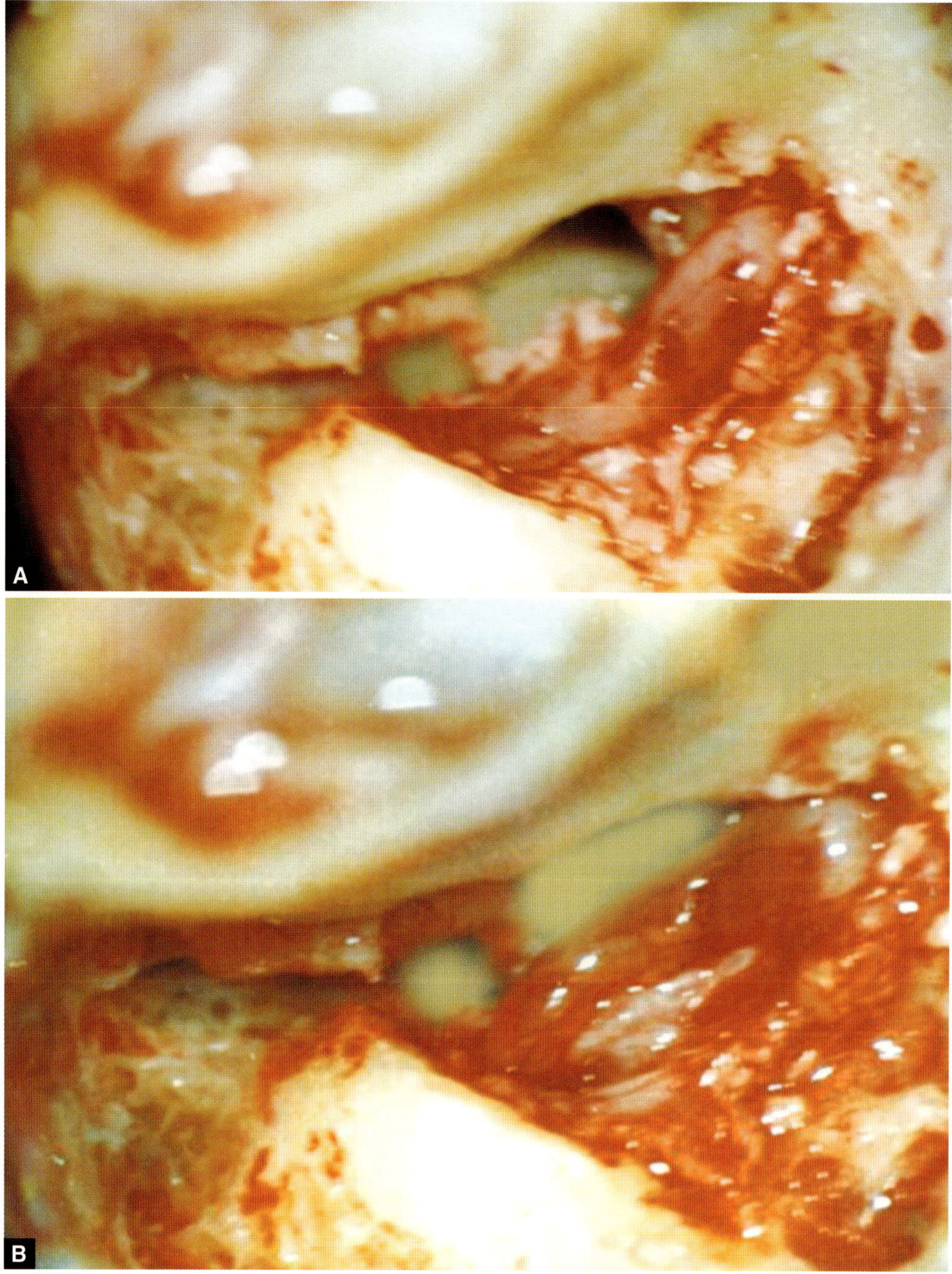

Figs 5.3A and B: (A) Intraoperative photograph of the facial nerve decompressed in a case of Bell's palsy with slitting of its sheath; (B) Intraoperative photograph of the facial nerve decompressed in a case of Bell's palsy. The nerve is seen removed from its sheath. Note the edema at the stylomastoid foramen

on these, we start postoperative treatment (Fig. 5.5). The pathologies seen include: an edematous nerve, with indentation which may be due to one or more fibrous band or bands. When we start steroids postoperatively; a congested nerve where we start Acyclovir in addition to steroids postoperatively or a thinned out atrophic nerve due to fibrosis as a result of disuse atrophy.

There are certain unique anatomical and surgical factors, which if considered during the procedure make the operation much simpler.

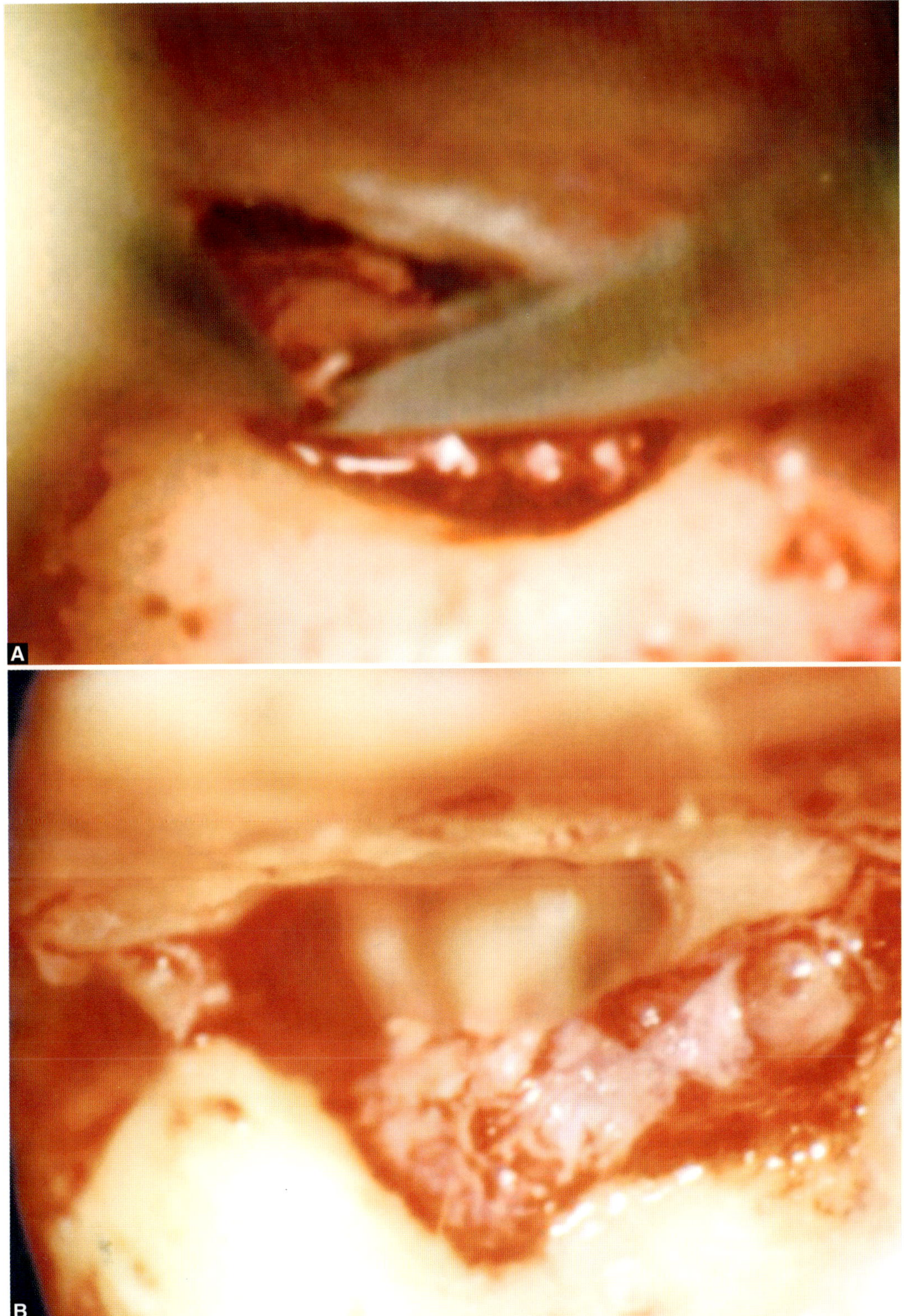

Figs 5.4A and B: (A) Intraoperative photograph showing the fibrosed and thickened facial nerve sheath in a decompression done for a case of Bell's palsy—a biopsy of its sheath being taken; (B) Intraoperative photograph showing the fibrosed and thickened facial nerve sheath in decompression done for a case of Bell's palsy-biopsy taken—note the nerve bulging out through the biopsy site

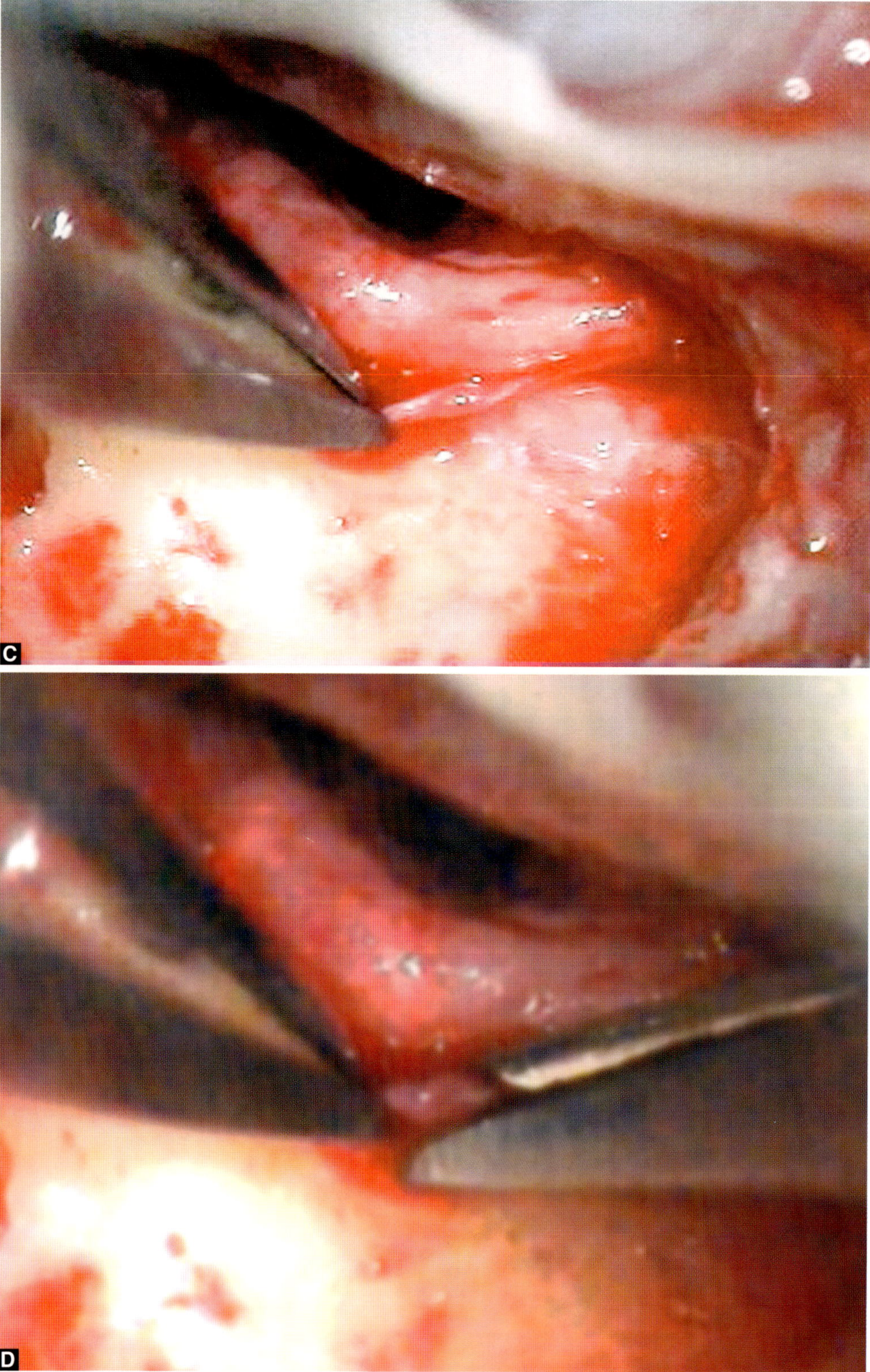

Figs 5.4C and D: (C) Intraoperative photograph of facial nerve decompression in another case of Bell's palsy, its sheath is caught with forceps for taking biopsy; (D) Intraoperative photograph of facial nerve decompression in the same case of Bell's palsy where biopsy of the thickened and fibrosed nerve sheath is being taken

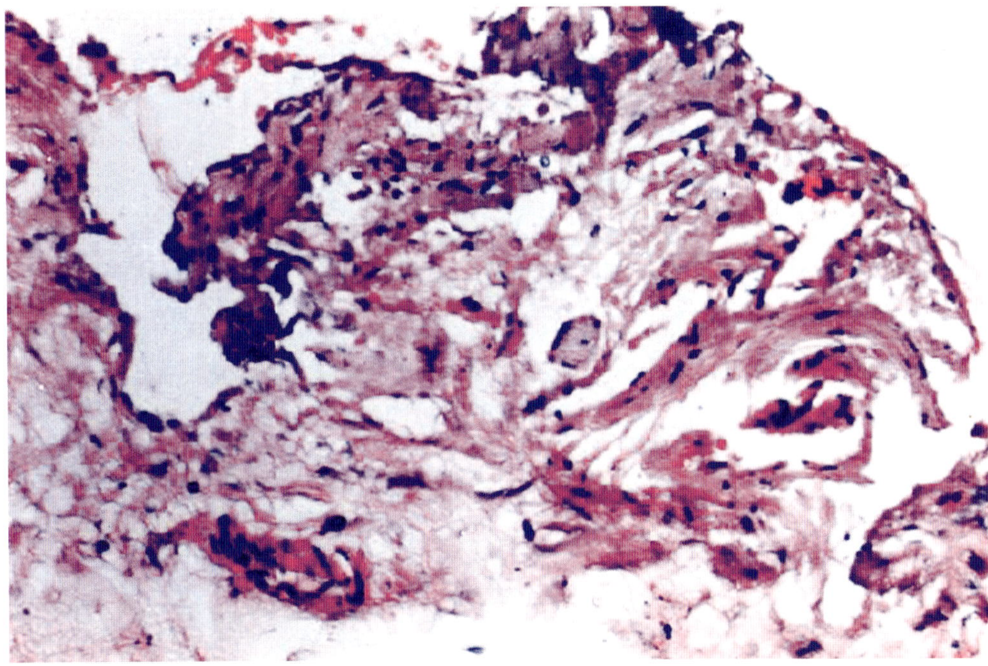

Fig. 5.5: Histopathology of the facial nerve sheath showing bundles of facial nerve fibers with intervening fibrosis (H&E staining 20X) of the same patient (Figs 5.4 C and D)

Anatomical Factors

A thorough knowledge of the anatomy of the antrum threshold angle (Mihalkovics, 1892) and chorda facial angle (Plester, 1965) is important before performing the posterior tympanotomy. However, we have noticed certain important anatomical facts that will aid the surgeon in performing a posterior tympanotomy:

- The posterior canal wall takes a gentle natural curve in its deep part, an anatomical fact that aids a surgeon in performing a posterior tympanotomy. A simple mastoidectomy is performed and the posterior meatal wall is thinned as much as possible. After this the opening of the facial recess can be commenced. An imaginary tangent drawn medially from the start of curve in the posterior meatal wall leads us to the facial nerve. Drilling anteriorly to this in the shaded area (Fig. 5.6) comprises posterior tympanotomy. Also, due to this natural curve of the deep part of the external auditory canal, the chorda tympani lies more anteriorly and the facial nerve lies posteromedially, thus facilitating posterior tympanotomy.

- The facial nerve, in its mastoid segment, takes a gentle turn anteriorly as it approaches the

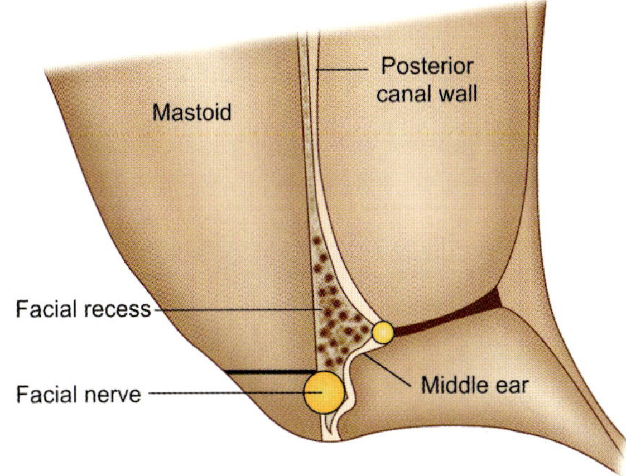

Fig. 5.6: Diagrammatic representation of the relation of facial nerve to the posterior canal wall and floor of the mastoid

stylomastoid foramen. This is a consistent feature found in all the cases and we have termed this as the third genu of the facial nerve (Fig. 5.7A and B).

This peculiar anatomical course of the facial nerve defines the lower limit of posterior tympanotomy. During surgery, if an imaginary line is drawn from the floor of the middle ear in the antero-posterior axis,

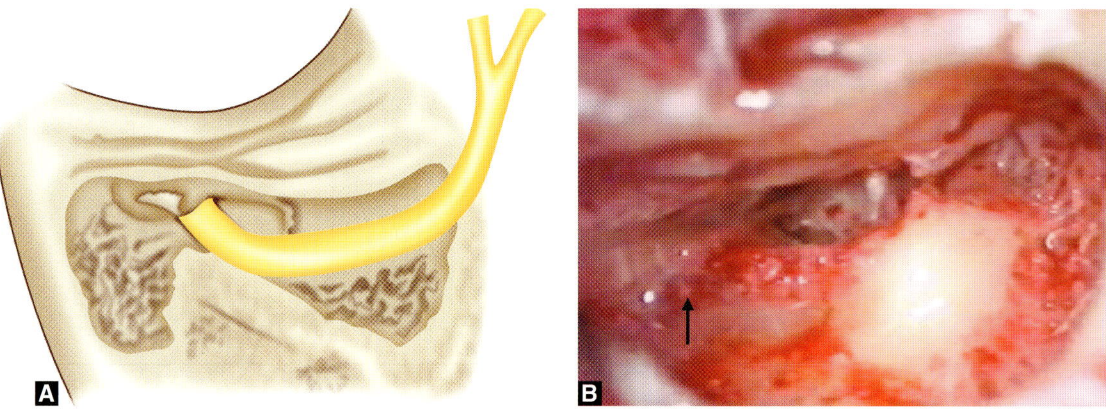

Figs 5.7A and B: (A) Diagrammatic representation of the third genu of the facial nerve; (B) Third genu of facial nerve which is lower limit of facial nerve decompression. It is a point at which nerve leaves the mastoid to exit at the stylomastoid foramen and turns anteriorly

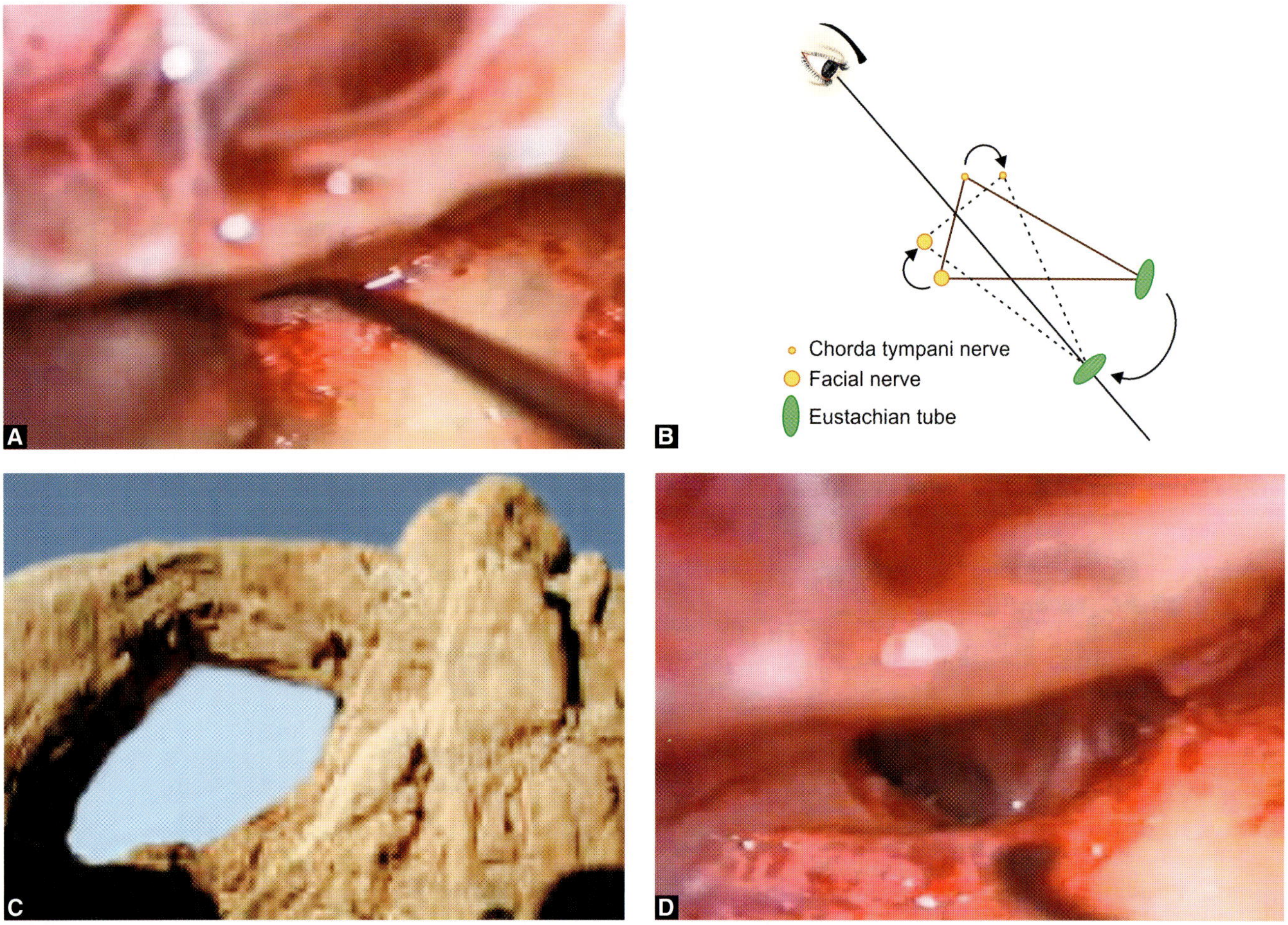

Figs 5.8A to D: (A) Posterior tympanotomy; a mere extension of simple mastoidtectomy, sickle knife is pointing the facial nerve which forms its postero-medial boundary; (B) Diagrammatic representation showing tilting of the patient's head away from the surgeon, bringing the chorda tympani nerve and the facial nerve in a horizontal plane, perpendicular to the surgeon's visual axis, thus improving visibility— "open window effect"; (C and D) Improved visibility of structures through a posterior lympanotomy on tilting the patient's head away from the surgeon—"open window effect"

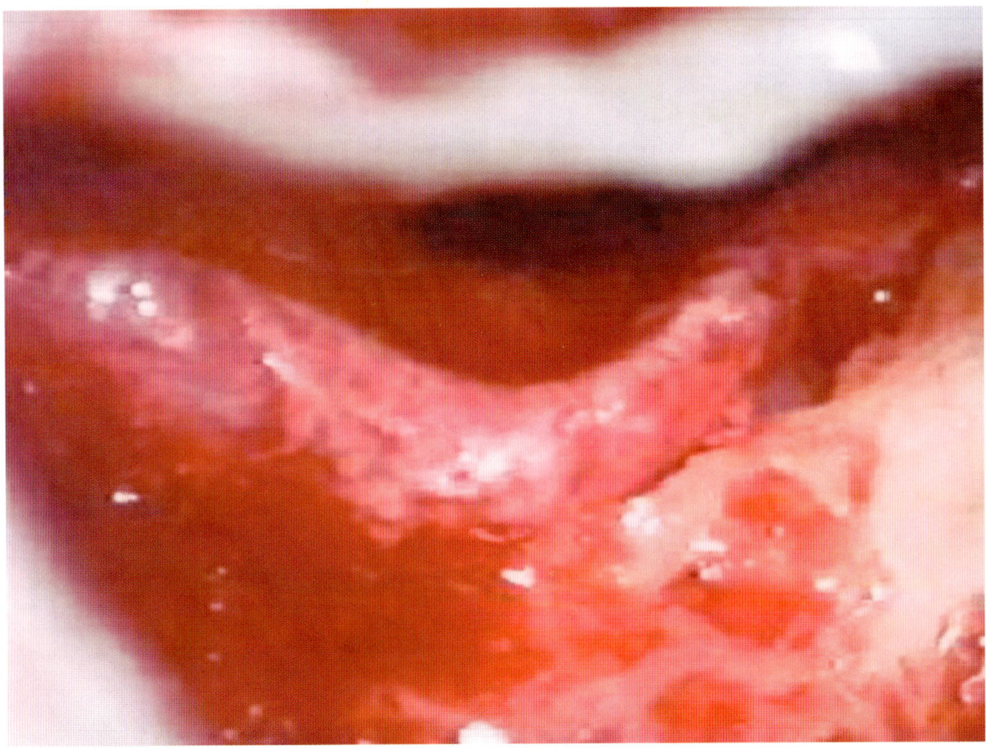

Fig. 5.9: Postero-superior tympanotomy done for facial nerve trauma

the third genu begins at the point where this line meets the facial nerve (Fig. 5.10). The third genu starts in the mastoid segment of the facial nerve and continues in its extra-temporal portion. We feel that the facial nerve should be identified by the third genu itself near the area of its exit through the stylomastoid foramen as it forms a consistent landmark. This, if identified can be considered as a more reliable landmark than the more conventional landmarks for the facial nerve in this region viz. the digastric ridge in its mastoid segment and the tragal pointer in its extratemporal segment.

Surgical Factors

The following surgical factors are very useful during posterior tympanotomy in our experience:

- Posterior tympanotomy is a very simple procedure as it as a mere extension of a simple mastoidectomy. After completing a cortical or simple mast-oidectomy, the posterior canal wall is thinned and the facial recess is opened. The posterior tympanotomy finally assumes a bean shaped opening in the posterior canal wall. However, with the standard surgical position of the patient, this bean shaped opening gives a limited view of the middle ear structures. This difficulty can be eliminated by tilting the head of the patient downward, i.e. away from the operating surgeon. This will apparently increase the working distance and thus the area under vision. In such a position, the chorda tympani and the facial nerve lie in approximately the same horizontal plane, which lies perpendicular to the visual axis of the surgeon. As a result, certain important middle ear structures such as the tympanic part of the facial nerve, the eustachian tube opening and the hypotympanum are now clearly visible and easily accessible. We have termed this as the **open window effect** (Figs 5.8A to D).

- The posterior tympanotomy can be extended superiorly upto the 12 O'clock position or a little beyond anteriorly and hence the term **postero-superior tympanotomy** appears more appropriate when used in this context. (Fig. 5.9).

Therefore, although some may not advocate surgical decompression in a case of Bell's palsy, I prefer decompression provided there is a definite indication

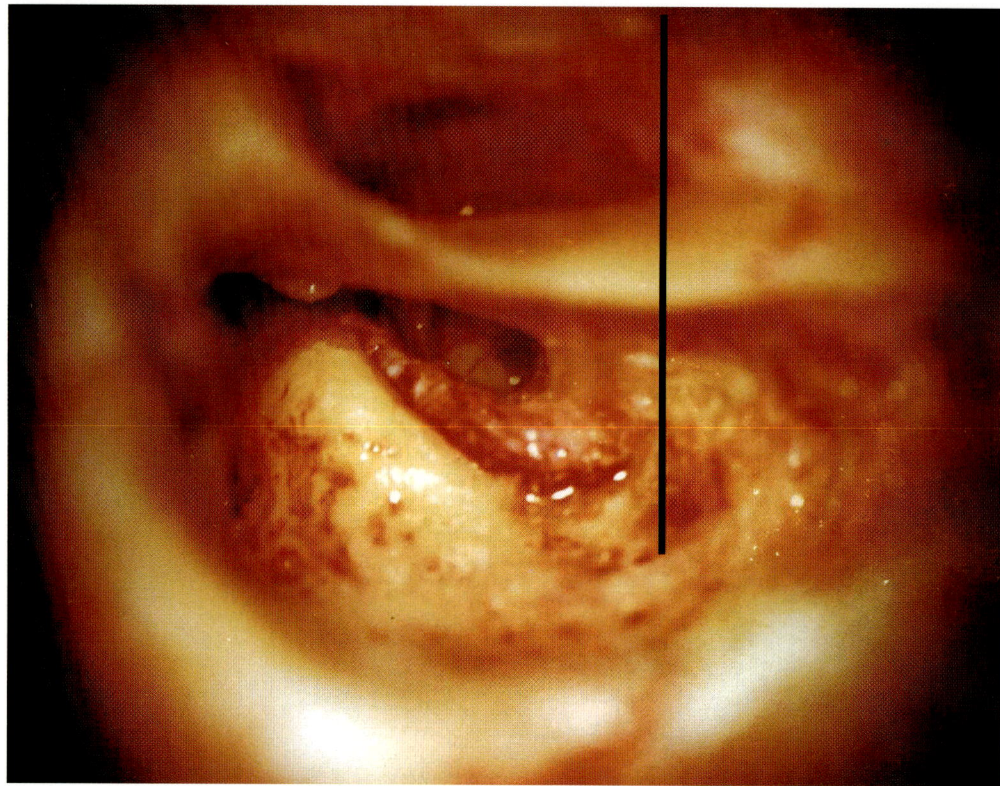

Fig. 5.10: Third genu is at an imaginary line drown from the floor of middle ear in the antero-posterior axis joining the facial neve

for the same. If indicated, I feel that transmastoid decompression is a safe and an easy approach to decompress the facial nerve and the above-mentioned factors should be considered by an otologic surgeon to facilitate the procedure of decompression via posterior tympanotomy. Medical treatment is adjuvant to the surgical treatment and both are incomplete without physiotherapy. Physiotherapy still remains most undisputed and simplest form of treatment.

BIBLIOGRAPHY

1. Adour KK. Medical Management of Idiopathic (Bell's) Palsy. The Otolaryngologic Clinics of North America. 1991;24:663-72.
2. Adour KK, Byl FM, Hilsinger RL, et al. The true nature of Bell's palsy: Analysis of 1000 Consecutive Patients. Laryngoscope. 1978;89:787-801.
3. Blunt MJ. The Blood supply of the Facial nerve. Journal of Anatomy. 1954;888:520.
4. Brackmann DE Bell's palsy incidence etiology and results of medical treatment. Otolaryngologic Clinics of North America Jun 1974;7:357-68.
5. Calcaterra TC, Rand RW, Bentson JR. Ischaemic paralysis of facial nerve: a positive etiological factor in Bell's palsy. Laryngoscope. 1976;86:92-7.
6. Dalton GA. Bell's palsy: some problems of prognosis and treatment. British Medical Journal. 1960;1:1765-70.
7. Donath T, Lengyel I. The vascular structure of the intrapetrosal section of the facial nerve, with special reference to peripheral facial palsy. Acta Med Acad Sci Hung. 1957;10:249.
8. Djupesland G, Berdal P, Johannessen JA, et al. Viral infection as a cause of acute peripheral facial palsy. Archives of Otolaryngology. 1976;102:403-6.
9. Drachman D. Bell's palsy. a neurological point of view. Archives of Otolaryngology. 1969;89:147.
10. Fisch U. Surgery for Bell's palsy. Archives of Otolaryngology. 1981;107:1-11.
11. Grewal DS, Hathiram BT, Walvekar R, et al. Surgical Decompression in Bell's palsy—Our viewpoint. Indian Journal of Otolaryngology and Head and Neck Surgery. 2002;54:198-203.
12. Grewal DS, Hatiram BJ, Saraiya S. V canal wall down Tympano mastoidectomy, the "on-disease" approach for retraction pockets and cholesteatoma. The journal of laryngology and otology. 2007;121:832- 9.

13. Hilger JA. The nature of Bell's palsy. Laryngoscope. 1949;59:228.

14. Kakar PK, Sawhney KL, and Saharia PS. Familial Bell's palsy (Case report) Journal of Laryngology and Otology 1996;80:628-30.

15. Kettel K. Pathology and surgery of Bell's palsy. Laryngoscope. 1963;73:837.

16. Korkis FB. Treatment of recent Bell's palsy by cervical sympathetic block. Lancet. 1961;1:255-7.

17. Marsh MJ, Coker NJ. Surgical Decompression of Idiopathic Facial Palsy. Otolaryngologic Clinics of North America. 24:675-90.

18. May M, Hardin WB. Facial palsy: interpretation of neurological findings. (Trans.) Am Acad Ophthalmol Otol. 84:ORL. 1977;710-22.

19. May M. Total facial nerve exploration: transmastoid, extralabyrinthine, subtemporal: indication and Results. Laryngoscope. 1976;89:906.

20. McGovern FH, Thompson E, Link N. The experimental production of ischaemic facial paralysis. Laryngoscope. 1966;76:1138.

21. Mihalkovics G. The Morphology of the central nervous system and sensory organs. (Hungarian) Franklin Co.:Budapest. 1892.

22. Minowski. Zur pathologischen Anatonnie der rhurriatischen Facialislahmung. Archives of General Psychiatry. 1891;23:586.

23. Murakami S, Mizobuchi M, Naakaashiro Y, et al. Bell's palsy and herpes simplex virus: identification of viral DNA in endoneural fluid and muscle. Annals of Internal Medicine. 1996;124:27-30.

24. Peiterson E. The Natural History of Bell's palsy. American Journal of Otology. 1982;4:107-11.

25. Plester (1965). Cited by Jako CJ: The posterior route to the middle ear: Posterior tympanotomy. Laryngoscope. 1967;77:306-16.

26. Proctor B. The Anatomy of the facial nerve. otolaryngologic clinics of North America. 1991;24:479-529.

27. Sade J, Levy E, Chaco J. Surgery and pathology of Bell's palsy. Archives of Otolaryngology. 1965;82:594.

28. Schaitkin B, May M. Disorders of the facial nerve. (6th edn). Scott-Brown's Otolaryngology. 1977;3:24:1-38.

29. Seddon HJ. Three types of nerve injury. Brain. 1943;66:237-88.

30. Sunderland S. Blood supply of the peripheral nerves. Archives of Neurology and Psychiatry. 1945;54:280.

31. Sunderland S. Nerve and Nerve Injuries. (2nd edn). London:Churchill Livingstone; 1978.pp.88-9:96-7, 133.

32. Taverner D. Lancet. Cortisone treatment of Bell's palsy 1954;2:1052.

33. Tomita H. In: Facial Nerve Surgery. (Ed). By U Fisch. Amsterdam:Kugler Medical Publication; 1977.

34. Weiss PA. Neuronal dynamics and neuroplasmic ('axonal') flow. New York: Academic Press; 1969. p. 8.

35. William Gowers as cited by: Cawthorne T and Wilson, T. Indications of Intratemporal Facial Nerve Surgery, Archives of Otolaryngology. 1963;78:429-34.

6

Medical Treatment of the Facial Nerve

Guy Kenyon

INTRODUCTION

Disorders of the facial nerve present with a variety of different functional and aesthetic problems which include the direct effects of the palsy as well as secondary effects such as synkinesis and hemifacial spasm. In many cases, medical management alone will be insufficient or inappropriate and surgical treatment of the palsy or its sequelae, will be required. However in certain instances, most notably in Bell's palsy and patients infected with the herpes virus (Ramsay Hunt syndrome), medical management will be the first priority with surgery reserved for a minority of specialized cases. This chapter will concentrate on the medical treatment of these two conditions.

BELL'S PALSY

Incidence and Prevalence

The incidence and prevalence of Bell's palsy is around 23 per 100,000 people per year or about 1 in 60-70 people in a lifetime (Victor, Martin, 1994). It affects men and women more or less equally, with a peak incidence between the ages of 10 and 40 years and occurs with equal frequency on the right and left sides of the face (Prescott, 1988).

Etiology

In the past the condition has thought to be idiopathic, although ischemia and hereditary influences have also been suggested. In the recent past, a viral etiology has become popular with the discovery of herpes simplex virus-1 genome from facial nerve endoneural fluid in people with Bell's palsy (Murakami, Mizobuchi, Nakashir, et al. 1996).

Management

The aim of any management strategy is to maximize the chances of recovery of facial function and to reduce the risk of sequelae, with minimal adverse treatment effects. The success or failure of treatment is normally rated by the grade of recovery of motor function of the face, the presence of sequelae (synkinesis, autonomic dysfunction and hemifacial spasm) and the time to full recovery.

Two-thirds of people achieve a full recovery spontaneously. The largest series of people with Bell's palsy who received no specific treatment (n = 1,011) found the first signs of improvement within three weeks of onset in 85%, and in the other 15% some improvement occurred 3-6 months later (Pietersen E, 1982). The same series found that 71% of people recovered normal function of the face, 13% had insignificant sequelae and the remaining 16% had permanently diminished function with contracture and synkinesis (involuntary movement accompanying a voluntary movement). It is against this background of spontaneous improvement that any therapeutic strategy must be assessed.

Corticosteroid Therapy

There is circumstantial evidence that the nerve is edematous when it is surgically decompressed and this knowledge has suggested that steroids might be helpful in aiding recovery. As recently as 2004 a Cochrane meta-analysis concluded that there was insufficient evidence to support the use of steroids in these patients (Salinas, Alvarez, Ferreira, 2004), but the results of several recently completed studies (Sullivan, Swann, Donnan, et al. 2007; Engström, Berg and Stjernquist- Desatnik, et al. 2008; Hato, Yamad, Kohno, et al. 2007; Kawaguchi, Inamura, Abe, et al. 2007; Minnerop, Herbst, Fimmers, et al. 2008; Yeo, Lee, Park, et al. 2008) have confirmed that there is substantial data to support their use.

In the first of these, Sullivan et al. performed a double-blinded, randomized, placebo-controlled trial involving 752 patients with Bell's palsy (Sullivan, Swann, Donnan, et al. 2007). Patients were randomized twice prior to receiving either steroids or acyclovir alone or in combination. The combinations offered were:

- Prednisolone (50 mg daily) and placebo for 10 days
- Acyclovir (2000 mg/day) and placebo for 10 days
- Prednisolone (50 mg daily) and acyclovir (2000 mg/ day) for 10 days
- Placebo for 10 days.

Randomization and initiation of treatment occurred within 72 hours following the onset of symptoms and outcomes were measured using the House Brackman grading system. Of the 251 patients who received prednisolone alone, 83% (205) at three and 94.4% (237) at nine months exhibited a complete recovery of function whereas in the patients receiving placebo 64.7% (91) and 85.2% (120) demonstrated complete recovery at three and nine months. The results of steroid therapy were significantly better than placebo (P < 0.001) and the study concluded that the administration of prednisolone increased the chances of complete facial function recovery.

Engström et al. also completed a randomized double-blinded placebo-controlled study that provided evidence that the administration of corticosteroids is effective in patients with Bell's palsy (Engström, Berg and Stjernquist-Desatnik et al. 2008). In this study 839 patients between the age of 18 and 75 years were treated within 72 hours from the onset of symptoms, by a protocol that divided them into one of four groups. These were:

1. Placebo and placebo
2. Prednisolone (60 mg/day) and placebo daily for five days which was then reduced by 10 mg each day for an additional five days
3. Valacyclovir (3000 mg/day) and placebo for seven days
4. Prednisolone (60 mg/day) for 10 days and valacyclovir (3000 mg/day) for seven days.

Six months after initiation of therapy the prednisolone and placebo group had a significantly shorter time to recovery when compared with placebo. Complete recovery was achieved in 150 patients (71%) in the prednisolone and placebo group compared to only 58% (120 patients) in the valacyclovir and placebo group, 72% (149 patients) in the prednisolone and valacyclovir group (P < 0.003) and 62% (127 patients) in the placebo and placebo group.

The efficacy of steroids and antiviral agents in Bell's palsy was also examined by Hato et al. (Hato, Yamad, Kohno, et al. 2007). In a single-blinded, randomized placebo-controlled trial, 221 patients were randomized to receive either:

- Prednisolone (60 mg daily for five days with a 5-day taper) and placebo (107 patients)
- Prednisolone (60 mg daily for five days with a 5-day taper) and valacyclovir (1000 mg/day) for five days (114 patients).

At six months, 89.7% (96 patients) in the prednisolone and placebo group achieved complete recovery of facial function in comparison with 96.5% (110) of those who received prednisolone and valacyclovir (P < 0.05). The patients in this study had a more severe facial palsy (House Brackman 4-5) than those who were included in the Sullivan study (mean

House Brackman score 3.6) and it is possible that this explains the apparent effectiveness of the addition of an antiviral agent.

Prednisolone and valacyclovir were also utilized in a study reported by Kawaguchi and others (Kawaguchi, Inamura, Abe, et al. 2007). This study randomized 150 patients and found that the administration of an antiviral agent provided no advantage when compared with prednisolone alone. The patients in this unblended, prospective trial were randomized into one of two groups which were:

1. Prednisolone (20 mg three times daily alone for five days with a 5-day taper)
2. Prednisolone (20 mg three times daily for five days with a 5-day taper) and valacyclovir (1000 mg/day) for five days.

The clinical results were reported as the cumulative recovery rate based on the Yanagihara 40-point facial grading system. Out of 66 patients treated with pednisolone alone, the mean time for complete recovery was 70.7 days as compared with 76.4 days in the prednisolone/valacyclovir group (84 patients). This difference did not achieve statistical significance (P = 0.977) but the study also found a statistically significant difference in the cumulative recovery rate based on the initial severity of the palsy.

In a study by Minnerop et al., 167 consecutive patients of whom 117 completed a full follow-up, received either prednisone alone or a combination of prednisone and famcyclovir within 2.4 or 2.6 days respectively after the onset of symptoms (Minnerop, Herbst, Fimmers, et al., 2008). The regimen used was:

1. Prednisone (1 mg/kg body weight for four days followed by an 8-day taper: 67 patients)
2. Prednisone (1 mg/kg body weight for four days with an 8-day taper) and famcyclovir (750 mg/day) for seven days (50 patients).

Three months after initiation of therapy 12% (8 patients) of the prednisone alone group exhibited at least a four-grade House-Brackman grade improvement as compared with 28% (14 patients) given prednisone and famcyclovir in combination (p 0.028). Interestingly herpes simplex virus-1 (HSV-1) antibody status was also reported, but was not found to correlate with recovery of facial function.

Finally, in a final double-blind randomized prospective trial comparing prednisolone with acyclovir Yeo et al. randomized 91 patients to receive either acyclovir together with prednisone or prednisone alone (Yeo, Lee, Park, et al., 2008). In this study, the combinations of drugs utilized were:

1. Prednisone 1 mg/kg/day (maximum 80 mg/day) for four days followed by a 6-day taper (44 patients)
2. Acyclovir (2400 mg/day) for five days and 1 mg/kg/day of prednisone (to a maximum of 80 mg/day) for four days followed by a 6-day taper (47 patients).

After six months, 85.1% (40 patients) in the prednisolone group demonstrated a complete recovery of function as compared with 93.1% (41 patients) in the acyclovir and prednisone group. However, the results were not statistically significant.

Antiviral Therapy

To date no controlled study has provided sufficient clinical evidence supporting the use of antiviral therapy alone in the treatment of Bell's palsy. A Cochrane meta-analysis of seven trial totalling 1987 patients found no data in favor of antiviral agents in Bell's palsy (Lockhart P, Daly F, Pitkethly M, et al. 2009). Several of the studies outlined above have reached similar conclusions and it is currently thought that antiviral therapy in isolation is ineffective when used for treating Bell's palsy.

Combinations of Antiviral and Corticosteroid Therapy

The reports of Sullivan and Engström (Sullivan, Swann, Donnan, et al. 2007; Engström, Berg and Stjernquist-Desatnik, et al. 2008) have shown that outcomes from the use of steroid therapy in Bell's palsy are better than placebo alone, but the same studies have also shown that the addition of an antiviral agent is ineffective. These authors concluded that there was no additional benefit conferred by using combination therapy when compared to the use of steroids alone. The studies of Kawaguchi et al. and Yeo et al. (Kawaguchi, Inamura, Abe, et al. 2007; Yeo, Lee, Park, et al. 2008) appear to support this conclusion.

However, in the study by Minnerop et al. (Minnerop, Herbst, Fimmers, et al. 2008) a subgroup of patients with severe palsies appeared to have had additional benefit conferred from the use of an antiviral agent. Eighteen of 35 patients with House Brackman grade 5 or 6 palsies were treated with a combination of famcyclovir and prednisone and were compared to

17 who were treated with prednisone alone. Seventy-two percent (13) of the combination therapy group achieved normal function whereas only 47% (8) of those receiving prednisone alone recovered completely. Moreover, the study by Hato et al. also found that the combination of antiviral and corticosteroid therapy could provide added benefit in severe cases (Hato, Yamad, Kohno, et al., 2007). In this instance, 114 patients who received 1000 mg daily of valacyclovir for five days and 60 mg/day of prednisolone for five days (with a 5-day taper) were compared with 107 patients who received steroid only (60 mg/day of prednisolone for five days with a 5-day taper). Among the patients with an initially complete or severe palsy who received the combination of valacyclovir and prednisolone, 95.7% (92) experienced complete recovery within six months as compared with 86.6% (82) who received prednisolone alone. These differences were significant ($p < 0.05$).

Some have questioned the validity of these findings suggesting that the high dropout rate and unblinded design of these trials may have yielded flawed and biased results.

In conclusion the additional role of antiviral agents in Bell's palsy remains confusing. It could be that patients with profound palsies benefit from combination therapy but a recent systematic review and meta-analysis comparing eighteen trials and involving a total of 2789 patients showed that the addition of antiviral agents was associated with a risk reduction of borderline significance when compared to corticosteroids alone (De Almeida, Al Khabori, Guyatt, et al. 2009).

Other Management Modalities

Acupuncture: Isolated case reports have reported the successful treatment of Bell's palsy with acupuncture (Rosted and Wooley, 2007; Wong and Wong, 2008). However, a Cochrane review involving 537 patients with Bell's palsy who were treated with acupuncture found that the lack of quality studies raised serious questions about the efficacy of such an approach (He, Zhou and Zhou, 2007). The role of this therapy is therefore not confirmed.

Botulinum toxin: Dyskinesia and synkinesis as result of effective nerve regeneration can be reduced effectively by botulinum toxin injections and this

therapy had reduced the necessity for selective myectomies or neurectomies. In areas with permanent weakened movements the asymmetry of the contralateral side may be amplified and in such cases botulinum toxin can also be applied on the healthy side to reduce the muscle movements in the overused mimic areas (Salles, Toledo and Ferreira, 2009; Chen and Tang, 2007). It is possible that botulinum toxin may also be effective when introduced into the lacrimal gland for the treatment of crocodile tears (Montoya FJ, Riddell CE, Caesar R, et al. 2002), although no substantive studies of this therapy are available.

Physical therapy: Systematic controlled studies on the role of physical therapy and also on the role of electrostimulation therapy are lacking. It is certainly possible that physical therapy could help to reduce the degree of muscle atrophy associated with palsy and it is also possible that patients who have had a muscle transfer procedure might be helped to train the transferred muscle for its new function (Teixeira, Soares, Vieira and Prado, 2008; Lindsay, Robinson and Hadlock, 2010). However, clinical benefits of such treatments remain uncertain.

Neurotrophic factors, growth factors and stem cells: A number of other agents have been used in laboratory trials in attempts to facilitate nerve repair and recovery after neural injury. These include neurotrophic factors, growth factors and stem cells. When used as adjuncts to nerve repair after transection these agents have shown promise in some laboratory studies but, at this stage, they have not been adopted in clinical practice since the outcomes of the available experimental work are mixed.

For example, in one study it was found that pituitary adenylate cyclase activating polypeptide (PACAP), which promotes release of the glial cell line derived neurotrophic factor (GDNF), facilitated the recovery of latency of compound muscle action potentials and promoted the formation of myelinated axons as well as raising local GDNF levels after nerve injury (Kimura H, Kawatani M, Ito E, Ishikawa K, 2003). However, other work suggested a contrary conclusion since GDNF also seems to inhibit a positive outcome in immediate nerve grafting (Barras FM, Kuntzer T, Zurn AD and Pasche P, 2009).

Experiments using stem cell therapy have also shown mixed results. In one study looking at both platelet rich plasma and neural-induced human mesenchymal stem cells the single use of one or other of these factors appeared to produce better outcomes after nerve transaction than controls, and their combined use was better than either agent alone (Cho HH, Jang S, Lee SC, Jeong HS, et al. 2003). However, in another study the use of mesenchymal stem cells in collagen appeared to promote overgrowth and an excess of collateral nerve branching in facial motor endplates (Grosheva M, Guntinas-Lichius O, Arnhold S, et al. 2008). This experimental study also used manual stimulation of the facial muscles, which the authors had previously shown to be effective in reducing the numbers of multiply innervated end plates during regeneration. However, such stimulation failed to improve the uncontrolled axonal branching patterns that resulted from the application of stem cells, and the study concluded that the resultant poly-innervation of motor end plates means that stem cells are unlikely to prove clinically beneficial in promoting facial nerve repair.

It, therefore, seems that we will need a number of additional studies, and perhaps a novel method of application, if stem cells and other topically applied neural stimulants are to be useful in promoting organized facial nerve regeneration in clinical practice. But, since severe degrees of facial injury frequently results in residual weakness and synkinesia—even after an apparently successful nerve repair—the use of these agents appears to offer some real hope for future research as to how outcomes after nerve injury might be enhanced.

HERPES ZOSTER

Introduction

Herpes zoster oticus is a viral infection of the ear that manifests as severe otalgia and an associated cutaneous vesicular eruption, which is usually within the external canal and on the pinna. When this is also associated with a facial paralysis the condition is called Ramsay Hunt syndrome.

Incidence and Prevalence

The incidence of Ramsay Hunt syndrome is about 5 per 1,000,000 of the population in the United States with a significant increase in prevalence in those aged over 60 years (Murakami, Hato and Horiuchi, 1997).

Such infections generally cause more severe symptoms and have a worse prognosis than a Bell's palsy (Uri, Greenberg, Kitzes-Cohen and Doweck, 2003) and an additional complication is that of postherpetic neuralgia, which carries significant morbidity. There is often severe pain at the onset of the disease and there may also be pain in the eye, excessive lacrimation and dysgeusia (alteration in taste). It is thought that individuals with decreased cell-mediated immunity resulting from carcinoma, radiation therapy, chemotherapy or HIV infection are at greatest risk but physical and emotional stress are also often cited as precipitating factors.

Etiology

The pathophysiology of this syndrome is thought to involve the re-activation of varicella-zoster virus (VZV) within the nerves innervating the ear with the associated symptoms occurring either as a result of transmission of the virus due to either proximity of the nerves at the cerebellopontine angle or through the vasa vasorum.

Management

Antiviral Agents

The standard first line treatment for herpes zoster infections at sites other than the ear is acyclovir, either given orally or intravenously. Other antiviral agents which have been tried include valacylovir, famcylovir and brivudin (Beutner, Friedman, Forszpaniak, et al., 1996; Tyring, Barbarash, Nahlik, et al. 1995; Dworkin, Johnson, Breuer, et al. 2007). The rationale for such treatment is that oral antiviral therapy is effective in reducing viral replication and that this prevents further proliferation and spread of the virus. Such drugs appear to reduce the duration of viral shedding and new lesion formation, thereby accelerating the healing of the concomitant rash and potentially diminishing the severity of any postherpetic neuralgia. (Jackson, Gibbons, Meyer, et al. 1997; Wood, Johnson, McKendrick, et al. 1994).

While there may be an empirical case for their use, the evidence in support of antiviral agents for infections in the ear is lacking. For example, Kinish et al. (2000) reported the use of acyclovir by infusion in combination with high dose prednisolone in treating

91 patients (Kinishi, Amatsu, Mohri, et al. 2001). Medication was started within seven days of the onset of the symptoms and the results were compared to 47 patients treated with steroid alone. Outcome was assessed by evaluation of facial movement and by nerve excitability testing. The results showed that patients receiving acyclovir and steroid had a statistically significant improvement in nerve recovery as assessed by nerve excitability with good function found in 69 (75%) who received combined therapy as opposed to the same outcome in only 25 (53%) who received steroid alone. In addition, a complete recovery of function to House Brackman grade 1 was found in 82 patients (90%) in those receiving steroid and acyclovir as compared to only 30 (64%) patients who had a similar grade of recovery when treated by steroids alone. However, this study was not randomized.

The same criticism can be leveled at the study of Uri, which also reported the use of acyclovir and prednisolone in patients with Ramsay Hunt syndrome (Uri, Greenberg, Kitzes-Cohen and Doweck, 2003). This study looked at 31 patients but was a retrospective review comparing outcome with 23 patients who had the same presentation but whose treatment was delayed beyond seven days: there was, therefore, no proper group for comparison and no control of the treatment group.

The only randomized study in the literature comparing treatments in Ramsay Hunt syndrome appears to be that of Ramos-Macias et al. who reported outcomes in only 15 patients (Ramos-Macias, De Miguel Martinez and Martin Sanchez, 1992). The subjects were all aged between 21 and 91 years old at the time of treatment but there is no report as to the duration of their symptoms at inclusion. At the onset of treatment seven had complete axontomesis (presumably a complete paresis) and eight had incomplete forms of neuropraxia. Seven patients were treated either with methylprednisolone 20 mg/8 hours (followed by a taper of oral prednisolone during the next 5-10 days) and eight were treated with methylprednisolone plus acyclovir (10 mg/kg/hr) for ten days in combination with an oral taper of prednisolone "for 5-10 days". It is not clear how the patients with differing grades of paresis were randomized to the two treatment groups, and it is also not clear whether the study was blinded. These failings severely limit the conclusions that can be drawn and

at present, while the role of an antiviral agent appears empirically correct, the evidence in favor of their use is lacking (Uscategui, Doree, Chamberlain and Burton, 2008).

Corticosteroids

The adjunctive use of systemic corticosteroids in herpetic infections in the ear appears to have been derived from the belief that is generally held that they relieve acute pain, decrease vertigo and limit the occurrence of postherpetic neuralgia. The prevailing wisdom is therefore that treatment with adjunctive steroids, by whatever route, has a beneficial effect— but there is, in fact, no evidence to support this conclusion at present (Uscategui, Doree, Chamberlain and Burton, 2008). Furthermore, no evidence exists to support the notion that the use of corticosteroids prevents development of postherpetic neuralgia.

The lack of clear-cut evidence in favor of such regimens does not mean that they should not be used or, indeed, that they are ineffective. However, these drugs are associated with a number of adverse side effects and in the uncomplicated cases it is salutary to realize that the evidence in their favor is lacking. There may be a stronger argument for using antiviral agents in particular cases, such as in treating herpes zoster in patients with HIV who are immunosuppressed— although the use of steroids is discouraged in such cases precisely because of their reduced immune status (Benson, Kaplan and Masur, 2004).

Vaccination

Prevention of herpes zoster by vaccination is recommended for all persons older than 60 years, even if they have had chickenpox or zoster in the past. This age group suffers significant morbidity from zoster and may, therefore, benefit from the vaccine (Harpaz, Ortega-Sanchez and Seward, 2008). Contraindications to vaccine administration include those patients who are younger than 60 years, current use of antivirals, pregnancy and certain immunosuppressive conditions.

Supportive Therapy

Supportive therapy for herpes zoster oticus included warm compresses, narcotic analgesics and antibiotics for any secondary bacterial infection. Nausea and vomiting may also require specific treatment in certain instances. Cyclic antidepressants, anticonvulsants, opioids and topical analgesics are sometimes used in the treatment of postherpetic neuralgia. These agents are more appropriately started by a pain management specialist in an outpatient setting (Parvan-Langstone, 2008).

CONCLUSION

The most recent evidence shows that there is an observable benefit from the early use of steroids in Bell's palsy and there is a reduced risk of synkinesis and autonomic dysfunction. The observed benefit of steroids and the low adverse affects of relatively short courses of these drugs leads to the conclusion that corticosteroid therapy confers significant benefit when compared to therapeutic inaction and suggests that steroids should be offered in most cases of Bell's palsy seen within 72 hours of the onset of symptoms.

In cases of severe Bell's palsy the addition of an antiviral agent may be warranted but the evidence behind such a recommendation in the routine case is certainly not strong.

In herpetic infections of the ear the evidence base for treatment is even less secure. The use of antiviral agents seems empirically appropriate and seems justified by their efficacy in reducing viral replication and shedding. However, these drugs have a number of adverse side effects and there is no prospective data to advance in support of their clinical use in the ear. In like manner the use of steroids, although widespread, is not proven. That does not mean these drugs are not appropriate or effective, but it is certainly the case that there is no evidence base in their favor. Properly conducted and randomized prospective trials are needed and, until these are available the risks and benefits of treatment are not known for certain.

BIBLIOGRAPHY

1. Barras FM, Kuntzer T, Zurn AD, Pasche P. Local delivery of glial cell line-derived neurotrophic factor improves facial nerve regeneration after late repair. Laryngoscope. 2009; 119(5): 846-855.
2. Benson CA, Kaplan JE, Masur H. Treating opportunistic infections among HIV-exposed and infected children: recommendations from CDC, the National Institutes of Health, and the Infectious Diseases Society of America. MMWR Recomm Rep. 2004;53(RR-15):1-112.
3. Beutner KR, Friedman DJ, Forszpaniak C, et al. Valacyclovir compared to acyclovir for improved therapy for herpes zoster in immunocompromised adults. Antimicrob Agents Chemother. 1996;39:1546-53.
4. Chen CK, Tang YB. Myectomy and botulinum toxin for paralysis of the marginal mandibular branch of the facial nerve: a series of 76 cases. Plast Reconstr Surg. 2007;120:1859-64.
5. Cho HH, Jang S, Lee SC, Jeong HS, Park JS, Han JY, Lee KH, Cho YB. Effect of neural-induced mesenchymal stem cells and platelet-rich plasma on facial nerve regeneration in an acute nerve injury model. Laryngoscope. 2003;113(6):1000-6.
6. De Almeida J R, Al Khabori M, Guyatt G H, et al. Combined corticosteroid and antiviral treatment for Bell's palsy: a systematic review and meta-analysis. JAMA. 2009;302(9):985-93.
7. Dworkin RH, Johnson RW, Breuer J, et al. Recommendations for the management of herpes zoster. Clin Infect Dis. 2007;44(Suppl1):S1-26.
8. Engström M, Berg T, Stjernquist-Desatnik A, et al. Prednisolone and valacyclovir in Bell's palsy: a randomised, double-blind, placebo-controlled, multicentre trial. Lancet Neurol. 2008;7:993-1000.
9. Grosheva M, Guntinas-Lichius O, Arnhold S, Skouras E, Kuerten S, Streppel M, Angelova S K, Wewetzer K, Radtke C, Dunlop S A, Angelov D N. Bone marrow-derived mesenchymal stem cell transplantation does not improve quality of muscle reinnervation or recovery of motor function after facial nerve transection in rats. Biol Chem. 2008;389(7):873-88
10. Harpaz R, Ortega-Sanchez IR, Seward JF. Prevention of herpes zoster: recommendations of the Advisory Committee on Immunization Practices (ACIP). MMWR Recomm Rep. 2008;57:1-30.
11. Hato N, Yamada H, Kohno H, et al. Valacyclovir and prednisolone treatment for Bell's palsy: a multicenter, randomized, placebo-controlled study. Otol Neurotol. 2007;28(3):408-13.
12. He L, Zhou MK, Zhou D, et al. Acupuncture for Bell's palsy. Cochrane Database Syst Rev. 2007:CD002914.
13. Jackson J L, Gibbons R, Meyer G, et al. The effects of treating herpes zoster with oral acyclovir in preventing postherpetic neuralgia: a meta-analysis. Arch Intern Med. 1997;157(8):909-12.
14. Kawaguchi K, Inamura H, Abe Y, et al. Reactivation of herpes simplex virus type 1 and varicella-zoster virus and therapeutic effects of combination therapy with prednisolone and valacyclovir in patients with Bell's palsy. Laryngoscope. 2007;117:147-56.
15. Kimura H, Kawatani M, Ito E, Ishikawa K. Effects of pituitary adenylate cyclase activating polypeptide on facial nerve recovery in the guinea pig. Laryngoscope. 2003;113(6):1000-6.

16. Kinishi M, Amatsu M, Mohri M, et al. Acyclovir improves recovery rate of facial nerve palsy in Ramsay Hunt syndrome. Auris, Nasus, Larynx. 2001;28(3):223-6.

17. Lockhart P, Daly F, Pitkethly M, et al. Antiviral treatment for Bell's palsy (idiopathic facial paralysis). Cochrane Database of Syst Rev. 2009;4:CD001869.

18. Lindsay RW, Robinson M, Hadlock TA. Comprehensive facial rehabilitation improves function in people with facial paralysis: a 5-year experience at the Massachusetts Eye and Ear Infirmary. Phys Ther. 2010;90:391-7.

19. Minnerop M, Herbst M, Fimmers R, et al. Bell's palsy: combined treatment of famciclovir and prednisone is superior to prednisone alone. J Neurol. 2008;255:1726-30.

20. Montoya FJ, Riddell CE, Caesar R, et al. Treatment of gustatory hyperlacrimation (crocodile tears) with injection of botulinum toxin into the lacrimal gland. Eye. 2002;16:705-9.

21. Murakami S, Hato N, Horiuchi J. Treatment of Ramsay Hunt syndrome with acyclovir-prednisone: significance of early diagnosis and treatment. Ann Neurol. 1997;41(3):353-7.

22. Murakami S, Mizobuchi M, Nakashiro Y, et al. Bell's palsy and herpes simplex virus: identification of viral DNA in endoneurial fluid and muscle. Ann Intern Med. 1996;124(pt 1):27-30.

23. Pavan-Langston D. Herpes zoster antivirals and pain management. Ophthalmology. 2008;115(2 Suppl):S13-20.

24. Peitersen E. The natural history of Bell's palsy. Am J Otol. 1982;4:107-11.

25. Prescott CAJ. Idiopathic facial nerve palsy (the effect of treatment with steroids). J Laryngol Otol. 1988;102:403-7.

26. Ramos Macias A, De Miguel Martinez I, Martin Sanchez A M, et al. Adding acyclovir to the treatment of facial palsy. A study of 45 cases. Acta Otorhinolarigol Espanol. 1992;43(2):117-20.

27. Rosted P, Woolley DR. Bell's palsy following acupuncture treatment: a case report. Acupunct Med. 2007;25:47-8.

28. Salinas RA, Alvarez G, Ferreira J. Corticosteroids for Bell's palsy (idiopathic facial paralysis). Cochrane Database Syst Rev. 2004;CD001942.

29. Salles AG, Toledo PN, Ferreira MC. Botulinum toxin injection in long-standing facial paralysis patients: improvement of facial symmetry observed up to 6 months. Aesthetic Plast Surg. 2009;33:582-90.

30. Sullivan FM, Swan IR, Donnan PT, et al. Early treatment with prednisolone or acyclovir in Bell's palsy. N Engl J Med. 2007;357:1598-607.

31. Teixeira LJ, Soares BG, Vieira VP, et al. Physical therapy for Bell's palsy (idiopathic facial paralysis). Cochrane Database Syst Rev. 2008;CD006283.

32. Tyring S, Barbarash RA, Nahlik JE, et al. Famciclovir for the treatment of acute herpes zoster: effects on acute disease and postherpetic neuralgia. A randomized, double-blind, placebo-controlled trial. Collaborative Famciclovir Herpes Zoster Study Group. Ann Intern Med. 1995;123(2):89-96.

33. Uri N, Greenberg E, Kitzes-Cohen R, et al. Acyclovir in the treatment of Ramsay Hunt syndrome. Otolaryngol-Head Neck Surg. 2003;129(4):379-81.

34. Uscategui T, Doree C, Chamberlain IJ, et al. Corticosteroids as adjuvant to antiviral treatment in Ramsay Hunt syndrome (herpes zoster oticus with facial palsy) in adults. Cochrane Database Syst Rev. 2008;CD006852.

35. Uscategui T, Doree C, Chamberlain IJ, et al. Antiviral therapy for Ramsay Hunt syndrome (herpes zoster oticus with facial palsy) in adults. Cochrane Database Syst Rev. 2008;CD006851.

36. Victor M, Martin J. Disorders of the cranial nerves. In: Isselbacher KJ, et al. (Eds). Harrison's Principles of Internal Medicine (13th edn). New York:McGraw-Hill. 1994. pp. 2347-52.

37. Wood MJ, Johnson RW, McKendrick MW, et al. A randomized trial of acyclovir for 7 days or 21 days with and without prednisolone for treatment of acute herpes zoster. N Engl J Med.1994;330(13):896-900.

38. Wong CL, Wong VC. Effect of acupuncture in a patient with 7-year-history of Bell's palsy. J Altern Complement Med. 2008;14:847-53.

39. Yeo SG, Lee YC, Park DC, et al. Acyclovir plus steroid vs steroid alone in the treatment of Bell's palsy. Am J Otolaryngol. 2008;29:163-6.

7

Facial Palsy in Infection

DS Grewal

INTRODUCTION

Infratemporal lesions are by far the most common cause of facial paralysis. In a series of 322 cases, Cawthorne found that 8% (26 patients) were due to chronic suppurative otitis media (CSOM). Of all cases of otitis, 1% (Tonndorf, 1924), 1.8% (Lund, 1929) or 2% (Kettel, 1943) show a facial palsy.

The various infections, which can cause facial palsy, include:
1. Acute suppurative otitis media (ASOM)
2. Acute mastoiditis
3. Chronic suppurative otitis media
   - Cholesteatoma
   - Granulations
   - Tuberculous otitis media
   - Aural polyp
   - Tympanosclerosis
4. Malignant otitis externa
5. Herpes zoster oticus
6. Otogenic abscesses
   - Citelli's abscess
   - Luc's abscess
   - Bezold's abscess

ACUTE SUPPURATIVE OTITIS MEDIA AND ACUTE MASTOIDITIS

Facial palsy can occur secondary to ASOM and acute mastoiditis, if the treatment is inadequate or if the organisms are very virulent or if the host immunity is low. This is commonly seen in children.

In ASOM, particularly in children, early facial palsy is seen occasionally (0.5% Vogt, 1899; Kettel, 1943). Such early paralysis is thought to be due to toxic neuritis (Lund, 1929), a collateral hyperemia (Burger, 1925) or edema of the loose fibrous tissue of the nerve. According to Pollack (1928), this edema may be due to a toxic vasomotor paresis of the epineural vessels. It has been assumed, not without controversy (Fremel, 1931; Lange, 1917) that toxins may reach the nerve via dehiscence in the fallopian canal (Nuhsmann, 1926; Mayer, 1932) or via the fine bony canals of the chorda tympani and the stapedius nerve (Rudinger, 1932; Sade, 1965).

The cause of facial palsy in ASOM is usually due to severe infection affecting the facial nerve in the presence of congenital dehiscences of the fallopian canal, usually in its tympanic segment.

The palsy usually responds well to antibiotics and myringotomy with a complete recovery. Rarely, a surgical decompression may be required in the presence of a coalescent mastoiditis.

CHRONIC SUPPURATIVE OTITIS MEDIA

Cholesteatoma

Facial palsy is 3-4 times more common in cholesteatoma than in ASOM. The facial palsy that occurs in a cholesteatoma is due to the erosion of the fallopian canal by the cholesteatoma matrix (Figs 7.1 A) following which the palsy is caused due to direct pressure on the nerve and the effect of various enzymes secreted by the cholesteatoma matrix. Involvement of the facial nerve is directly proportional to the size and extent of the cholesteatoma, which determines the intensity of infection, which in turn is responsible for the palsy. A number of cases have been described in which the intact nerve ran freely through the tympanum and the substance of the cholesteatoma (Lund, 1929; Kettel, 1943). This seems to indicate that the real cause of facial palsy in such cases is compression, which is caused by inflammatory edema of the neurilemma (Eisinger, 1925; Hall, 1941; Lund, 1929; Neumann, 1906; Pollman, 1937) and by hyperemia and serous infiltration of the endosteum (Krischek, 1950; Neumann, 1906). Kettel emphasized that in his opinion it is not so much direct pressure on the axons but strangulation of epineural vessels, which produces paralysis. Postmortem findings of Darkeschewitsch (1893) as well as Flatau (1897), confirm this view.

Treatment is done by decompression of the nerve with removal of the matrix which drapes over the dehiscent nerve as it can be easily peeled off from the nerve sheath. The various methods by which the matrix can be peeled off include:

- Peeling it using a suction and sickle knife
- Gently peeling it off using a moist cotton ball
- I advocate, irrigating the cavity with water/saline which results in the floating of the edges of the matrix, now they can be easily demarcated and then removed by suction and instrumentation.

The outer layer of the nerve sheath is relatively thick because it is the periosteal layer and hence it offers protection to the nerve against infection and instrumentation. Antibiotics with steroids both locally as well as systemically are given postoperatively for 10 days.

Granulations

They tend to erode the bone of the fallopian canal and affect the bare nerve resulting in facial palsy.

Tuberculous Otitis Media

It usually presents with complications of CSOM such as facial palsy, labyrinthitis secondary to labyrinthine fistula, meningitis and intracranial abscess (Grewal and Hathiram, 1999). Facial palsy tends to occur early in tuberculous otitis media due to erosion of bone by the granulation tissue and formation of bony sequestra (Ormerod, 1931) (Fig. 7.1B). In advanced/late cases, there may be a huge tuberculoma in the mastoid causing facial palsy (Figs 7.2 A and B).

Treatment consists of decompression of the facial nerve with removal of granulations and the bony sequestra, which may press upon the nerve, followed by anti-tuberculous therapy.

Aural Polyp

Occasionally, an aural polyp may be adherent to a dehiscent facial nerve in its tympanic segment and on attempting to remove this polyp there may be facial twitching which should alert the surgeon to this possibility. Therefore, in such cases a polypectomy and mastoidectomy are planned as one-stage surgery (Fig. 7.3).

Tympanosclerosis

The tympanic cavity and the fallopian canal are common sites of tympanosclerosis. A tympanosclerotic plaque may be rarely adherent to a dehiscent facial nerve in its tympanic and/or labyrinthine segment and removal of tympanosclerosis from the attic region during surgery should be undertaken with due precaution to prevent damage to a dehiscent facial nerve. However, there is no pathology seen in the facial nerve in cases of tympanosclerosis (Fig. 7.4).

Association of Facial Palsy with Labyrinthine Fistulae in CSOM

I have observed in advanced cases of CSOM with cholesteatoma and/or retraction pockets the facial

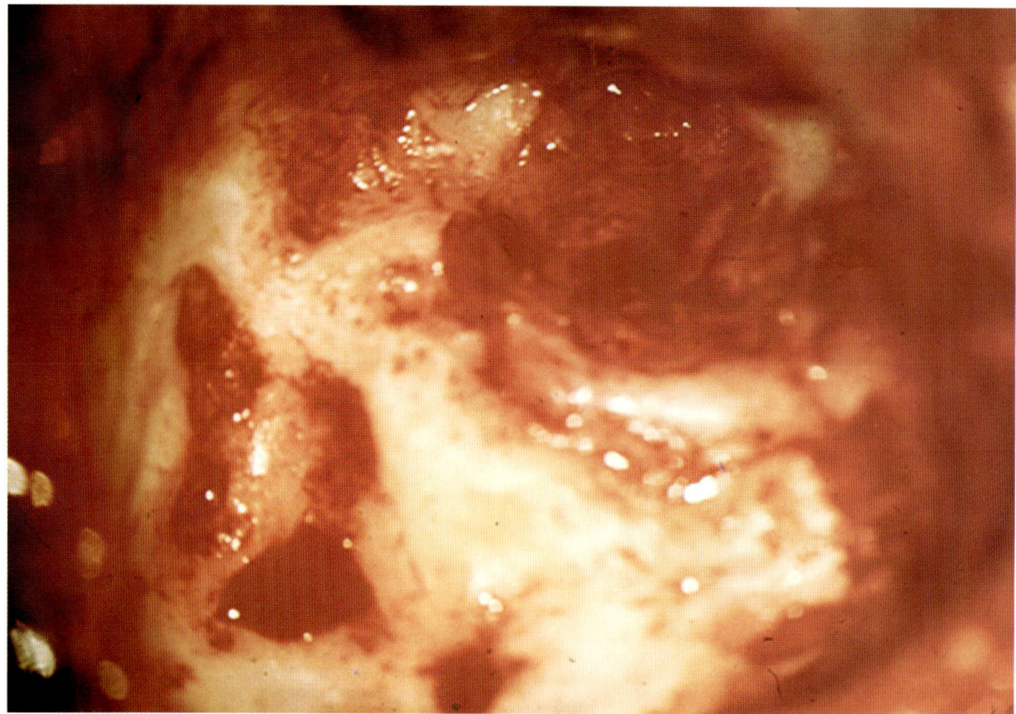

Fig. 7.1A: Tympanomastoid surgery with an exposed facial nerve as seen after removal of the cholesteatoma matrix. The edges of the eroded fallopian canal are ragged, due to the disease process

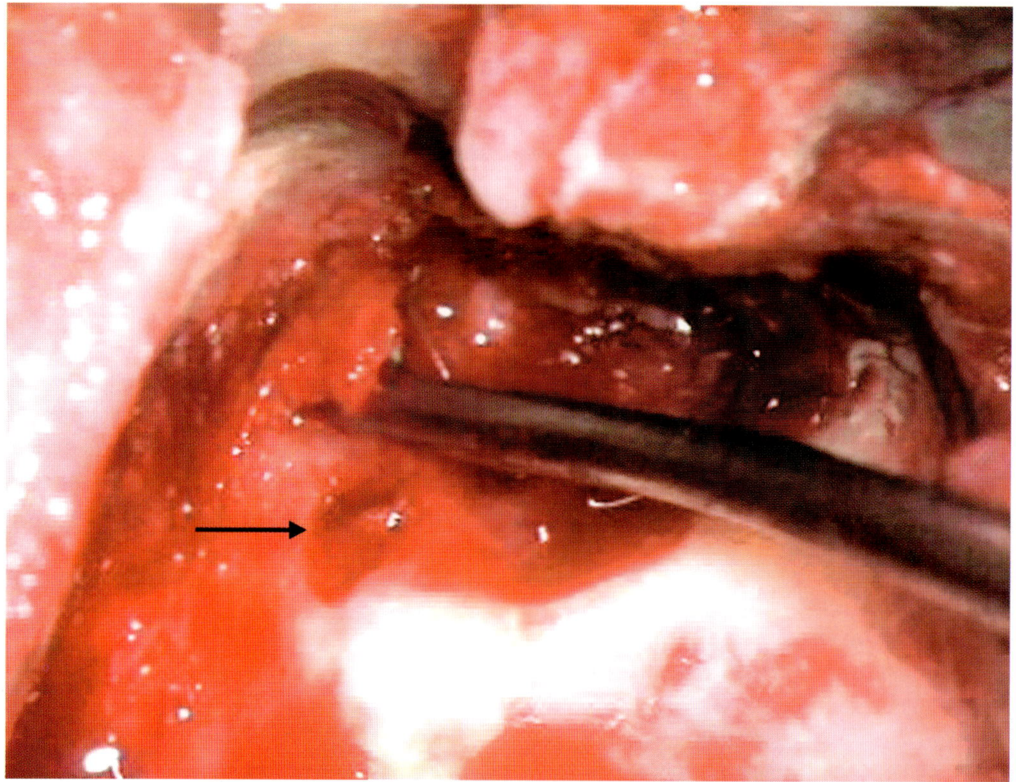

Fig. 7.1B: A case of labyrinthine fistula covered by a bony sequestrum. The patient also had facial nerve palsy

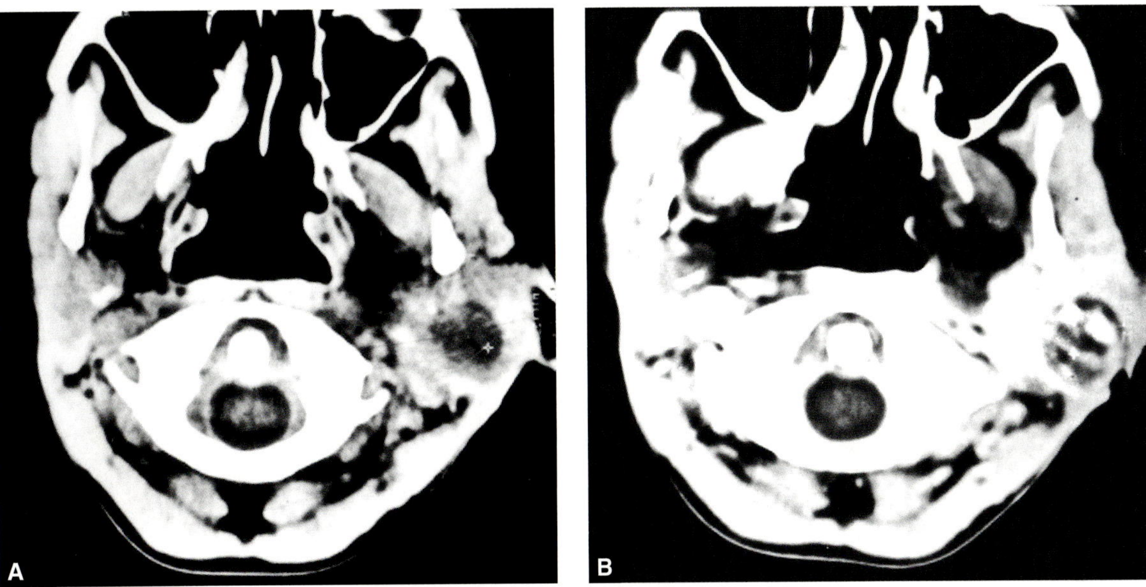

Figs. 7.2A and B: CT scan showing presence of a heterogeneous space occupying lesion in the temporal bone resulting in widening of the temporal bone. Histopathology revealed it to be a tuberculoma. (A) Plain; (B) Contrast showing enhancement

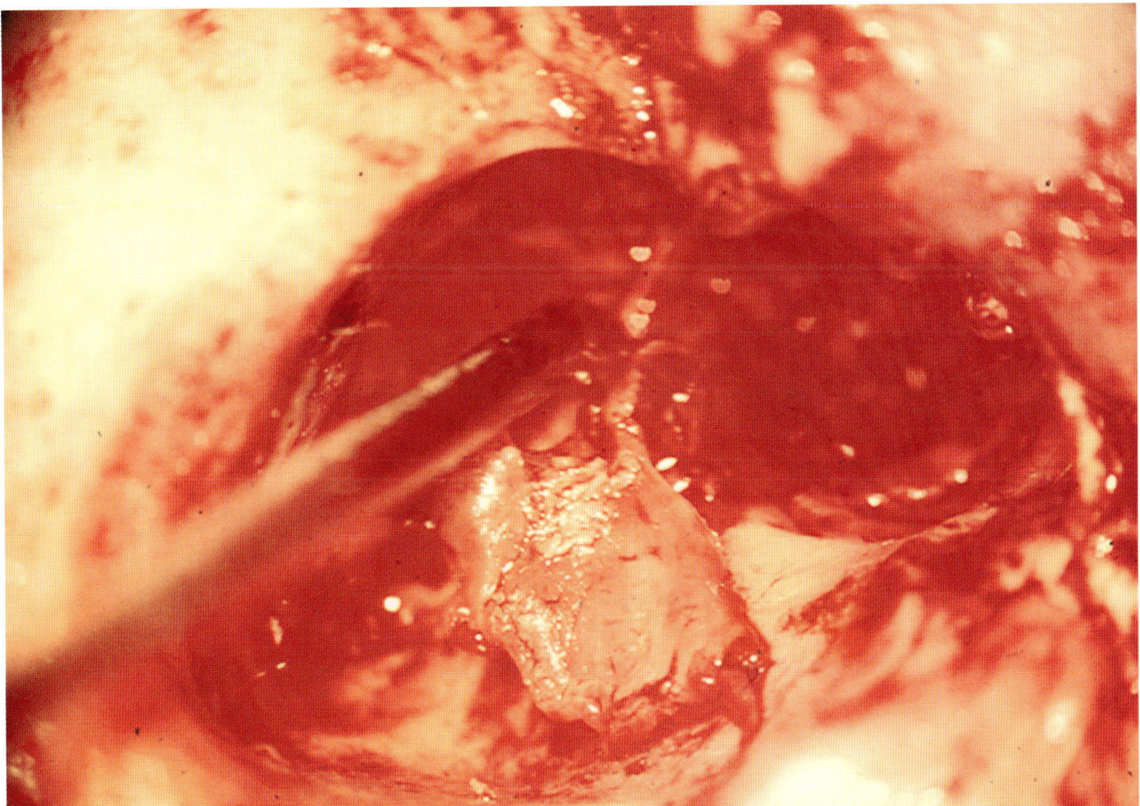

Fig. 7.3: A polyp of tuberculous origin arising from the fallopian canal. In this case, manipulation of the polyp resulted in facial twitchings hence, a canal wall down mastoidectomy was performed for removal of polyp and clearance of the mastoid air cell system

palsy may be associated with labyrinthine fistula or fistulae (Fig 7.5 A to F).

This is because of close proximity of the facial nerve to the lateral, superior semicircular canals and promontory in its course in the middle ear. When retraction pocket is fully formed, it's sac is related to medial aspect of labyrinth as under:

- The neck and body of the retraction pocket to the lateral semicircular canal
- The body of fully formed retraction pocket to the superior semicircular canal
- The tympanic membrane in grade IV atelectasis and mouth of the sac to the promontary.

The mastoid part of the facial nerve is more often

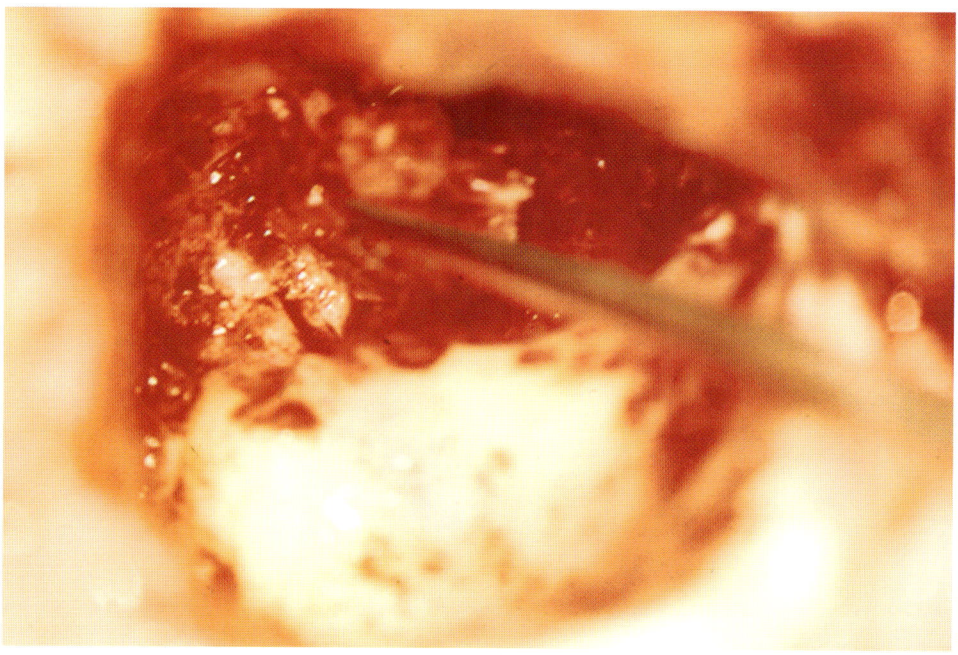

Fig. 7.4: Intraoperative photograph of tympanomastoid surgery showing a large plaque of tympanosclerosis which was covering the eroded fallopian canal and involving the facial nerve in its tympanic segment. The patient did not have facial palsy

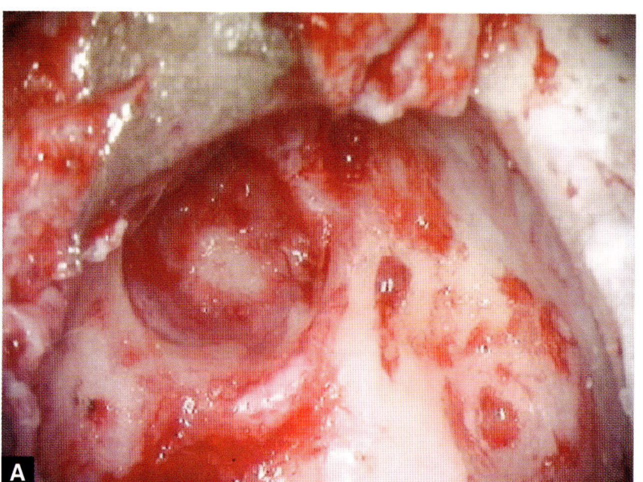

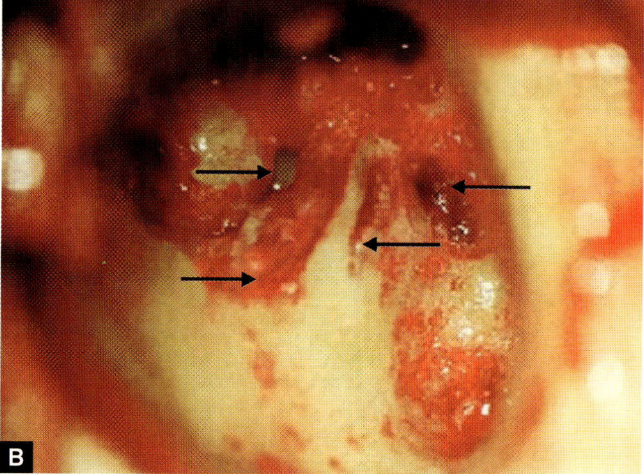

Figs 7.5A and B: (A) Canal wall down tympanomastoidectomy with lateral semicircular canal fistula with intact labyrinth and erosion of fallopian canal; (B) Intraoperative photograph of labyrinthectomy with huge fistula of lateral and superior semicircular canals, and erosion of entire fallopian canal. The facial nerve is swollen and congested

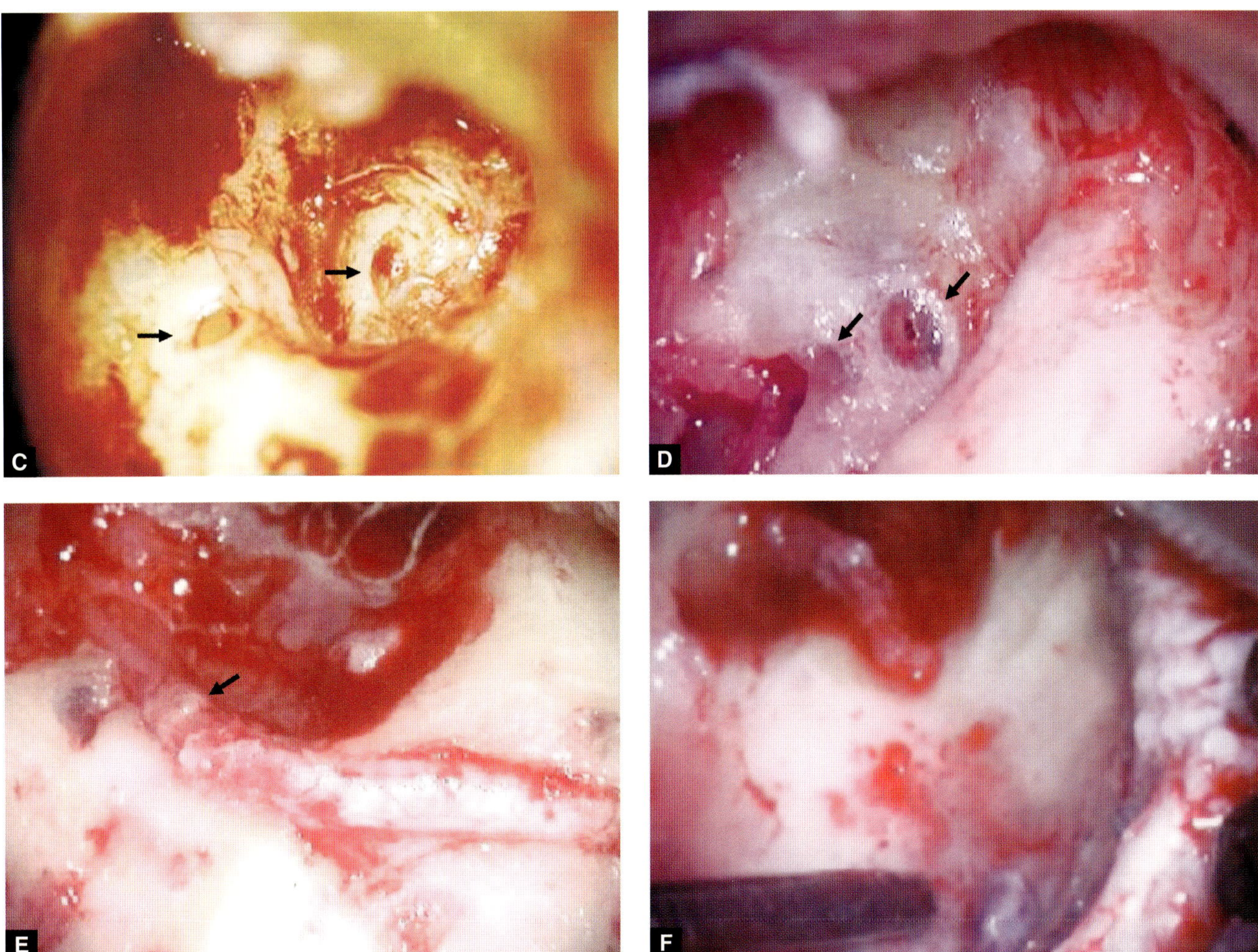

Figs 7.5C to F: (C) Intraoperative photograph showing the presence of two labyrinthine fistulae (arrows) on either side of the facial nerve—one on the promontory and one on the lateral semicircular canal. (D) Two fistulae over promontory (arrow) with facial nerve over hanged. There was grade IV atelectasis. (E) Canal wall down tympanomastoidectomy—there is a huge fistula of the lateral semicircular canal with intact endosteum with erosion of fallopian canal in its entire length with herniation of facial nerve (arrow). (F) Bone over the entire labyrinth is eroded resulting in autolabyrinthectomy. The facial nerve is edematous and congested. There is a dural herniation, the defect was closed by taking bone graft from the mastoid tip

involved than the tympanic part because of erosion of the fallopian canal due to infection.

In one case of CSOM with facial palsy, a facial nerve neuroma was found (Fig 7.6).

Surgical Treatment

We prefer to treat all cases of CSOM with facial palsy with canal wall down tympanomastoidectomy on disease approach (Grewal, et al. 2007).

It is an innovative three-dimension technique based on universally accepted surgical principles. We modified the technique to ensure complete exposure and thereby eradication of disease, with resultant small cavity working in three-dimensional field we began drilling at the posterior meatal wall lowering it while simultaneously widening the cavity as the mastoid was drilled to reach the antrum and the aditus. The ridge was lowered and incus removed to completely expose the entire disease. The facial ridge was debulked and a temporalis fascia graft placed so as to **simplify the middle ear cleft**, thereby dividing it into two with tympanic cavity draining via Eustachian tube and the mastoid cavity communicating with external auditory canal (Figs 7.7 A and B). After drilling the resultant

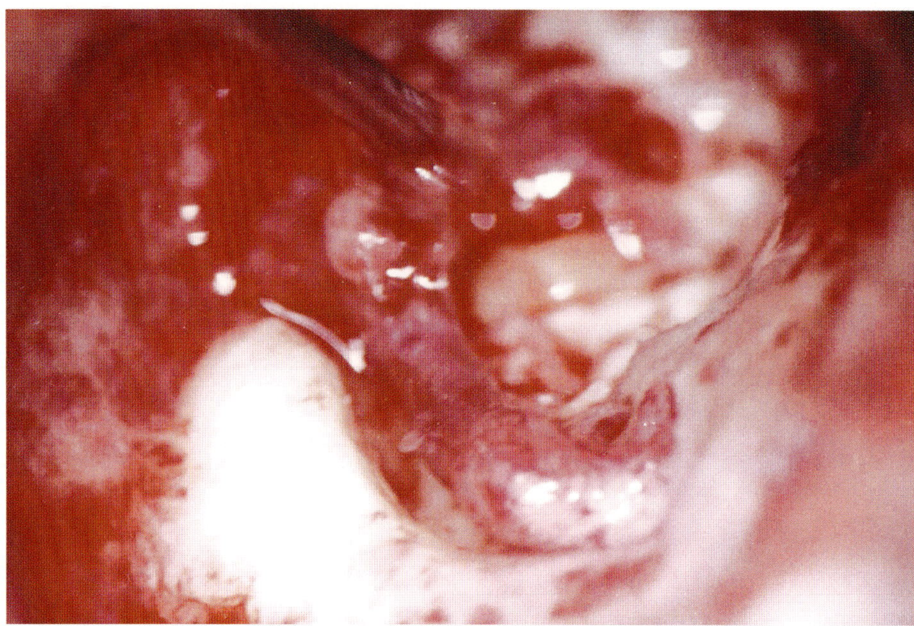

Fig. 7.6: Canal wall down tympanomastoidectomy for retraction pocket with cholesteatoma and facial paresis. There was a 3 mm neuroma at the mastoid segment

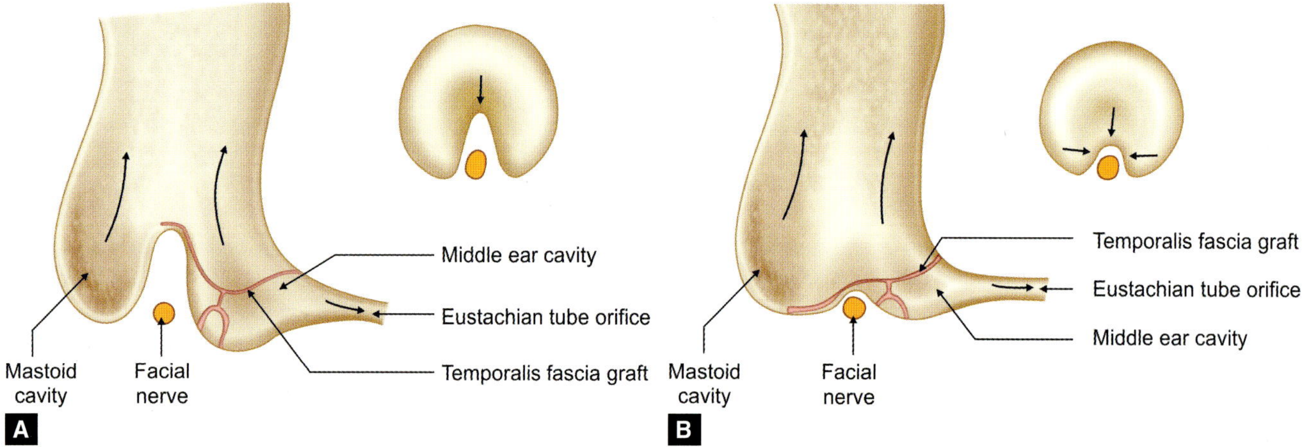

Figs 7.7A and B: (A) Diagrammatic representation of two communicating cavities (mastoid and EAC) due to a high and bulky facial ridge; (B) Diagrammatic representation of an ideal cavity. The tympanic cavity communicating with the Eustachian tube and the external auditory canal communicating with the mastoid cavity. A debulked facial ridge (Simplified middle ear cleft)

cavity is likened to the interior of sea shell, the external auditory canal being the smaller cavity within the larger drilled cavity (Figs 7.8 A and B).

Meatoplasty

A proper meatoplasty is absolute requirement of canal wall down tympanomastoidectomy. After the temporalis facia graft is placed meatoplasty retains the mastoid cavity and external auditory canal as one cavity and allows proper follow-up postoperatively. I prefer to perform meatoplasty first, thereafter, mastoid is explored, this helps in providing much wider and better access for surgery.

High points of meatoplasty:
- The postaural incision is taken, skin flap is elevated and temporalis fascia graft is taken

- The fibrofatty tissue over the mastoid bone is cut from 12 O'clock to 6 O'clock position right at the external auditory meatus right up to the bone. It is then extended posteriorly at the 3 O'clock position for about 2 cms till the postaural incision. Two flaps are then elevated to expose the mastoid cortex.
- Posterior meatal skin flap is now cut at the level of external auditory meatus from 12 to 6 O'clock positions and the upper flap is cut upwards from its free edge at 12 and 6 O'clock positions as much as required to form a meatoplasty flap.
- After placing the temporalis fascia graft, the gel foam is placed and fibrofatty tissue flaps are stitched together then the meatoplasty flap is shaped and stitched to their free edges or underneath them. The mastoid cavity is packed as required (Figs 7.9 A to D).

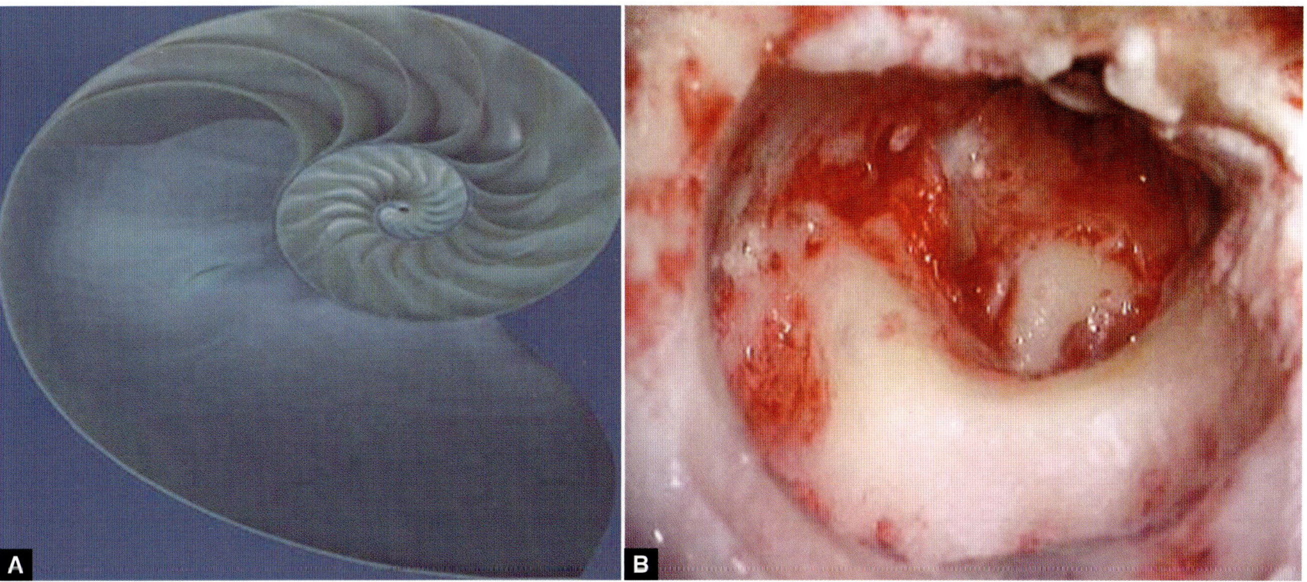

Figs 7.8A and B: An ideal cavity likened to the interior of a sea-shell

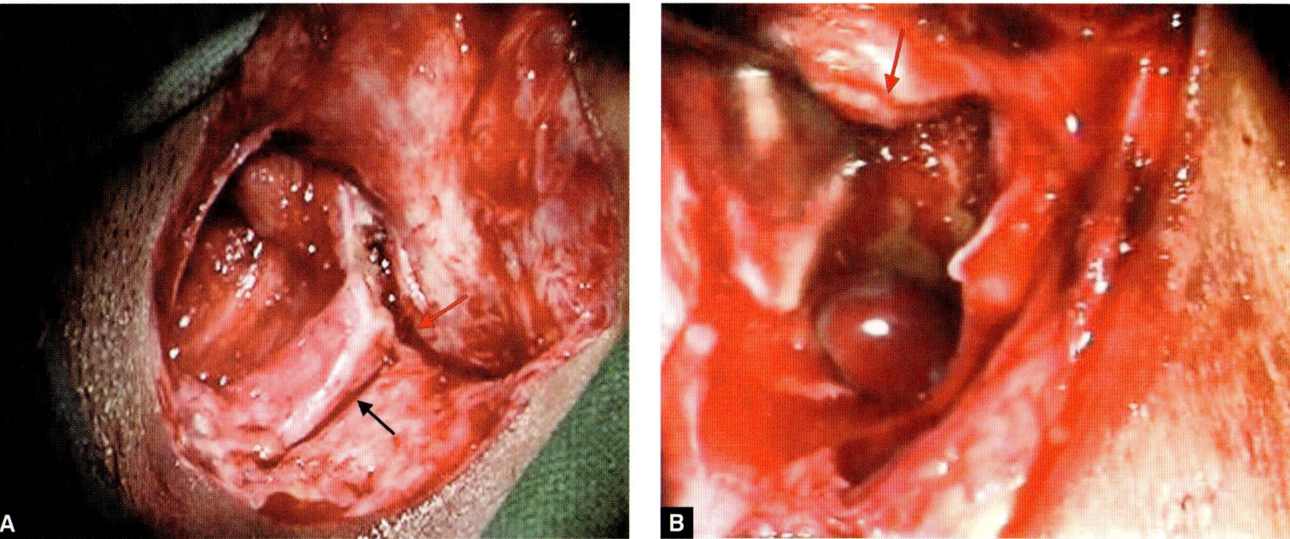

Figs 7.9A and B: Steps of meatoplasty (A) Incision; (B) Meatoplasty flap

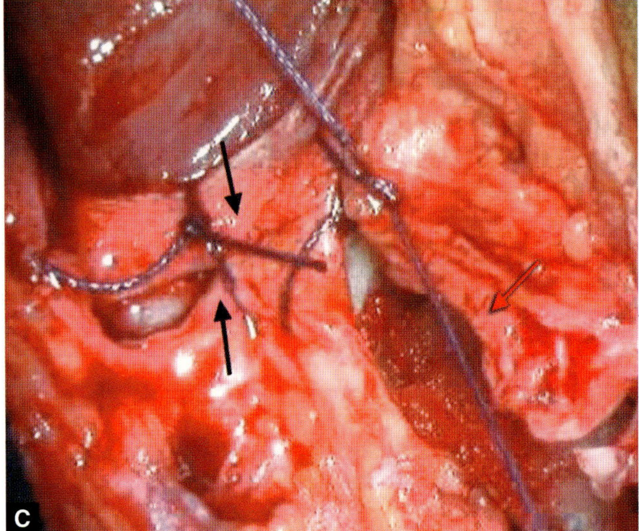

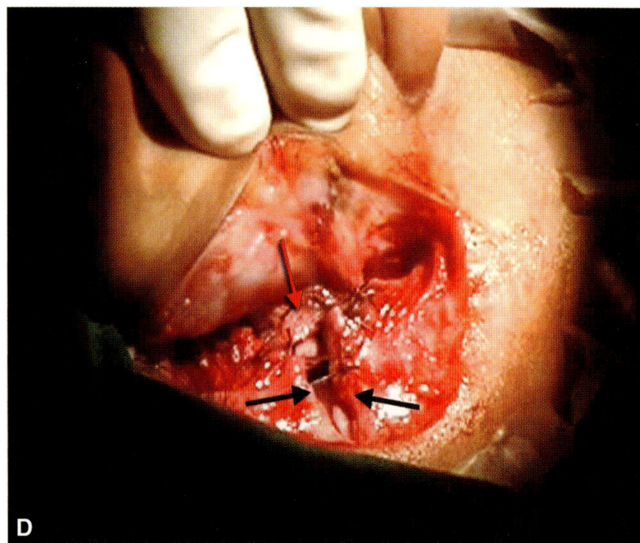

Figs 7.9C and D: (C and D) Meatoplasty closure (Black arrows shows mastoid flaps, red arrow shows meatoplasty flap)

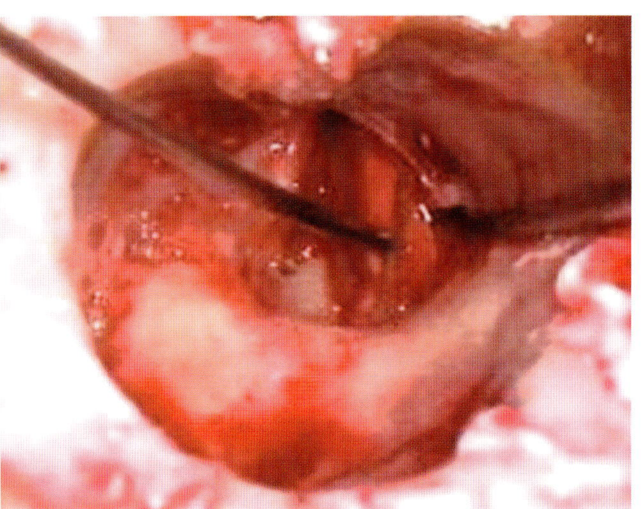

Fig. 7.10: Intraoperative photograph of an ideal shell shaped cavity. Chromic catgut is being placed to create a middle ear space

I prefer to use 1-0 or 2-0 chromic catgut to create an adequate middle ear space. Five to seven pieces of chromic catgut are placed parallel to each other in the middle ear from the Eustachian tube orifice to the sinus tympani region (Fig. 7.10). Chromic catgut has an advantage of being cylindrical and hence conforms to the contours of the Eustachian orifice. It has been well tested in the human body and not extruded. It is also atraumatic due to its cylindrical shape. Due to the use of this material, the surgery involved only one stage, which is an advantage especially in India where the majority of the patients do not attend regular follow-up.

In my opinion:

1. Canal wall down tympanomastoidectomy is not a series of steps given in the book or literature to be performed, in reality it is much more. One needs to sharpen one's technique, skill and understanding of the surgery constantly.

2. 'Problem cavity' emphasized by critics of canal wall down procedure is a result of improperly performed surgery. Canal wall down tympanomastoidectomy has stood the test of time and because of its life saving potential it is still being done. I strongly believe—**The mastoid cavity by itself is not a problem, in fact, it solves all problems of CSOM and its complications.**

One of the complications of CSOM is facial palsy and canal wall down tympanomastoidectomy offers best chances of its recovery.

MALIGNANT OTITIS EXTERNA

Pseudomonas infection is generally seen in debilitated or elderly and uncontrolled diabetics that begins in the external auditory canal to progressively involve the temporal bone and skull base is termed as malignant otitis externa. This infection is often associated with facial paralysis, due to bone erosion. Treatment is by extensive surgical debridement and antibiotics with steroids as well as control of diabetes mellitus.

HERPES ZOSTER OTICUS: (RAMSAY HUNT SYNDROME) (FIG. 7.11)

This is a multicranial nerve involvement by the herpes zoster virus. Typically, the individual manifests with sudden onset of facial paralysis associated with severe pain in the ear and mastoid region. The auricle and external auditory meatus are inflamed and red with painful vesicles filled with clear fluid. The facial palsy is probably due to edema of the nerve particularly in the area of the geniculate ganglion. Treatment is non-surgical usually with acyclovir orally 800 mg 3-5 times a day for five days. Valacylovir 1 gm tds and famcylovir 500 mg tds are also recommended.

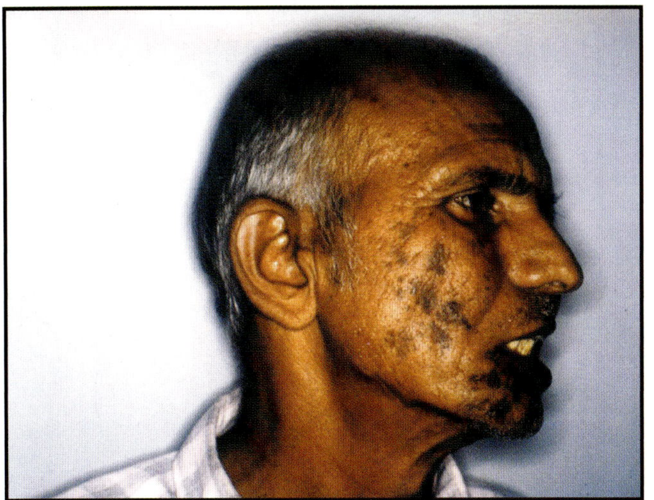

Fig. 7.11: Clinical photograph of a patient of herpes zoster oticus with facial palsy

OTOGENIC ABSCESSES

Extracranial abscesses such as Bezold's, Citelli's and Luc's abscesses secondary to unsafe CSOM (Tuberculous otitis media, cholesteatoma or granulations) cause facial palsy due to erosion of bone with necrosis of the fallopian canal, in the region of the stylomastoid foramen in case of Bezold's abscess and in the mastoid segment due to Luc's abscess or a Citelli's abscess. The facial palsy is probably due to both necrosis of bone of the fallopian canal as well as severe infection and inflammation of the facial nerve (Figs 7.12 to 7.14).

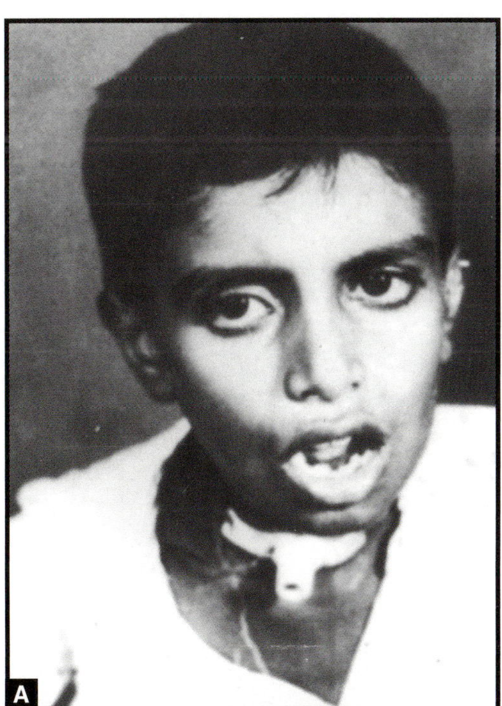
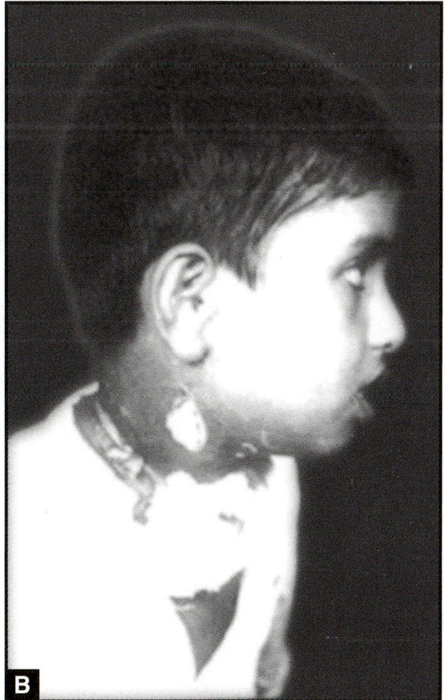

Figs 7.12A and B: (A) An 8-year-old boy 4 days after draining of parapharyngeal space abscess (Citelli's) with marked cellulitis of the neck; (B) Same patient (Fig. 7.12A) lateral view showing ear discharge and gauze pack in the drained abscess cavity

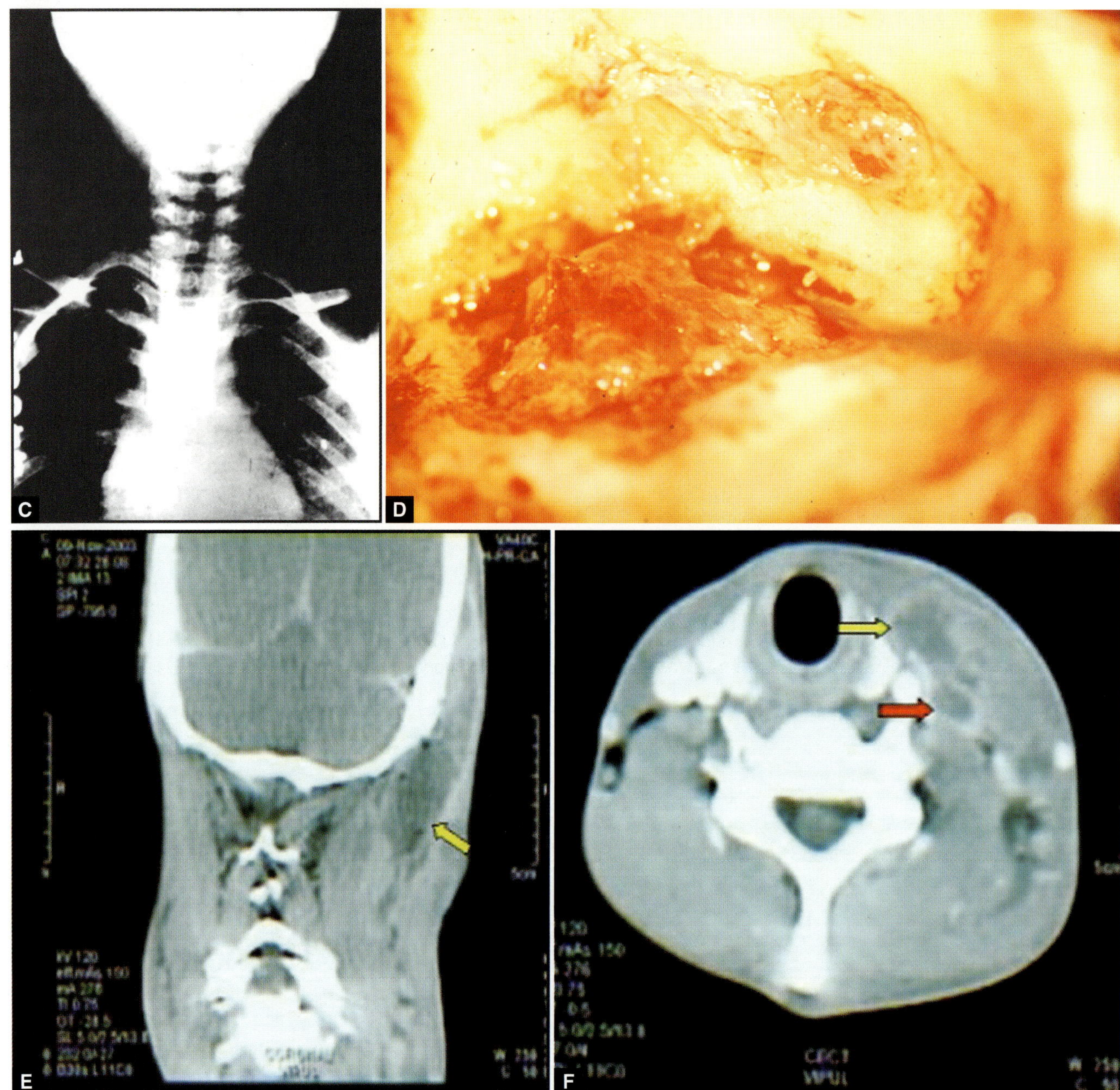

Figs 7.12C and F: (C) X-ray of the neck and chest of the same patient (Fig. 7.12A) showing soft tissue shadow on right side of the neck with marked shift of trachea to the left; (D) Radical mastoidectomy of the same patient (Fig. 7.12A). Note the cavity eroded at its base by tuberculous granulation tissue and the pick in the fistulous track under the exposed digastric muscle, which resulted in pus entering the parapharyngeal space to cause a Citelli's abscess; (E) Coronal CT scan showing Citelli's abscess in another patient; (F) Axial CT scan of same patient (Fig. 7.12E) showing Citelli's abscess with internal jugular vein thrombosis

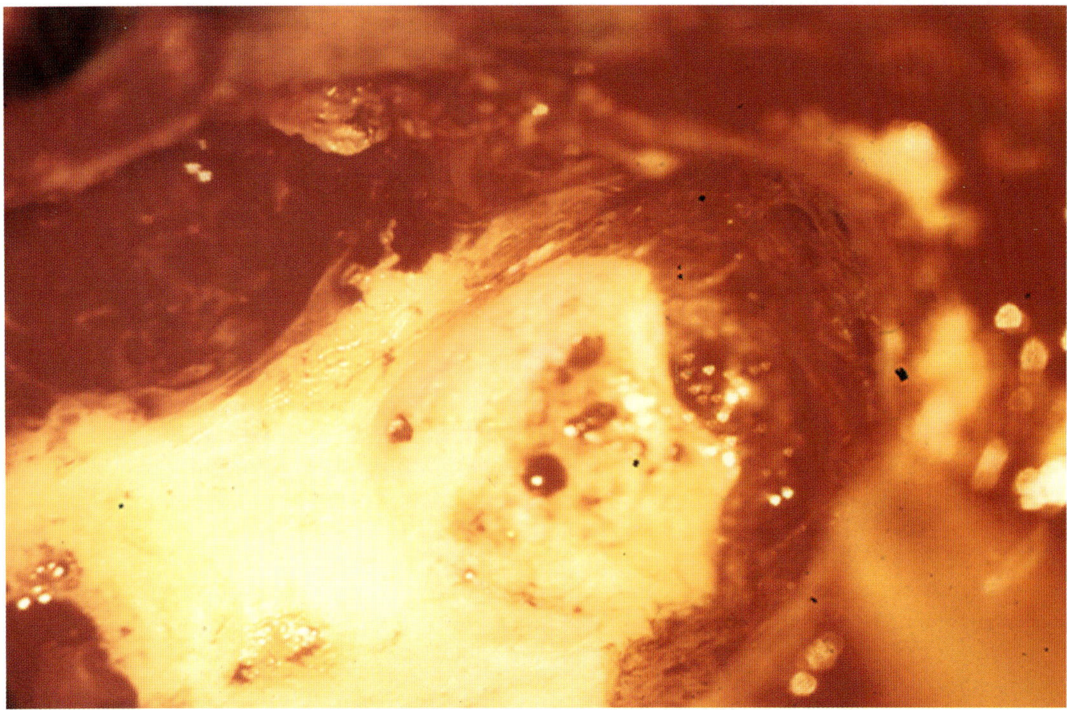

Fig. 7.13: Intraoperative photograph of tympanomastoid surgery in a case of Bezold's abscess. The entire bony tip is eroded by disease process including the stylomastoid foramen. This was tuberculous in origin as diagnosed from the histopathology report of granulation tissue

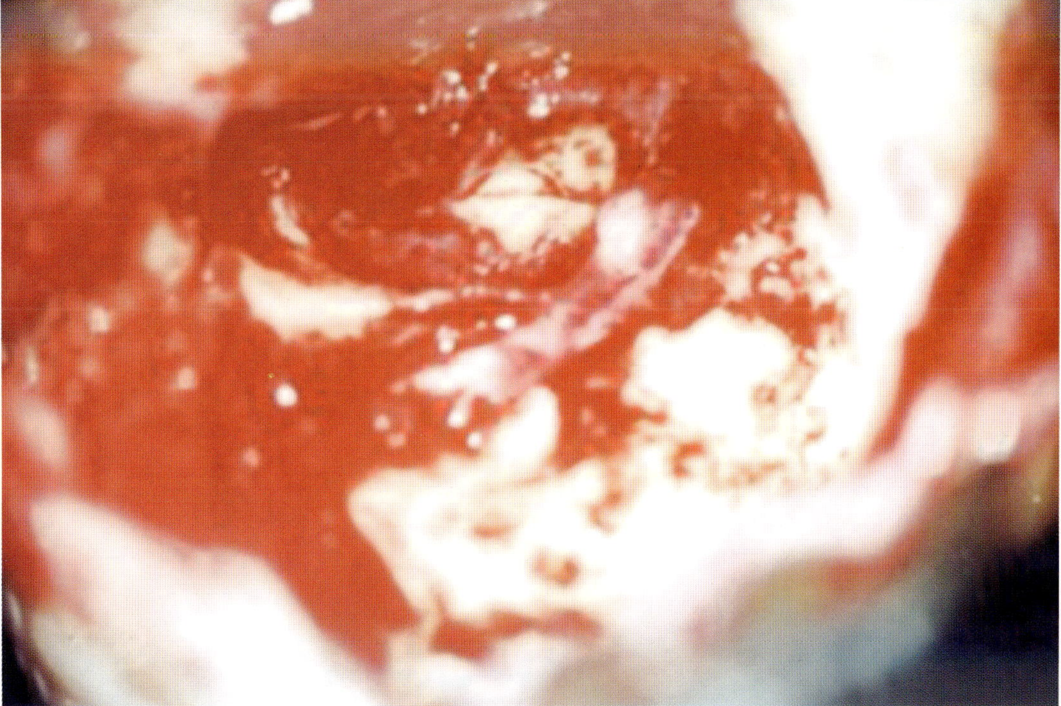

Fig. 7.14: Intraoperative photograph showing Luc's abscess of tuberculous origin. This patient presented with facial palsy

BIBLIOGRAPHY

1. Burger H. Lahmung des Gesichtsnerven bei akuter Mittel-ohrentzundung. Ndld. Tschr. Geneesk. 1925, quoted from Pollak.
2. Darkeschewitsch L. Zur Frage von den pathologisch-anatomischen Veranderungen bei peripherer Facialis-lahmung nicht spezifischen Ursprungs Neur Zbl. 1893;12:329.
3. Eisinger K. Bezoldmastoiditis mit Facialislahmung in allen drei Asten Mschr Ohrenhk. 1925;59:863.
4. Flatau E. Peripherische Facialislahmung mit retrograder Neurondegeneration; ein Beitrag zu der normalen und pathologischen Anatomie der Nn. facialis, cochlearis und trigeminus. Z Klin Med. 1897;32:280.
5. Fremel F. Zur Pathologie der otogenen Gesichtslahmung. Mschr Ohrenhk. 1931;65:950.
6. Grewal DS, Hathiram BT. Tuberculous Otitis Media in ENT disorders in a tropical environment (2nd edn). Prof S Kameswaran, Prof Mohan Kameshwaran (Eds). MERF publications: Chennai, India. 1999. pp. 65-77.
7. Grewal DS, Hatiram BJ, Saraiya S. V canal wall down Tympanomastoidectomy, the "on-disease" approach for retraction pockets and cholesteatoma. The journal of laryngology and otology. 2007;121:832-9.
8. Hall A. Pathology of Bell's palsy. Archives of Otolaryngology. 1941;54:475.
9. Kettel K. Facial palsy of otitic origin. Arch. Oto-laryng (Am) 37(1943), 303.Ormerod, F.C "Tuberculous disease of the middle ear". Journal of Laryngology and Otology. 1931;46:449-59.
10. Krischek J. Facialislahmung und Poliomyelitis. Arztl Wschr. 1950;6:421.
11. Lange W. Pathologie der Taubstummheit. In: MANASSE: Handbuch der pathologischen Anatomie des menschlichen Ohres, Bergmann:Wiesbaden. 1917.
12. Lund R. Die Facialisparese bei den suppurativen Mittelohr-leiden mit besonderem Hinblick auf ihre Verbindung mit labyrintharen Komplikationen and ihre Bedeutung als Operationsindikation. Z. Hals-usw. Hk. 1929;23:296.
13. Mayer O. Quoted from Szende. Szende, B.: Herpes zoster oticus mit Facialislahmung. Mschr Ohrenhk. 1932;66:814.
14. Neumann H. Die otitischen Facialisparesen. Wien. Med. Wschr. 1906;56:1233/1306-355.
15. Nuhsmann T. Diagnose, Prognose und Therapie der otogenen Facialislahmung. In: Handbuch der Hals-Nasen-Oherenheilkunde vii/2 Bergmann, Munchen; Springer:Berlin. 1926.
16. Ormerod F C. "Tuberculous disease of the middle ear". Journal of Laryngology and Otology.1931;46:449-59.
17. Pollak E. Affektionen im Gebiete des Trigeminus und Facialis. In: Alexander und Marburg: Handbuch der Neurologie des Ohres ii/I. Urban and Schwarzenberg, Berlin-Wien. 1928.
18. Pollmann L. Facialisparesen. Mschr. Ohrenhk. 1937;71:1068.
19. Rudinger. Quoted from SZENDE: Herpes zoster oticus mit Facialislahmung. Mschr. Ohrenhk. 1932;66:814.
20. Sade J. Retrograde facial paralysis. Annals of Otology (St. Louis). 1965;74:94.
21. Tonndorf W. Facialiskrampfe. Z Hals-usw Hk. 1924;8:98.
22. Vogt H. Die Paralyse des Nervus facialis im Anschlub an Otitis media acuta; ein Beitrag von derLehre der otogenen Gesichtslahmung. Dissertation Heidelberg. 1899 (quoted from Pollack).

8

Facial Nerve in Temporal Bone Fractures

DS Grewal

INTRODUCTION

The human race today faces an uncontrolled and mounting epidemic of severe injuries and death due to trauma. Since direct trauma to the ear in closed head injuries constitutes a major cause of correctable ear pathology, a particular discussion of fractures of the temporal bone desires the readers' closest attention (Hough and Stuart, 1968).

Temporal bone fractures are extremely common with head injuries. They present with a variety of symptoms including facial nerve paralysis, hearing loss, vertigo and leakage of the cerebro-spinal fluid (CSF) through the ear or the nose. Since the temporal bone is the domain of the otologist, he plays a major and important role in management of fractures along with the neurosurgeon.

Fractures involving the temporal bone can be classified depending on the relationship of the fracture line to the long axis of the petrous part of the temporal bone as:

1. Longitudinal (Fig. 8.1)
2. Transverse (Fig. 8.1)
3. Mixed.

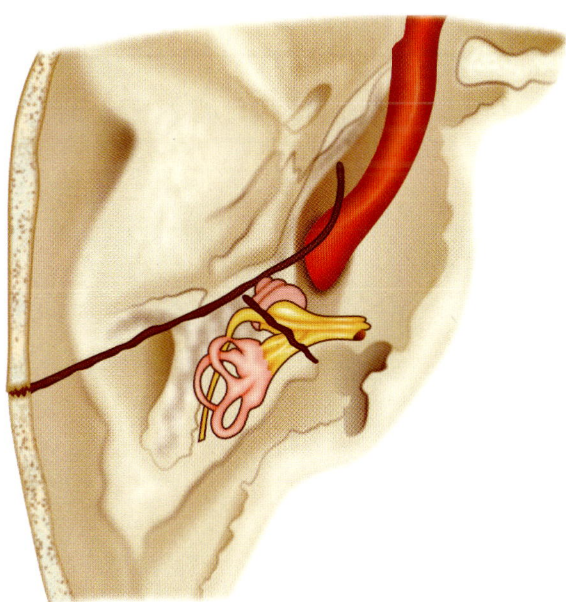

Fig. 8.1: Diagrammatic representation of longitudinal and transverse fractures of the temporal bone

The facial nerve is rendered functionless either temporarily or permanently in longitudinal fractures whereas the risk of permanent facial nerve palsy is much more in transverse fractures. Kettel (1950) believed that an immediate paralysis should be explored as soon as the patient's condition permits.

The facial nerve paralysis could be due to:

- An incomplete or complete transection of the nerve
- Bony fragments compressing on the nerve
- Edema of the nerve as a part of generalized inflammation due to trauma
- Compression due to the bands formed in the nerve sheath which is caught between the fractured fragments.

Often the diagnosis is made purely on clinical grounds as the fractures are not always seen on routine skull X-rays. Rarely, the diagnosis is delayed until the appearance of discoloration of the skin over the mastoid (Battle's sign).

Patients with temporal bone fractures may develop ear bleeding and occasionally CSF otorrhea with deafness, which may be conductive or sensorineural. These fractures may give rise to vertigo and facial paralysis, which, however, are commonly seen with transverse fractures.

In a case of vehicular accident or trauma to the head, these fractures often appear in combination with other skull fractures or brain injuries (contrecoup injuries), which may be associated with air in the cranium. In these cases, interdisciplinary co-operation with the neurosurgeon is required. Today, high resolution computed tomography of the temporal bone makes it possible to define priorities in the treatment of these patients.

Pathology

Longitudinal Fractures

Eighty percent of temporal bone fractures are longitudinal (Figs 8.2 and 8.3) and usually result from blows to the temporal or parietal areas (Proctor, Gurdjian and Webster, 1956). The fracture line usually runs anterior to the otic capsule and involves the external and middle ears resulting in bleeding from the ear with conductive hearing loss due to ossicular disruption. Since the fracture does not involve the otic capsule, sensorineural hearing loss is not seen. The

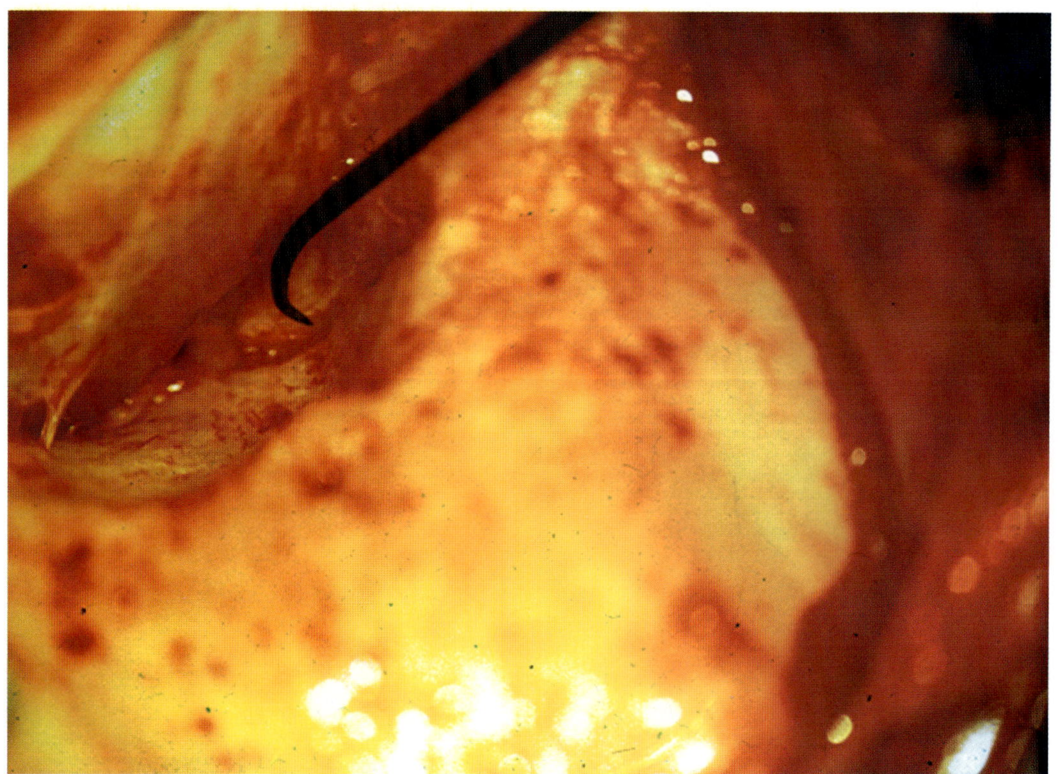

Fig. 8.2: Intraoperative photograph of longitudinal fracture of the temporal bone involving the external auditory canal and going towards the second genu of the facial nerve

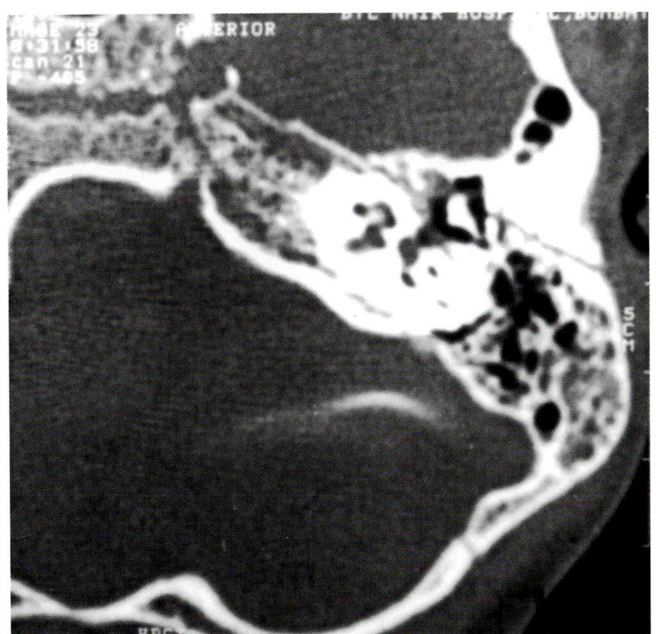

Fig. 8.3: CT scan axial view showing a longitudinal fracture of the temporal bone

facial nerve canal is usually spared and facial palsy occurring in longitudinal fractures is usually delayed in onset and is due to nerve edema in most of the cases (Figs 8.4A and B). Such cases can be conserved and medical line of management, which includes steroids, will result in improvement of the function of the facial nerve. Facial nerve exploration should be undertaken in well-selected cases only.

Transverse Fractures (Fig. 8.5)

Transverse fractures usually result from frontal or occipital blows and account for approximately 20% of temporal bone fractures (Proctor, Gurdjian and Webster, 1956). The fracture line passes through the otic capsule thus damaging the inner ear. A pure transverse fracture can result in a hemotympanum and since the tympanic membrane is usually intact, it is not associated with bleeding from the ear. It is characterized by sensorineural hearing loss, tinnitus, nausea, vomiting, vertigo and facial palsy on the

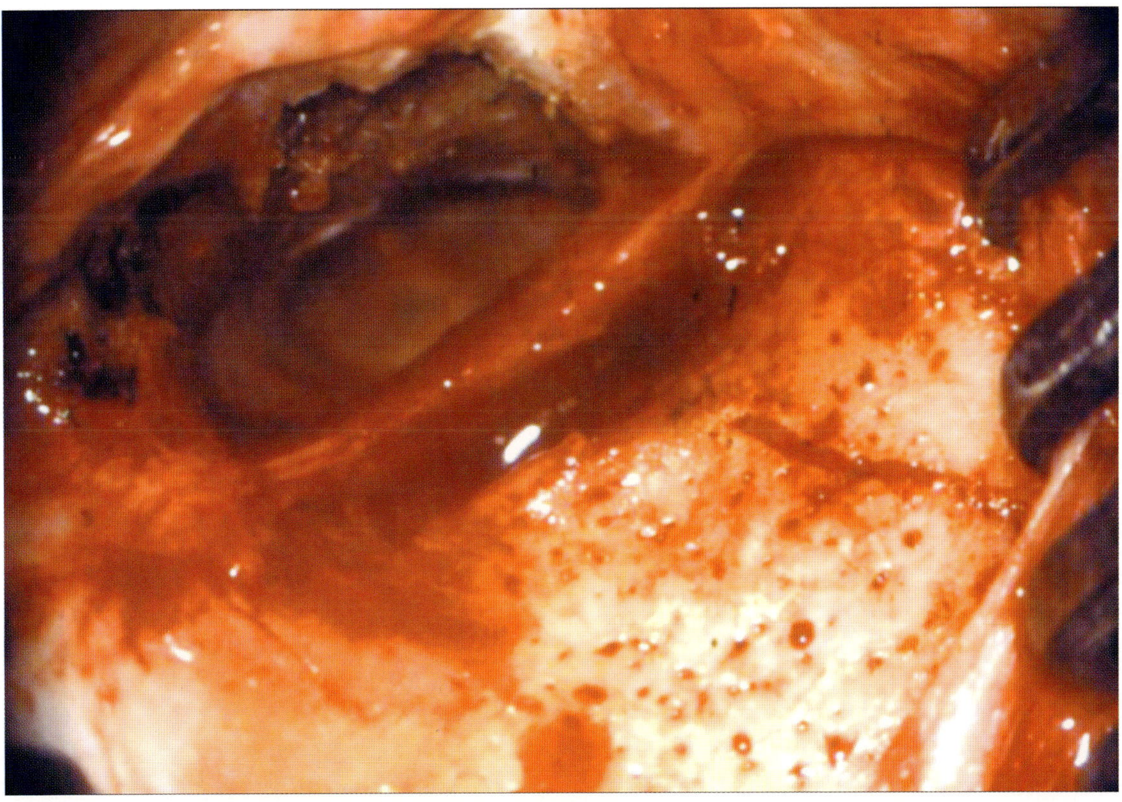

Fig. 8.4A: Intraoperative photograph showing fracture of the mastoid cortex, on exploration, it was involving the dura but there was no CSF leak

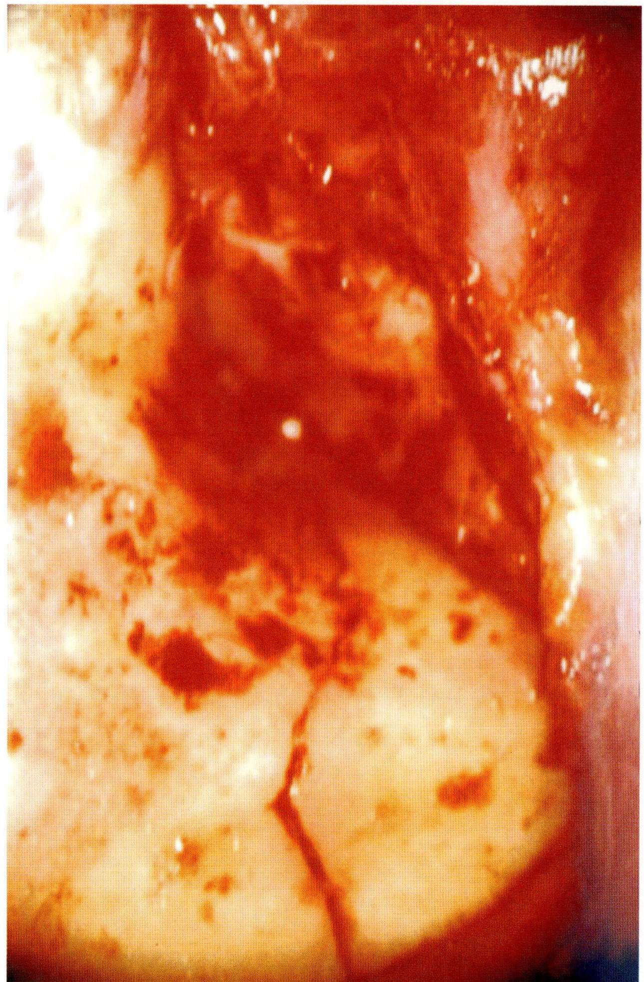

Fig. 8.4B: Intraoperative photograph showing fracture of the mastoid cortex and the posterior bony wall of the external auditory canal

affected side. However, in an unconscious patient with head injury, these signs may be missed until recovery occurs. Fifty percent of these patients develop facial nerve palsy, which is immediate in onset.

Mixed Fractures (Figs 8.6 and 8.7)

In severe head injuries, there may be a combination of the longitudinal and transverse fracture with a loose fragment of bone, which can result in facial palsy if it lies over the facial nerve. The facial palsy seen in these mixed (comminuted) fractures of the temporal bone, is usually immediate in onset. Also, the head injury resulting in such a massive complex fracture of the temporal bone is usually severe and associated with brain edema or pneumocranium and prolonged

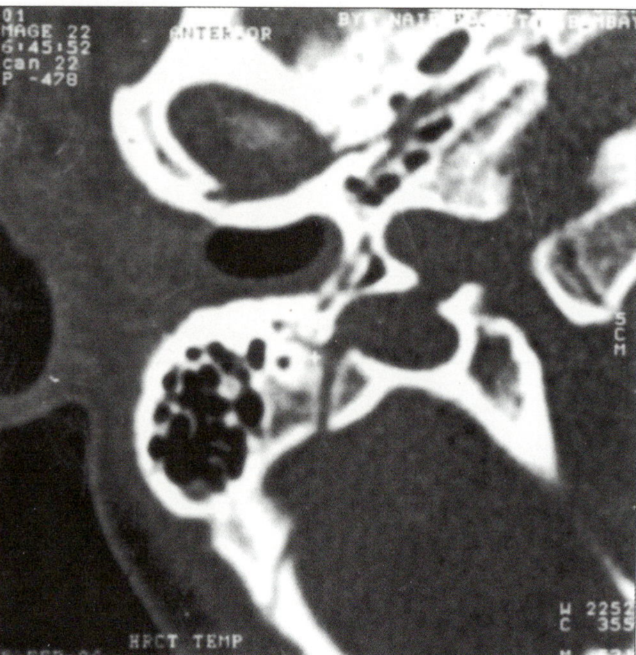

Fig. 8.5: CT scan axial view showing transverse fracture of the temporal bone

unconsciousness as well as other skull bone fractures with CSF leakage. Depending on the type of trauma, there may be fractures of other bones like those of the extremities.

CLINICAL FEATURES

- *Deafness*: Conductive, sensorineural or mixed
- Hemotympanum and bleeding from ear, which may become purulent at a later date. The bleeding from the ear may also be due to the laceration of the skin from the external auditory canal.
- *Facial palsy*: Lower motor neuron type. It may be immediate or delayed in onset.
- *Vertigo*: Severe initially but usually tends to subside on its own within 2 weeks. This is usually due to hemorrhagic labyrinthitis or leakage of the perilymphatic fluid through the fracture line.
- *Lateral rectus palsy*: This is usually on the side opposite to the fracture and is due to intraorbital hematoma secondary to contrecoup brain injury (Figs 8.8A to D)
- *CSF otorrhea and otorhinorrhea*: This is rarely seen and may occur in severe head injury resulting in fractures of skull bones other than the temporal bone. In the presence of an intact tympanic

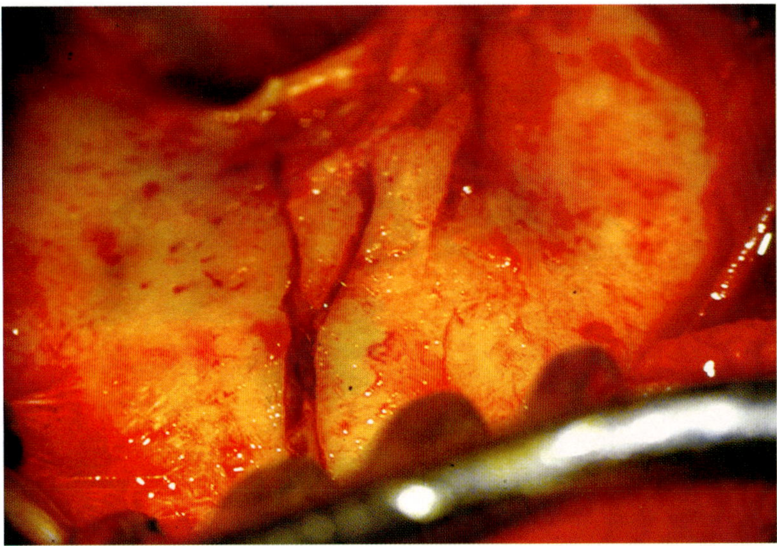

Fig. 8.6: Intraoperative photograph showing comminuted fracture of the temporal bone. One of the fragments of the fracture was pressing over the mastoid segment of the facial nerve

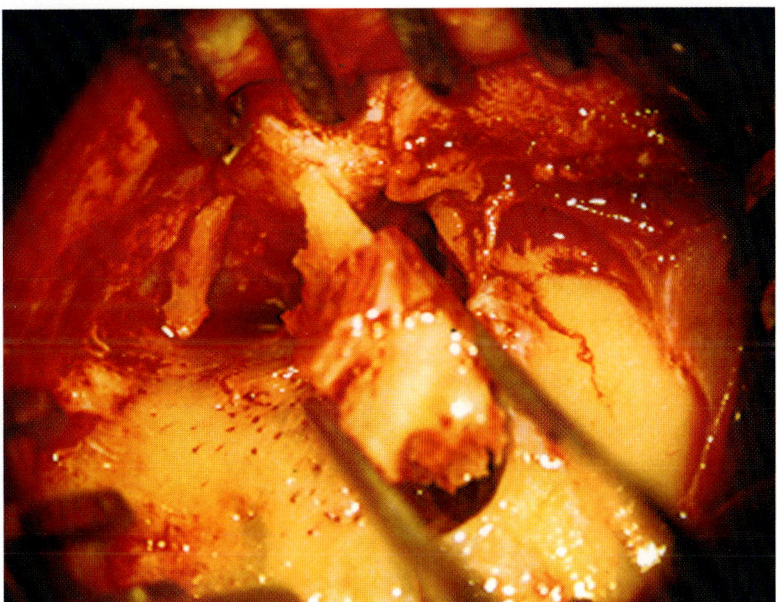

Fig. 8.7: Intraoperative photograph showing removal of a loose fractured segment of the mastoid bone in a case of temporal bone fracture of the same patient (Fig. 8.6) during facial nerve decompression

membrane, CSF may leak through the nose going via the Eustachian tube.

- Discoloration of the skin over the mastoid: Battle's sign
- Presence of other injuries to the skull may manifest themselves as unconsciousness, neurological deficit and bleeding from various sites
- CT scan will show evidence and type of fracture as well as associated fractures of other skull bones, hematoma, brain edema and pneumocranium (Figs 8.9 and 8.10).

MANAGEMENT

The priority in management of a patient of head injury with fracture temporal bone depends on the

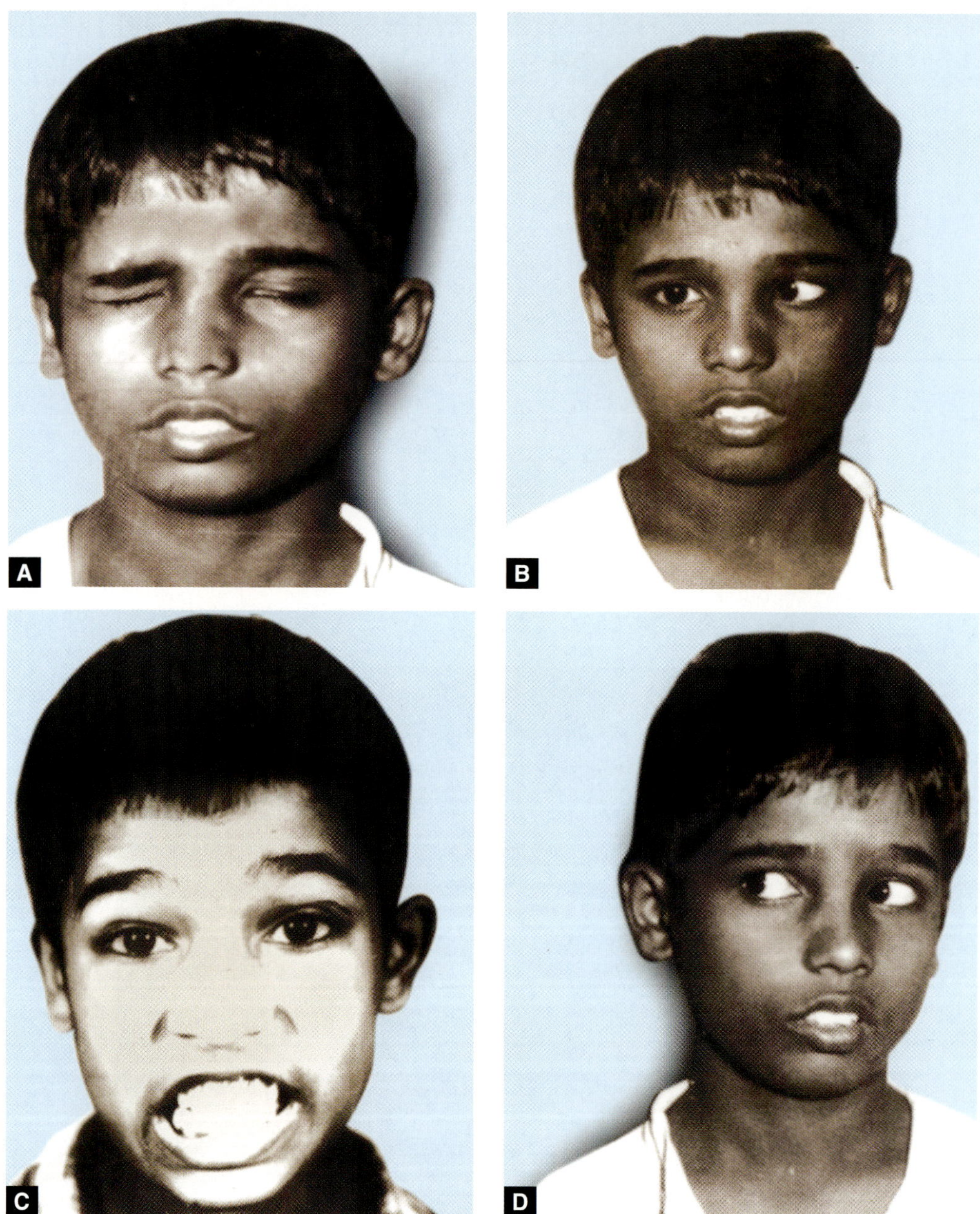

Figs 8.8A to D: Clinical photograph of a patient with left side facial palsy and right sided lateral rectus palsy due to vehicular accident causing fracture of the left temporal bone and hematoma in the right orbital cavity. Postoperative photograph of the same patient (Figs 8.8A and B) three months after decompression of the facial nerve. Note the improvement in facial function and recovery of lateral rectus palsy

general condition of the patient. Unconsciousness and vital parameters are stabilized first.

Investigations required should be done on emergency basis. For the diagnosis of fractures of the temporal bone, high resolution computed tomography (HRCT) of the temporal bone is the investigation of choice. Previously, X-rays of the mastoid like the Stenver's, Owen's and Schüller's views were done. However, they are very poor diagnostic indicators of temporal bone fractures.

Once the patient is stable, the conductive hearing loss and facial palsy are to be treated. Vertigo usually

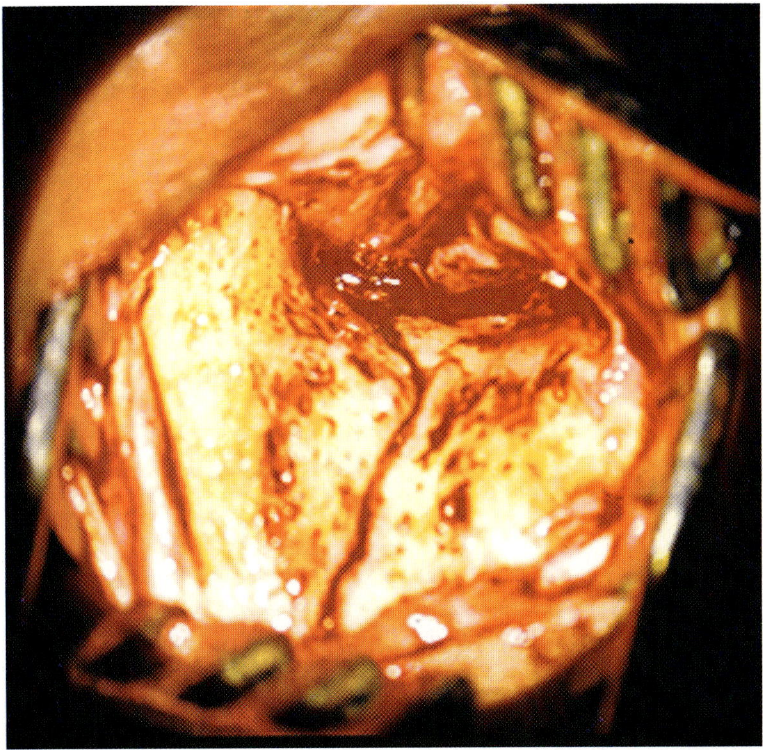

Fig. 8.9A: Intraoperative photograph showing an extensive longitudinal fracture of the right temporal bone involving the second genu anteriorly and the posterior cranial fossa posteriorly

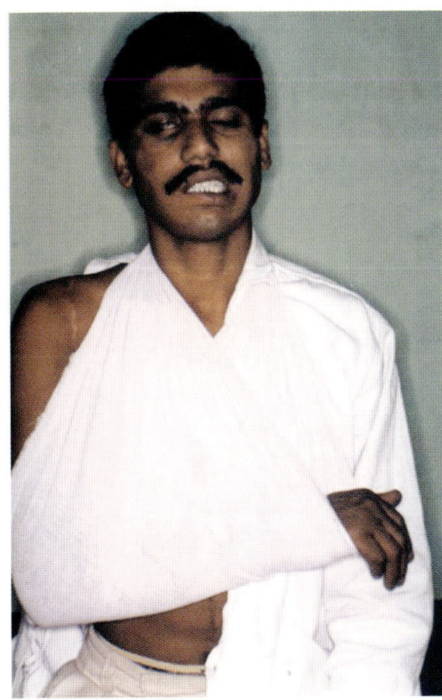

Fig. 8.9B: Clinical photograph of the same patient (Fig. 8.9A) with right facial palsy and upper limb fracture

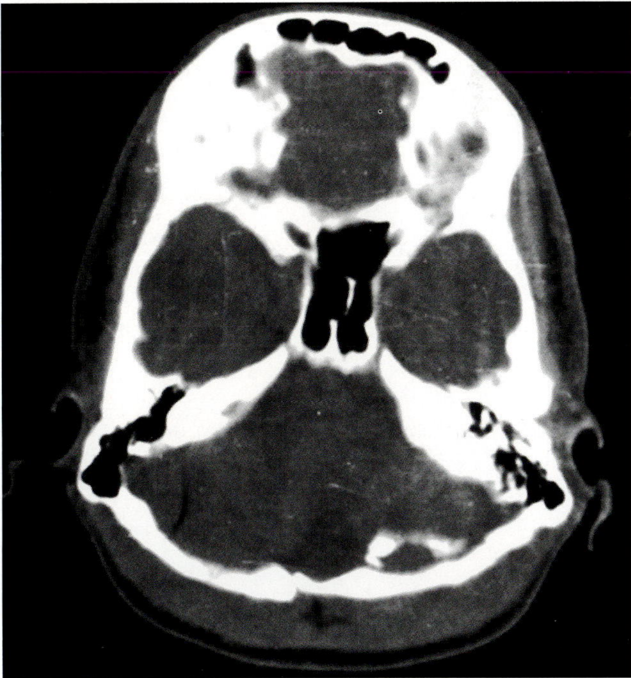

Fig. 8.10: CT scan axial view showing longitudinal fracture of the temporal bone with fractures of other cranial bones. Patient also had a fracture of the shaft of femur

subsides within 2-3 weeks and the sensorineural hearing loss is irreversible. Vertigo is either due to labyrinthine concussion or due to perilymph leakage. If it is due to concussion and edema, it tends to resolve with medical management. Whereas in case of a perilymph leakage, the vertigo subsides due to complete leakage of the middle ear fluid resulting in a dead ear followed by compensation.

In a case of conductive hearing loss, repair of the torn tympanic membrane and disrupted ossicular chain is performed.

Unusually, I have observed that in cases of facial palsy related to fractures of the temporal bone that present late, the facial nerve sheath may be caught between the fractured fragments and the fracture heals. This results in bands that are formed in the nerve sheath which compress the nerve. These bands have to be cut during the procedure of facial nerve decompression to relieve the nerve of its strangulating effects, thus improving the chances of a functional recovery (Figs 8.11 and 8.12).

In the case of facial palsy, a decompression of the facial nerve is performed in its entire length after the hematoma is evacuated from the mastoid antrum. If the fracture has involved the posterior meatal wall and there is associated anteriorly placed facial nerve, decompression may be performed by the canal wall down technique. We prefer to decompress the nerve in all its segments (labyrinthine, tympanic and mastoid) and then if required lift it out of its canal followed by widening of the fallopian canal and replacement of the nerve back in the widened canal (Grewal et al. 1998) (Figs 8.13 and 8.14). The exploration of the facial nerve should be preferably

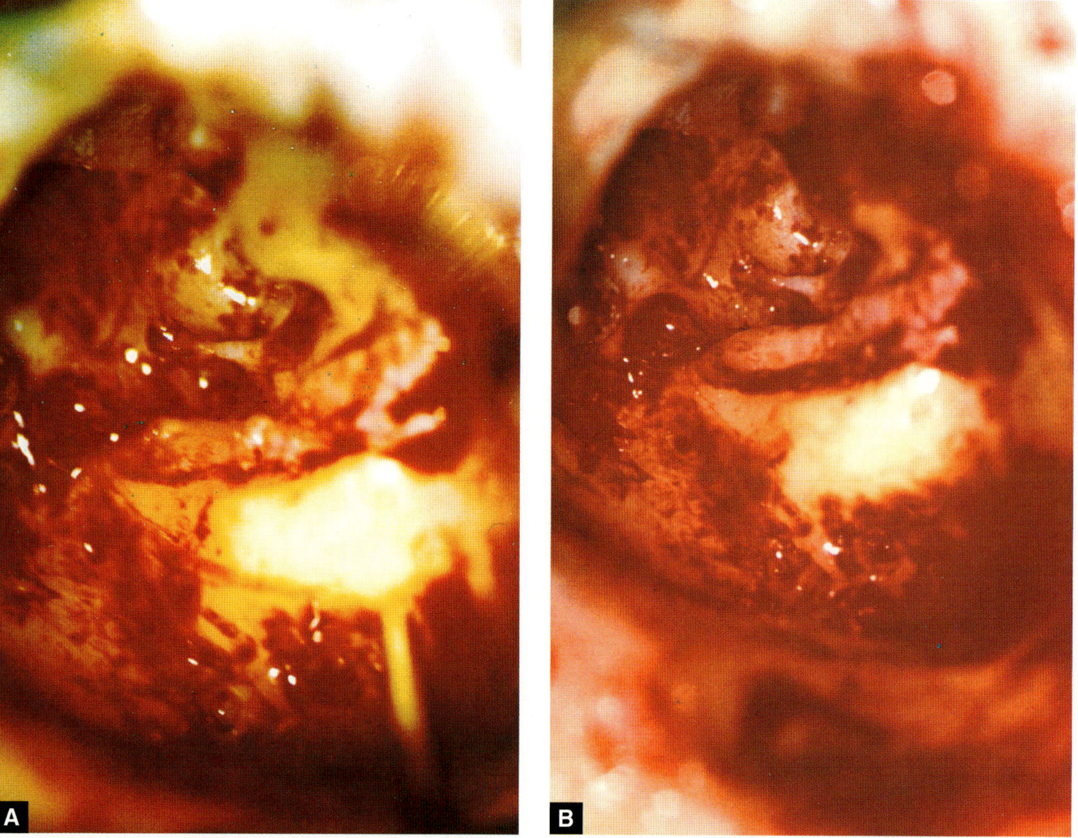

Figs 8.11A and B: (A) Intraoperative photograph of facial nerve decompression done in a case of long-standing facial palsy due to fracture temporal bone. There was no indication of the fracture line (probably healed as it was long-standing). The nerve sheath shows bands compressing the nerve leading to the nerve herniating in between; (B) Intraoperative photograph of the same patient (Fig. 8.11A) during facial nerve decompression. The compressing bands were cut and the nerve relieved of its strangulating effect

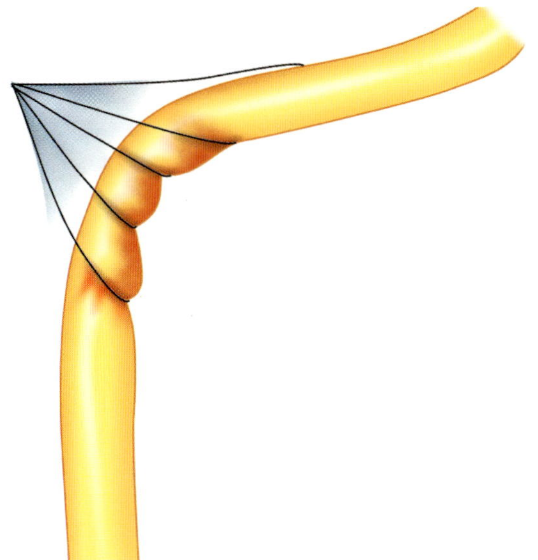

Fig. 8.12: Diagrammatic representation of the nerve sheath causing strangulation and herniation of the nerve when pulled by the fracture line

performed within 72 hours, as after that the process of Wallerian degeneration sets in. According to McCabe (1972), if 72 hours have passed, the optimum time for the repair of the facial nerve is on the 21st day, as the nerve cell body is maximally capable of passing the axoplasmic filaments across the neuronal gap. If decompression is carried out, we advocate not to perform any ossiculoplasty, since if the ossicle/prosthesis slips, it can damage the bare nerve (Fig. 8.15). Rarely, a combined management involving a neurosurgeon and ENT surgeon is required in extensive fractures.

I always like to state that blood in blood vessels is very good but when it collects outside blood vessels in human body forming hematoma, it has adverse effects like bluish discoloration of skin and necrosis of soft tissues. Therefore, when required hematoma in mastoid should be timely and surgically treated. This is helpful in promoting early recovery.

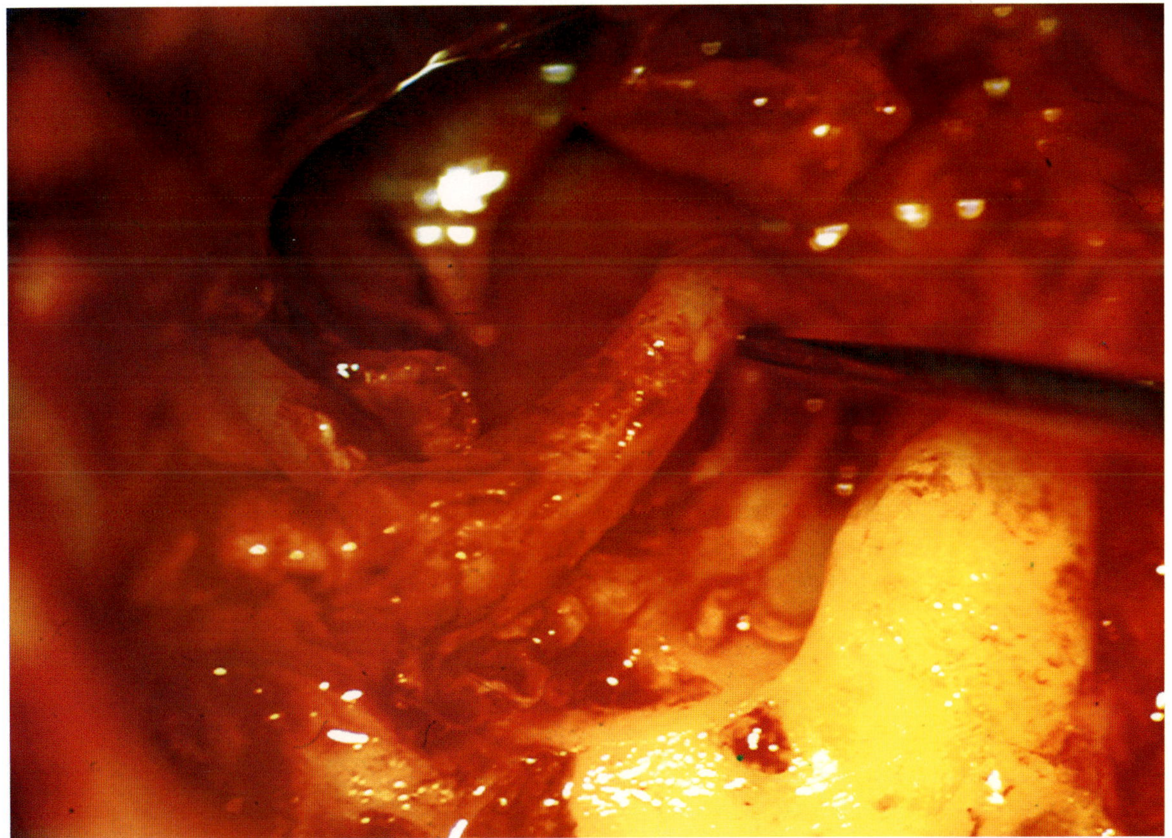

Fig. 8.13: A case of longitudinal fracture of the temporal bone in which the facial nerve was decompressed and taken out of the fallopian canal (High power). The canal was widened and nerve was replaced back

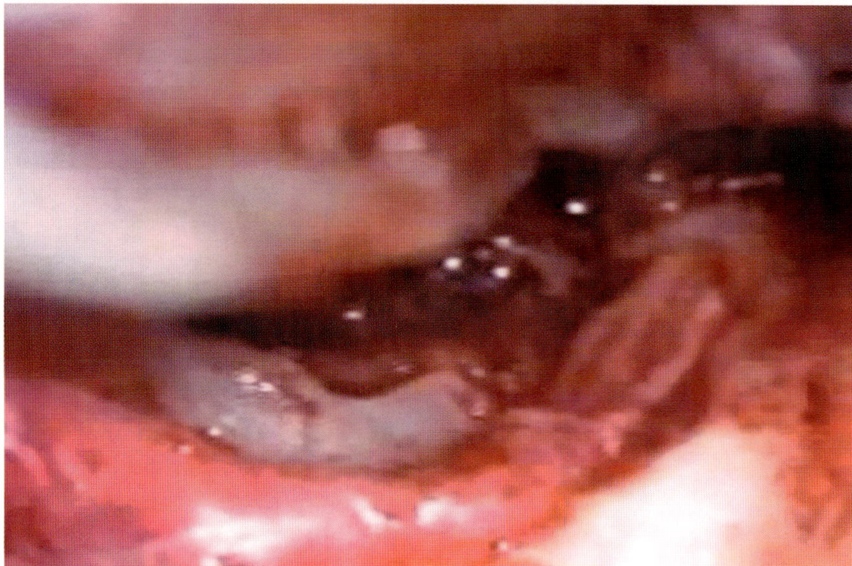

Fig. 8.14: Intraoperative photograph showing facial nerve decompressed in a case of fracture of the temporal bone. The fracture line was involving the fallopian canal leading to superficial trauma to the facial nerve

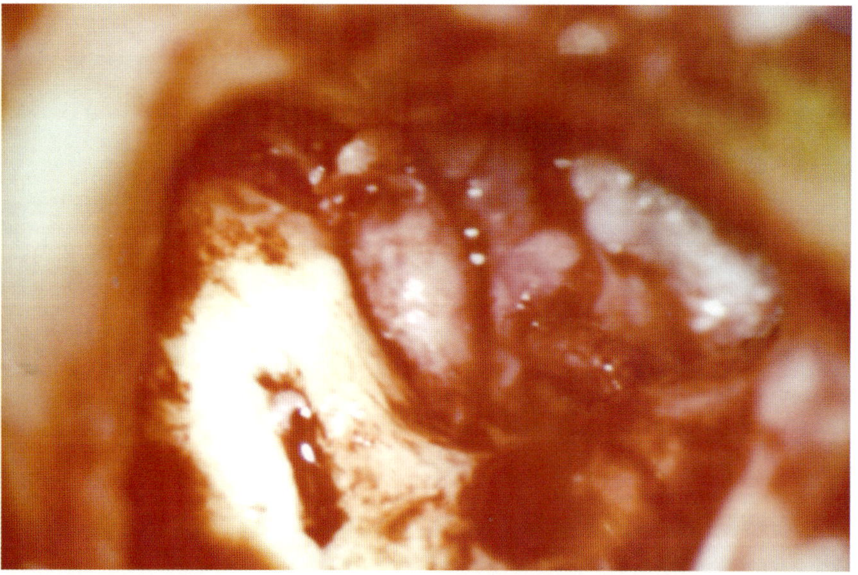

Fig. 8.15: Intraoperative photograph of the facial nerve where the nerve sheath is slit open and a markedly edematous nerve is observed. The patient had a fracture of the temporal bone, which resulted in facial palsy along with sudden hearing loss and giddiness. The patient presented late and on exploration the incus was compressing the facial nerve with edema of the nerve. The ossicle was removed and the nerve sheath was slit. The patient also had a lateral semicircular canal fistula

BIBLIOGRAPHY

1. Grewal DS, Hathiram BT, Manjrekar T, et al. Fractures of the temporal bone. Indian Journal of Otology. 1998;4:109-14.
2. Hough JVD, Stuart WD. Middle ear injuries in skull trauma. Laryngoscope. 1968;78:899-937.
3. Kettel K. Peripheral facial palsy in fractures of the temporal bone. Archives of Otolaryngology. 1950;57:25.
4. McCabe BF. Injuries to the facial nerve. Laryngoscope. 1972;82:1891-96.
5. Proctor B, Gurdjian ES, Webstar JE. The ear in head trauma. Laryngoscope. 1956;66:16-59.

9

Iatrogenic Injury of the Facial Nerve During Surgery of CSOM

DS Grewal

INTRODUCTION

An injury to the facial nerve represents the otologic surgeons' greatest fear. Surgeons are aware of not only the cosmetic and functional consequences of such a complication, but also related medicolegal aspects. Unfortunately, the fear of damage to the facial nerve may lead to avoidance of the nerve instead of positive identification. The best method of preventing iatrogenic injury to the facial nerve is to identify the nerve and use it as a landmark for finding other structures. When the surgeon can see the full course of the nerve in the operative field, he or she will not injure it (Shambaugh and Glasscock, 1990).

Although the normal anatomy of the facial nerve is familiar to most otolaryngologists, it may be distorted by prior surgery, granulation tissue (which may be tuberculus) or cholesteatoma. In rare instances, the facial nerve may follow an anomalous course, rendering the usual surgical landmarks unreliable (Mayer et al.1976). These circumstances challenge the most experienced otologic surgeon. In the days of the mallet and the chisel, and mastoidectomies without microscope, the incidence of iatrogenic facial injuries was high. Now, the use of micromotors, irrigation, suction and the operating microscope with an improved anesthetic technique has greatly reduced this complication of ear surgery (Grewal and Hathiram, 1999).

However, facial palsy still does occur due to some or the other reason, such as:

- Destruction or distortion of landmarks for identification of the facial nerve
- Anomalous course of the facial nerve
- Anomaly of the facial nerve
- Faulty operative technique—drilling and handling of sharp instruments
- Slipping of material used for reconstruction such as prosthesis, bone or cartilage.

Injury during otologic surgery is most likely to occur in the second genu and the tympanic segment (Green et al. 1994). The surgical landmarks for the tympanic segment include the cochleariform process, the oval window and the pyramidal process. The lateral semicircular canal and the cog are the landmarks while approaching the facial nerve (tympanic segment) through the mastoid. Landmarks for the mastoid segment include the lateral semicircular canal, the fossa incudis and the digastric ridge. The posterior semicircular canal may be a useful landmark in the well-pneumatized temporal bone (Green et al., 1994).

In cases of intact canal wall mastoidectomies and ossiculoplasties, the facial nerve may be damaged by:

- Inadvertent handling of incus which can injure the dehiscent second genu of the facial nerve
- Graft materials and prosthetic materials like PORP, TORP and synthetic materials kept for ossicular reconstruction might injure the dehiscent horizontal facial nerve and second genu
- While widening the aditus from the antrum, dehiscent second genu can be injured
- When antrum is exposed through Macewan's triangle, if the dural plate is low lying and the antrum is small and contracted, the surgeon may drill more anteriorly and inferiorly and can injure the nerve in the mastoid segment. This was the most important etiologic factor in my experience (Fig. 9.1).
- While performing a posterior tympanotomy, it may be preferable to identify the facial nerve first and then to do a posterior tympanotomy otherwise the mastoid segment of facial nerve can be injured.

In case of canal wall down mastoidectomies, the most common site injured was the second genu (Grewal, 1996).

- Second genu can be injured while operating in the floor of the fossa incudis and on removal of posterior buttress
- Mastoid segment can be injured while lowering the facial ridge especially when the nerve is dehiscent, malformed or its course is anomalous

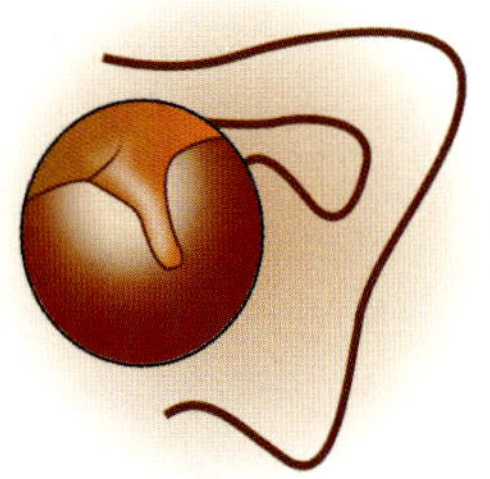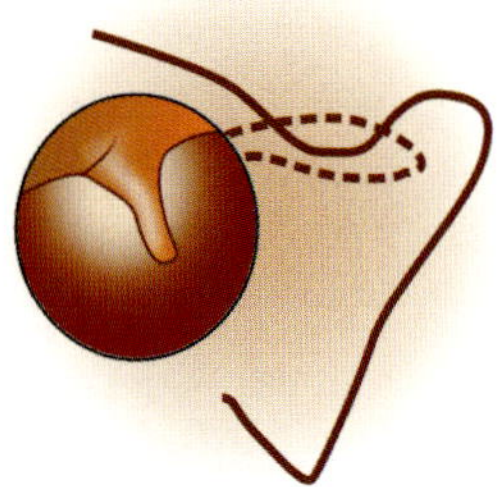

Fig. 9.1: Diagrammatic representation of the normal mastoid antrum and a narrow contracted and posteriorly placed mastoid antrum with a low lying dura which predisposes to facial nerve injury

- In children, post-auricular incision itself can cause facial palsy if it is extended inferiorly because of the absence of a well formed mastoid tip.

TESTS FOR FACIAL NERVE FUNCTION

1. A detailed history and facial nerve examination is essential. Important points in the history include:
   i. Onset of palsy
      - Time of onset
      - Completeness of the palsy at the onset.
   ii. Duration of palsy
   iii. Progress of palsy.
2. Schirmer's test and test for taste sensation of anterior 2/3rd of the tongue can be of value if properly performed, to identify the probable site of injury.
3. Electrodiagnostic tests are more reliable if available. Nerve conduction study helps to detect the type of injury and also helps in evaluating the post-operative conduction through the repaired nerve segment/graft. Electromyography helps in prognosis.

MANAGEMENT OF IATROGENIC FACIAL PALSY

Iatrogenic injury of the facial nerve represents a special problem, especially when there is an unexpected postoperative facial palsy.

After surgical exploration of the facial nerve, further management depends upon:

- Site of injury
- Extent of nerve section—partial or complete
- Cut nerve ends are in approximation or there is a loss of nerve segment
- Whether cut ends are fibrotic or not
- The time interval between onset of palsy and time of exploration.

It is imperative to ascertain whether the palsy is complete or incomplete and whether the nerve was identified by the surgeon during the surgery. If there is partial recovery after six hours of surgery, medical line of management is followed. However, if after six hours of surgery, there is no recovery or the palsy continues to worsen, early surgical exploration is merited. If the injured nerve is identified intra-operatively, the repair is carried out at the same time.

On early surgical exploration there may be either a cut injury or some compressing factors, which may be the cause of the facial palsy. If there are compressing factors present such as ossicle/cartilage/bone wax, they should be removed and the facial nerve should be decompressed (Figs 9.2 to 9.9). If there is a cut injury, it should be repaired by suturing and/or nerve grafting (Flow chart 9.1).

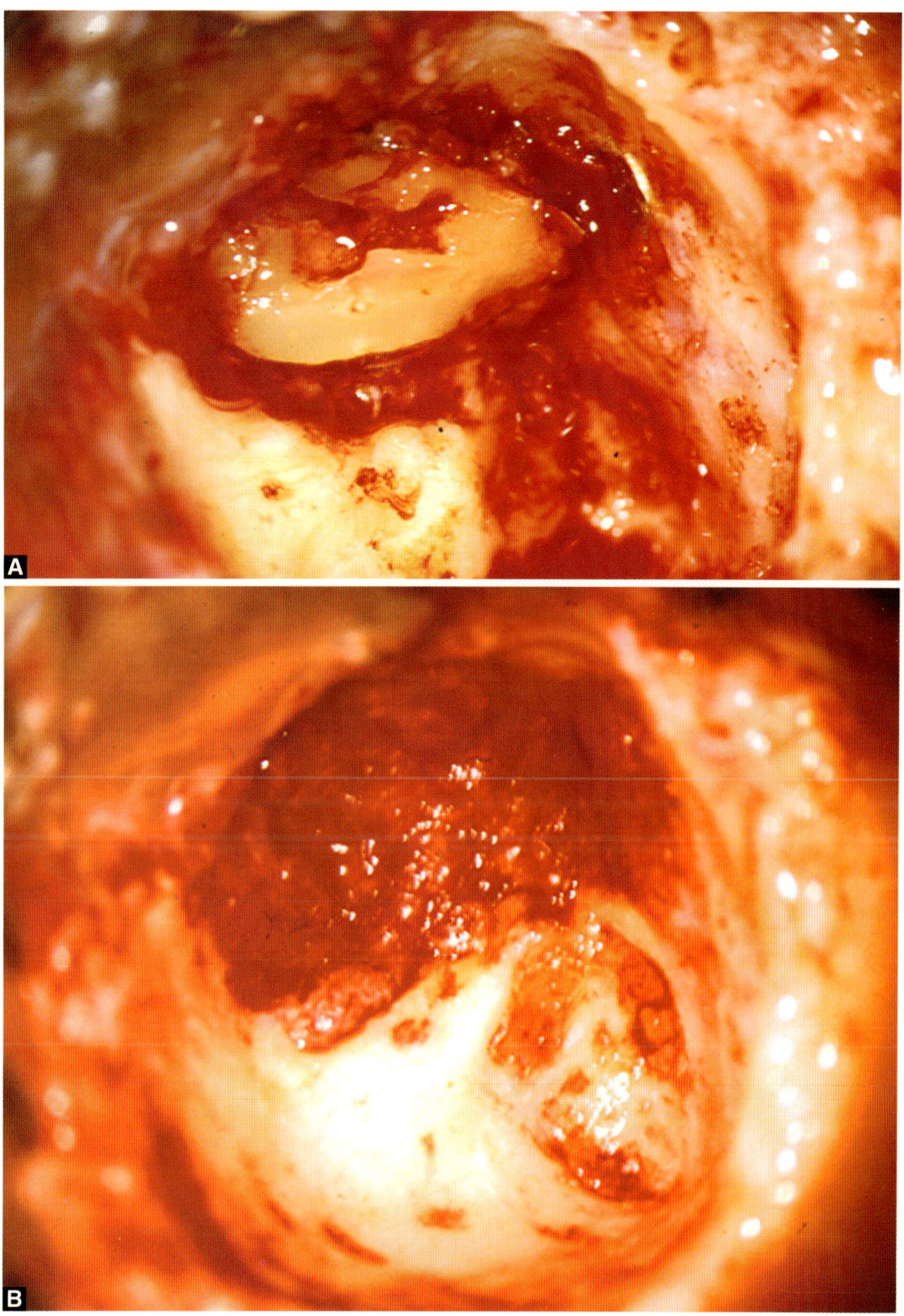

Figs 9.2A and B: (A) This patient underwent ear surgery when the surgeon had to abandon the operation as there was massive bleeding from a high jugular bulb. The tear in the jugular bulb was sealed by bone wax. Postoperatively there was complete facial palsy. The mastoid was explored at a later date and bone wax was removed; (B) On removal of bone wax, there was an anteriorly placed facial nerve running over the promontory

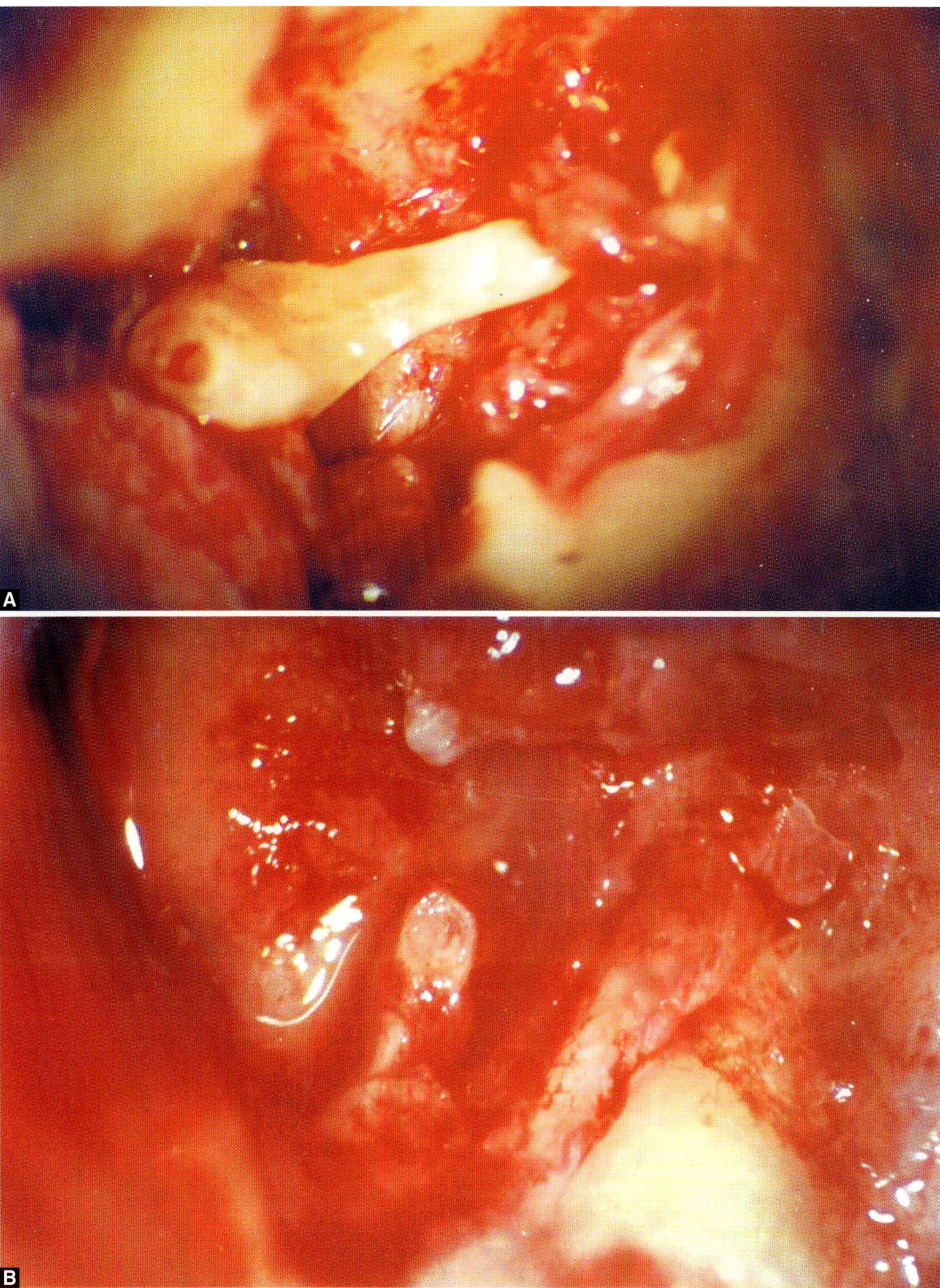

Figs 9.3A and B: (A) Intraoperative photograph showing injury to the dehiscent facial nerve in its tympanic segment due to the displaced refashioned incus used for reconstruction of the ossicular chain (seen on 10th postoperative day). Note the shallow socket which resulted in the ossicle graft slipping from the stapes head; (B) Note the lesion over the dehiscent facial nerve after removal of the displaced incus resulting in neuropraxia

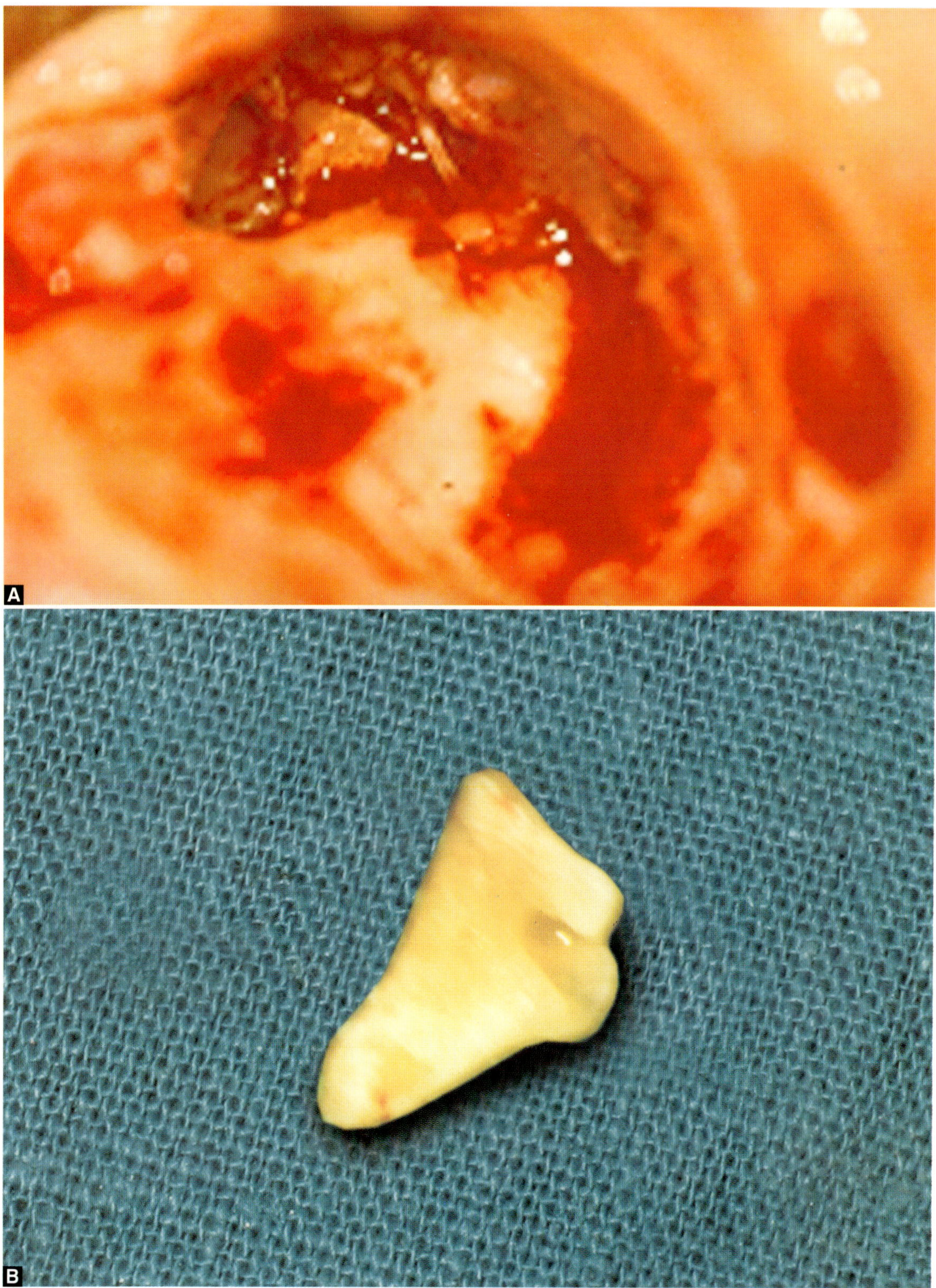

Figs 9.4A and B: (A) Intraoperative photograph showing the displaced (tilted) incus used for reconstruction of the ossicular chain resulting in injury to the dehiscent facial nerve in its tympanic segment; (B) Note the deep socket which is improperly fashioned on the incus which resulted in an unstable assembly with the stapes head resulting in tilting of the ossicle

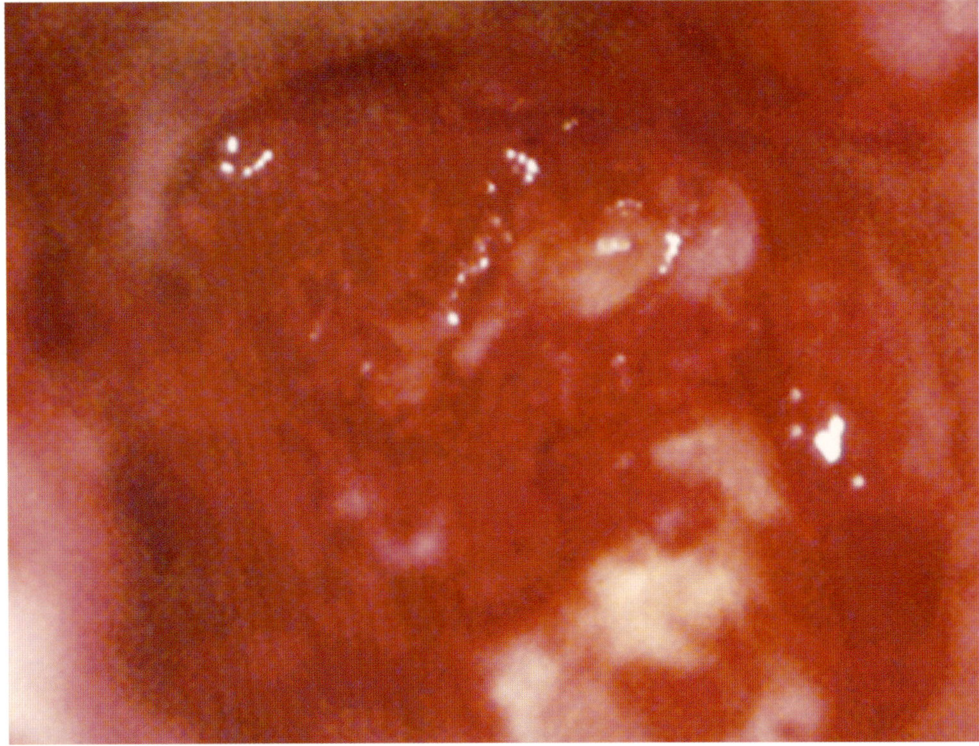

Fig 9.5: Malleus resting over facial nerve which was used for ossiculoplasty has caused palsy and it was removed and facial nerve was decompressed

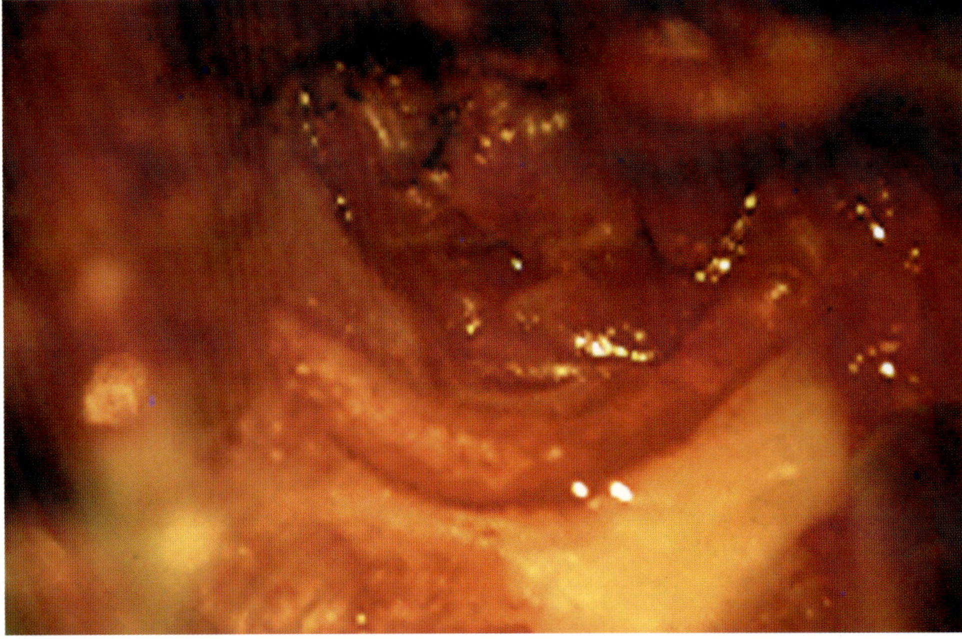

Fig 9.6: Intraoperative photograph of revision tympanomastoidectomy for facial palsy following type III tympanoplasty using incus showing a decompressed facial nerve in its tympanic and mastoid course. Note that the nerve is edematous, congested and running over the stapes foot plate. Also note the deep indentation at the site of trauma by the incus, where it pierced the nerve running over the stapes footplate

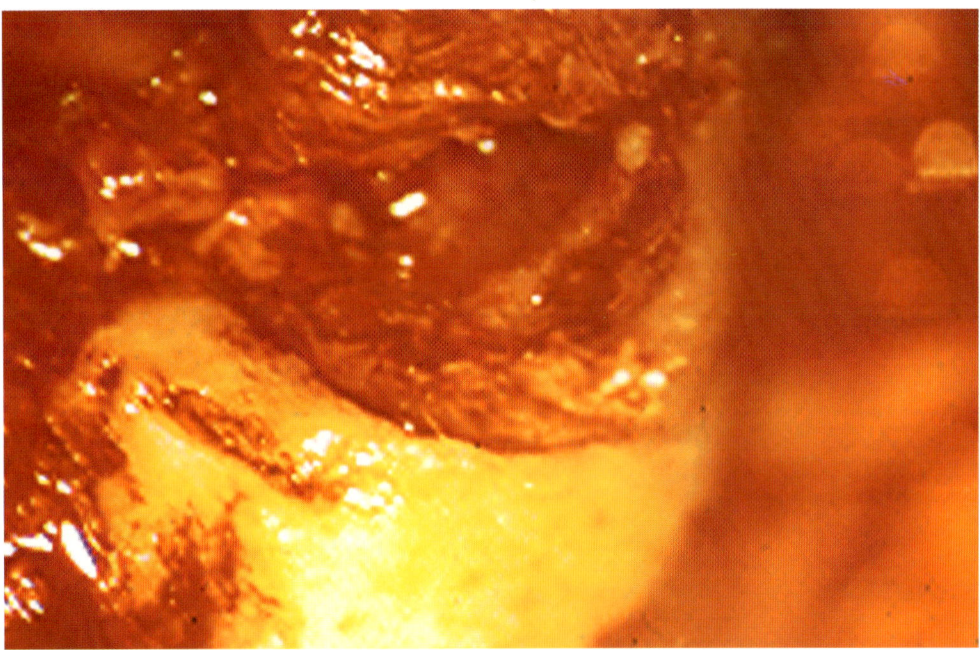

Fig. 9.7: Injury to the dehiscent facial nerve in its mastoid segment due to the jagged edges of a cartilage graft used to reconstruct the tympanic membrane during myringoplasty

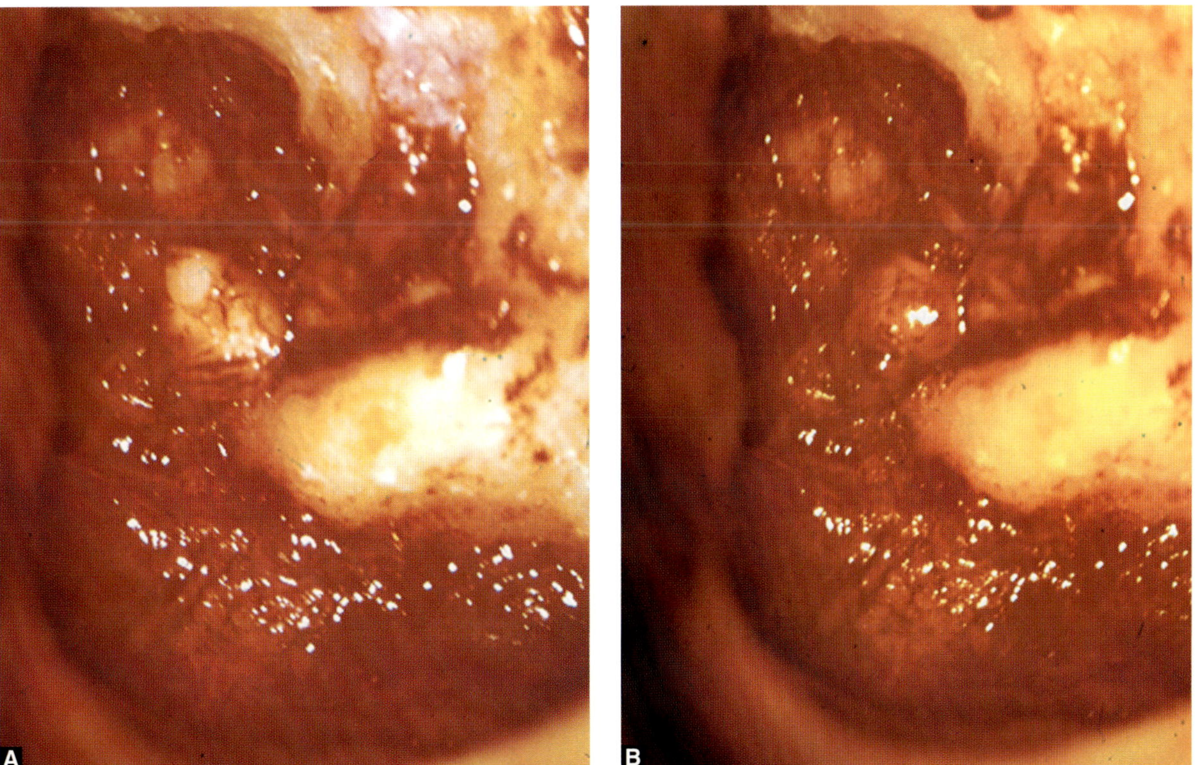

Figs 9.8A and B: (A) Cartilage used for ossiculoplasty causing facial nerve palsy in a patient. On exploration, the cartilage was seen lying directly over a dehiscent facial nerve causing compression; (B) Note the edematous injured facial nerve after removal of the cartilage

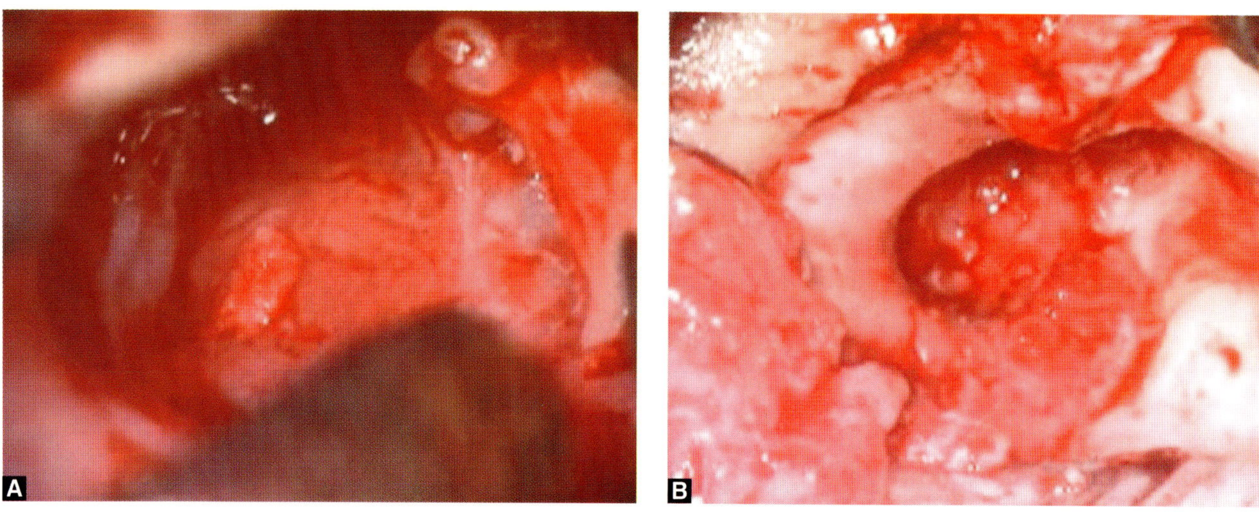

Figs 9.9A and B: (A)Revision surgery done after 1 year showing ossicular assembly done which was resting over second genu of facial nerve causing facial palsy; (B) Decompressed facial nerve showing formation of granuloma

Flow chart 9.1: Management of Iatrogenic facial palsy

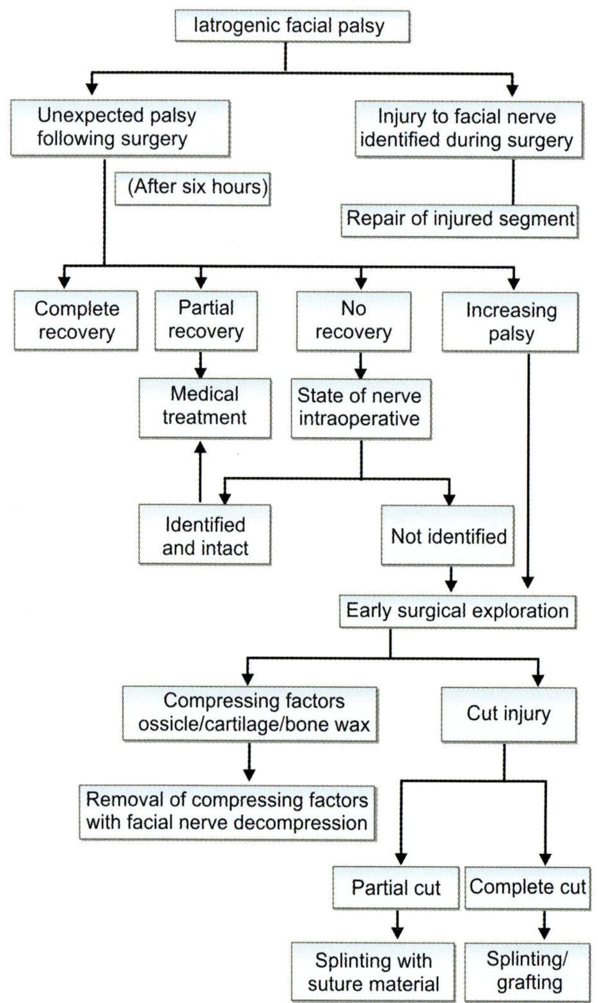

METHODS TO RESTORE FUNCTIONAL CONTINUITY OF THE FACIAL NERVE

- If the nerve is intact but edematous and congested, decompression of the nerve has to be done till healthy nerve is found on either side. The nerve decompression should be done by removing the fallopian canal all around with widening of the canal using diamond burrs. Slitting of the nerve sheath should be done only to drain a suspected intraneural hematoma.

- If there is a partial cut to the nerve early nerve suturing with 8-0 nylon/prolene gives best results.

- If there is complete transection of the nerve and length of nerve damaged is less than 5 mm re-routing and providing end-to-end anastomosis gives the best results. Although, in my experience, I did not perform re-routing.

- If there is complete transection and both cut ends are apart, not in approximation even after re-routing, nerve grafting preferably with greater auricular nerve gives the best results. It is preferable to take the nerve graft a little longer than the defect and the preferred anastomotic technique is natural self-adhesiveness without use of sutures. If the nerve graft is placed in the facial canal, sutures may not be necessary; but if fallopian canal is destroyed by excessive drilling then connective tissue should be placed underneath the graft and sutures should be taken. It is better to take only one suture with 8-0 nylon/prolene at each end. It is more important to keep upper end of anastomotic site more stable because axonal nerve regeneration is from above downwards. It is also important to remove approximately 1 mm of neurilemmal sheath at the anastomotic ends and to bevel the cut ends. The ideal time of nerve grafting is within 30 days of onset of palsy but it can be done as a re-innervation procedure up to 18 months following injury.

- If there is complete transection with the upper stump not being available for reinnervation and the duration of palsy is more than 18 months, the procedure of choice is facio-hypoglossal anastomosis. But this procedure has the disadvantage of mass movement, lack of emotion and paralysis of tongue muscles which may be over come by the facio-hypoglossal "jump" anastomosis technique.
- The main factors that influence the results following the nerve repair are the technical flaws that might down-grade recovery; these include:
  - Lack of suitable nerve ends
  - Tension at the suture line
  - Infection

Regeneration of an uninterrupted nerve occurs approximately at the rate of 1 mm per day. The first sign of returning of function is the improvement in tone of the paralyzed muscles. Other techniques of facial re-animation include:

- Sling operations using tendon or fascia
- Free neurovascular repair
- Muscle transposition—masseter or temporalis.

Protection of eye—mainly to prevent exposure keratitis includes:

- Wearing dark goggles
- Tarsorrhaphy
- Gold weight for upper eyelid
- Eyelid spring
- Lower eyelid tightening with temporalis muscle transfer.

Types of Nerve Injuries

The facial nerve may be injured during surgery either by a sharp instrument or by a cutting burr (Flow chart 9.2). When a sharp instrument injures, it usually leads to a cut injury of the nerve, which may be partial or complete. A partial cut usually results in palsy of the angle of the mouth and spares the eye (due to the representation of fibers in the nerve) whereas a total cut injury results in complete palsy involving the hemiface. However, we have seen that a partial cut injury, at times may present as a complete palsy especially when the patient comes late (after few months) and this fact is explained on the basis of intra-operative finding of a granuloma which is seen to completely encircle the injured nerve segment. This in my view, results in compressing the whole thickness of the nerve and a complete palsy occurs inspite of only a partial cut injury being present. Recovery is rapid once the granuloma is peeled off and nerve ends are approximated.

When the nerve is injured by a cutting burr, the damage depends on the surface of the burr, which comes in contact with the nerve:

- If the tip of the burr comes in contact with the nerve, the injury ranges from abrasion to transection of the nerve with a segment of nerve missing
- If the side of the cutting burr comes in contact with the nerve, it can lead to injury ranging from superficial abrasion to loss of a large segment of the nerve as the nerve is wrapped around the burr and torn out of its canal due to the impact of the rotating burr (Figs 9.10 to 9.14).

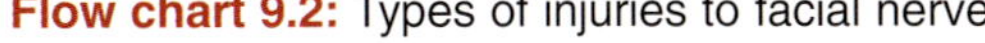

Flow chart 9.2: Types of injuries to facial nerve

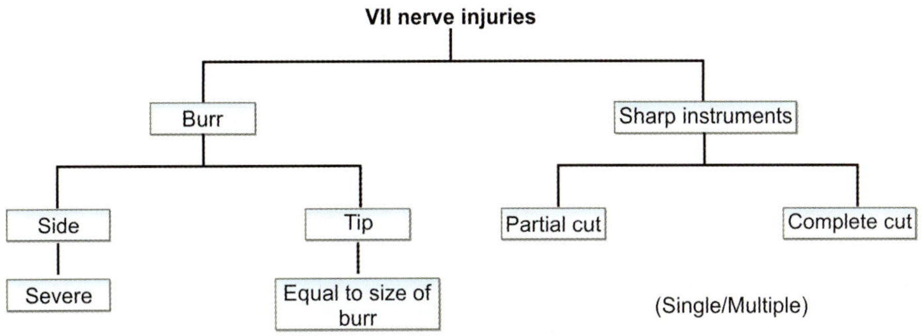

Technique of Nerve Repair

Suturing of the cut ends when there is no loss of facial nerve segment is not always possible as infection and granulation result in bleeding which makes identification of the cut ends difficult since the ends are also edematous, congested and friable. This also makes tying of a knot difficult since the sutures cut through the nerve ends. Also if a knot (of prolene or nylon) is tied I have observed that the cut ends tend to get inverted thus, impeding physiological nerve reunion and the knot being big as well as non-absorbable can result in pressure and neuropraxia once the graft is in place. Due to these reasons, I only pass an 8-0 nylon/prolene suture material through the cut ends of the nerve without tying a knot. The nylon/prolene is passed approximately 2 mm on either sides of the cut ends and the ends are approximated gently by sliding over the nylon in a manner similar to sliding of curtains over a rod. This helps to approximate the ends without damage to the nerve tissue. The ends of the suture material are tagged under the nerve sheath, which is reposited back over the nerve, thus helping the suture material to remain in place. This is then covered and supported by a temporalis fascia graft (Grewal and Hathiram, 1999).

In my opinion this technique works on the following principle:

- The suture material serves as a splint, keeping both nerve ends stable and in approximation, which aids in nerve healing and reunion
- This technique can be compared to a creeper, which requires the support of a stick to grow in a particular

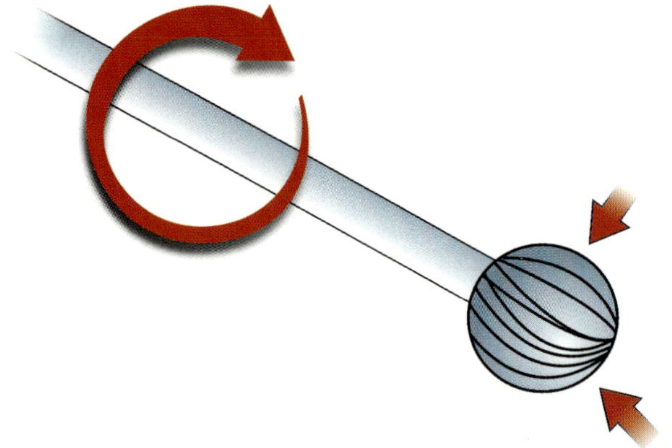

Fig. 9.10: Diagrammatic representation of a cutting burr. Note the tip and the side of the burr, which can cause different types of injuries to the facial nerve

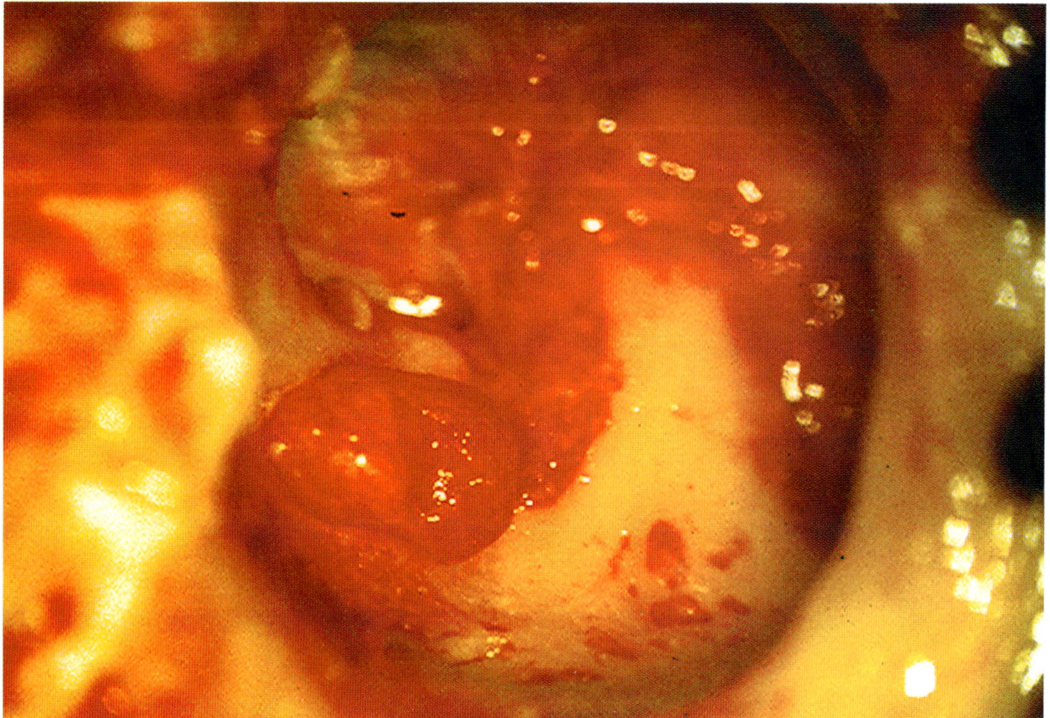

Fig. 9.11: Intraoperative photograph of a cut injury of the facial nerve (sickle knife)

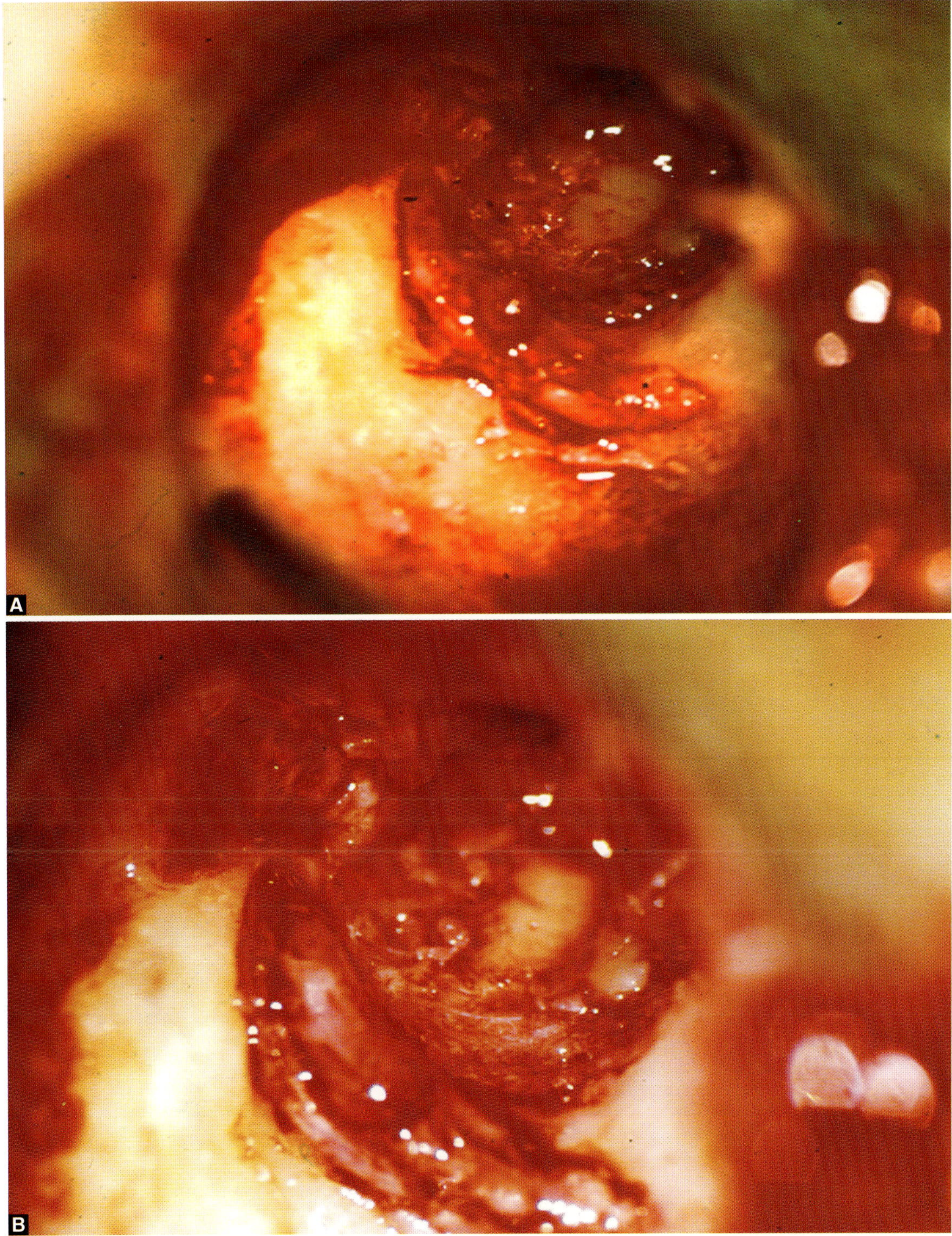

Figs 9.12A and B: (A) Intraoperative photograph showing herniation of the facial nerve through its sheath at the second genu; (B) The facial nerve sheath was slit open to reveal a partial cut injury to the facial nerve which was repaired

direction. Similarly, the suture material merely serves as scaffolding for guiding the cut ends of the nerve to unite in the correct and desired direction for recovery of nerve function (Figs 9.13 to 9.19).

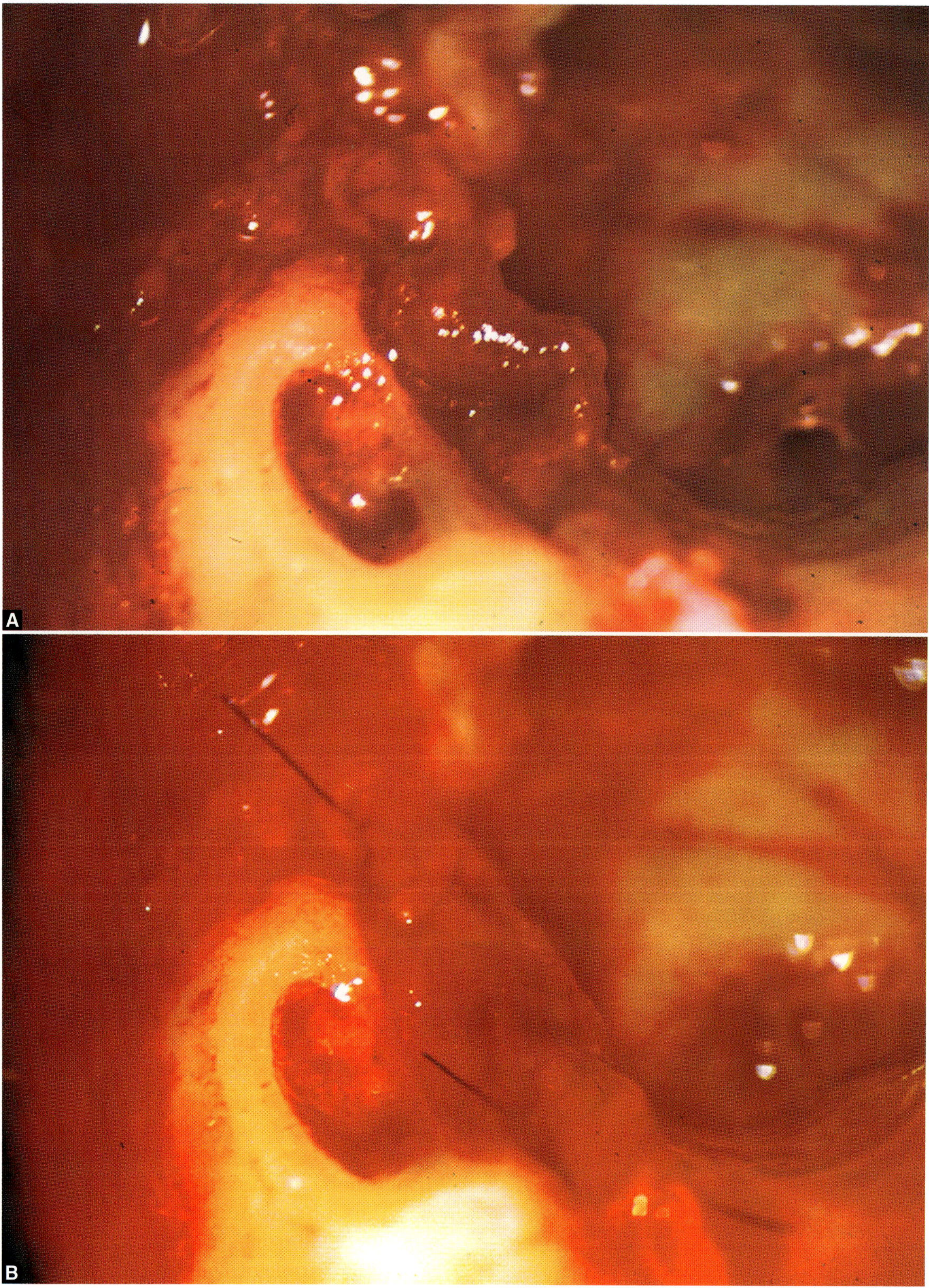

Figs 9.13A and B: (A) Note the iatrogenic injury to the facial nerve as well as the lateral semicircular canal resulting in a facial palsy and labyrinthine fistula with the membranous labyrinth clearly seen through the fistula; (B) Repair of the facial nerve at two sites using 8-0 prolene and closure of the fistula using a temporalis fascia graft

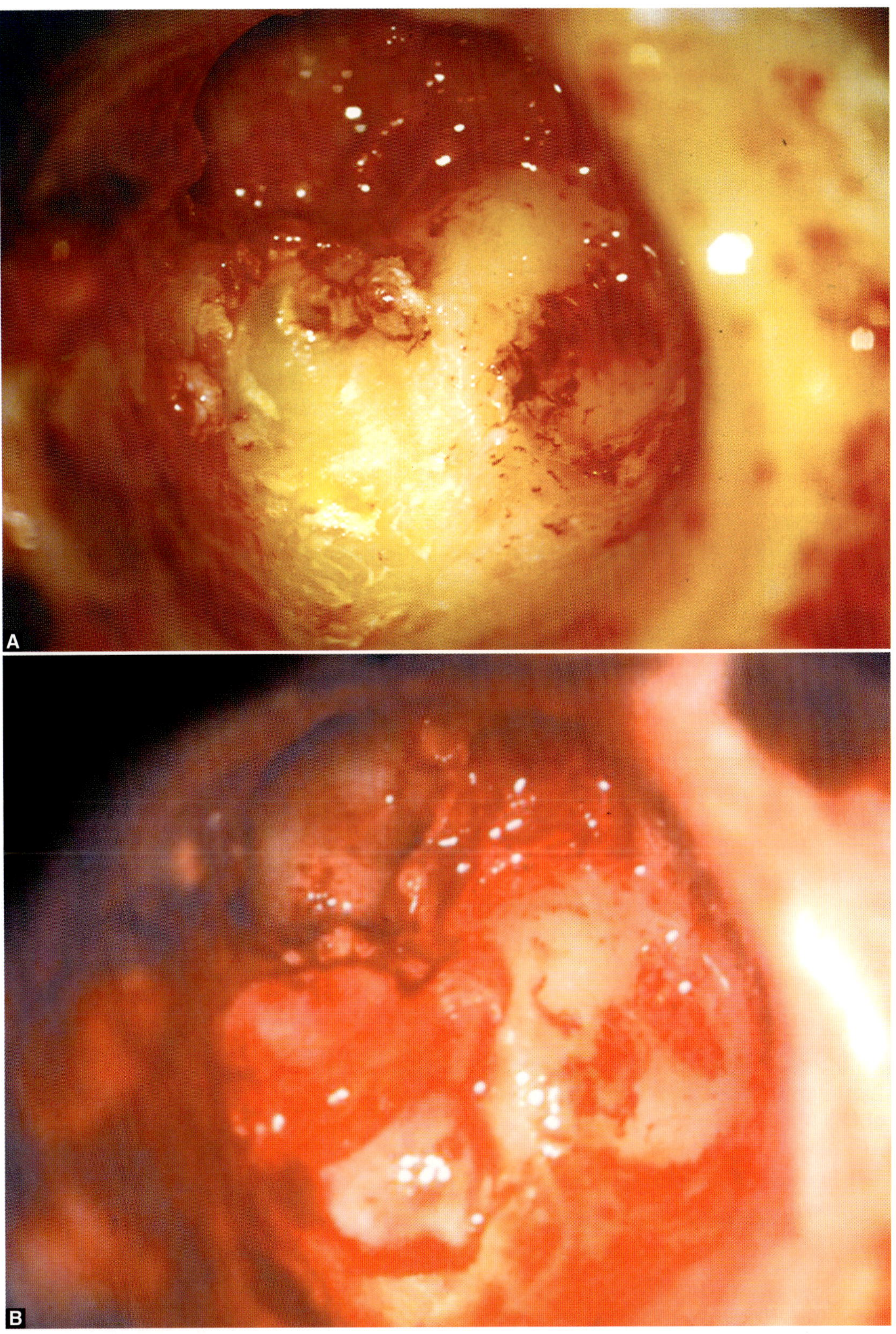

Figs 9.14A and B: (A) This patient had immediate facial palsy following tympano-mastoidectomy. On exploration, a low lying dura and cut ends of the facial nerve due to faulty and excessive drilling are seen; (B) Cable grafting by using greater auricular nerve

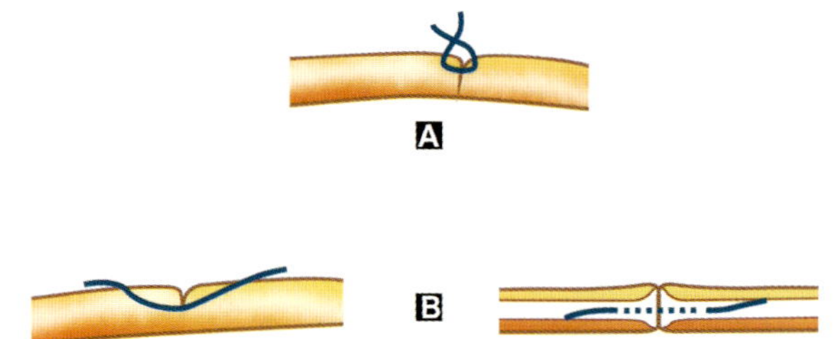

Fig. 9.15: Diagrammatic representation of (A) the inversion of the cut ends of the nerve after tying a knot and (B) the maintenance of the nerve ends in anatomical approximation when a suture material is passed through the cut ends without tying a knot therefore acting as a splint. Subsequently nerve sheath is placed over the suture ends

Location of Site of Nerve Injury

In a revision mastoid surgery, all the landmarks are destroyed and the usual warning signs indicating that the nerve is being approached such as decrease in size of mastoid air cells, bone becoming whiter and denser and the bleeding from the perineural vessels, are absent. Also there is granulation tissue due to faulty mastoid surgery, which bleeds during revision surgery.

Therefore, in my experience during previous surgery the nerve was always exposed and then injured. Now on opening the mastoid and clearing the granulations, we see a red inflamed site along the course of the facial nerve, which is the site of injury. We initially identify this **"red spot"** and proceed to decompress the nerve on either side of this trauma. I use this sign for identification of site of injury since it is most consistent in the absence of usual anatomical landmarks and easy to detect once the eye is trained to look for it.

PREVENTION OF IATROGENIC INJURY

Facial nerve trauma can be avoided by (Grewal, 1996):
- Making the surgeon competent to identify the nerve in its anatomical and anomalous course
- To identify important landmarks during surgery.

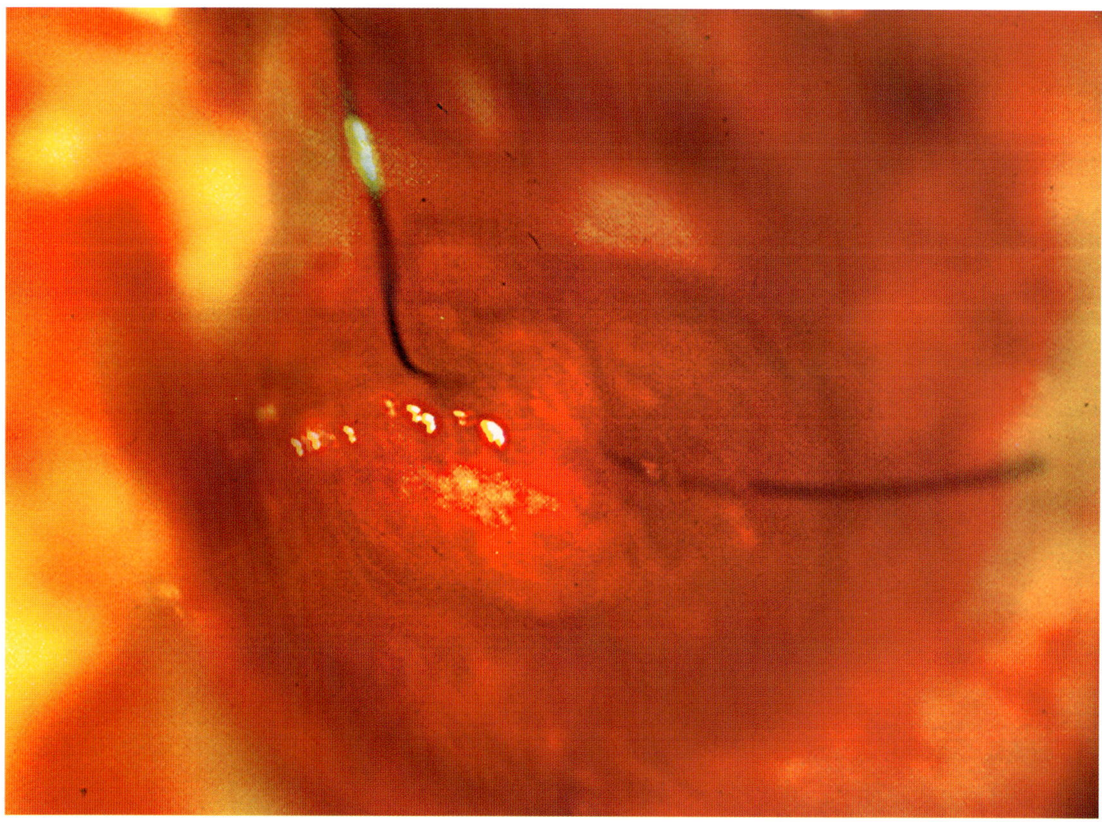

Fig. 9.16: Intraoperative photograph of a suture material in position holding the cut ends stable and in approximation acting as a splint. Note the absence of the knot

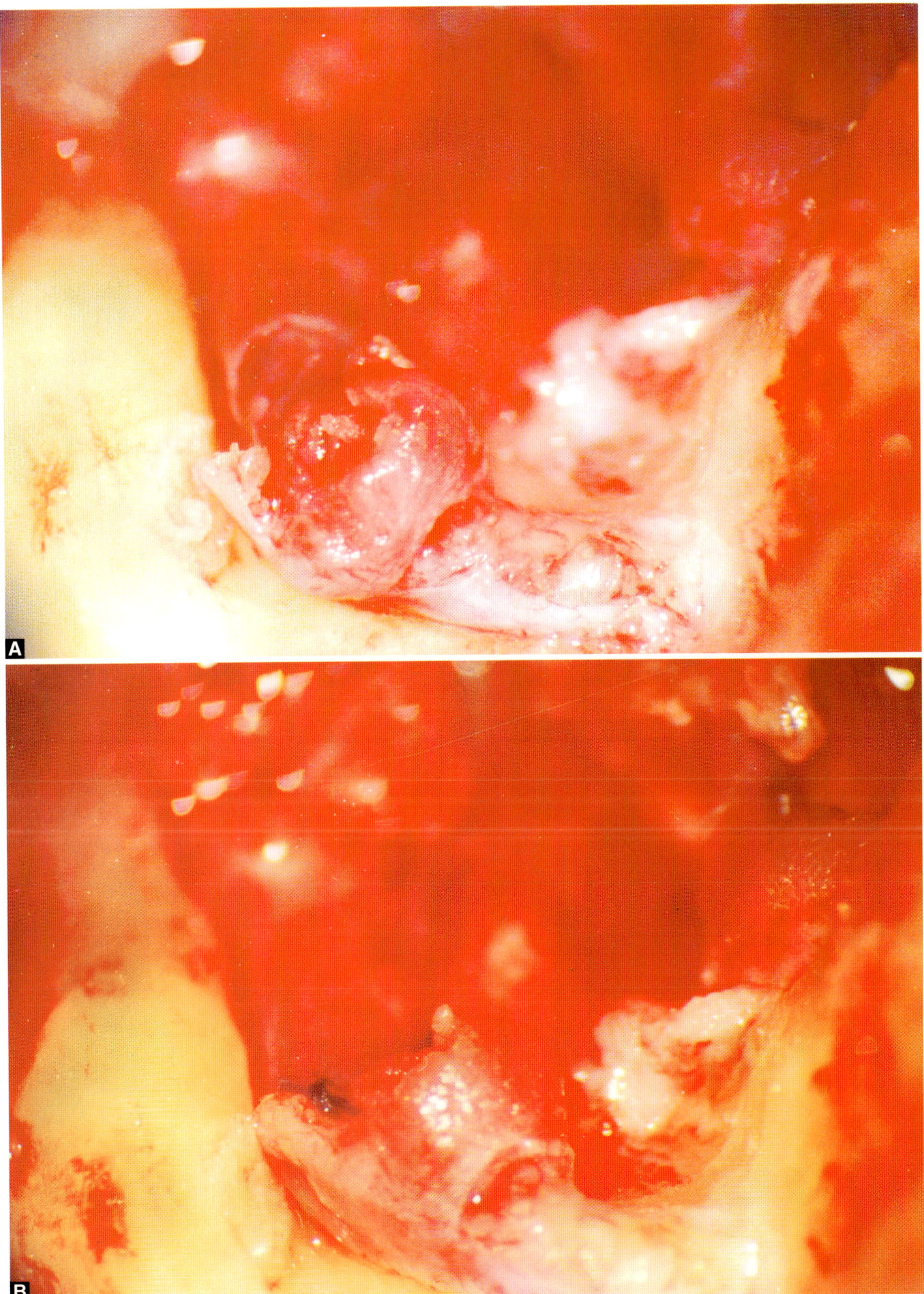

Figs 9.17A and B: (A) Long standing cut injury to the facial nerve showing formation of a granuloma; (B) The cut edges were refashioned and sutured

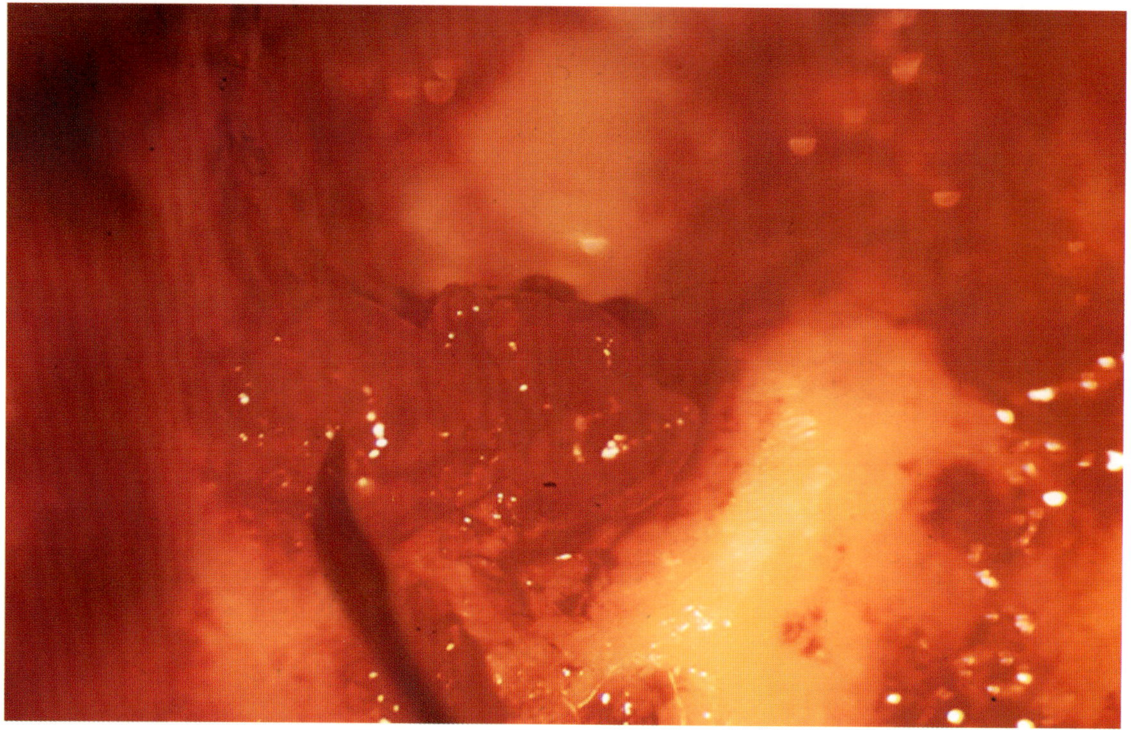

Fig. 9.18: Intraoperative photograph of a decompressed facial nerve. The sickle is pointing towards the granuloma formed following previous surgery

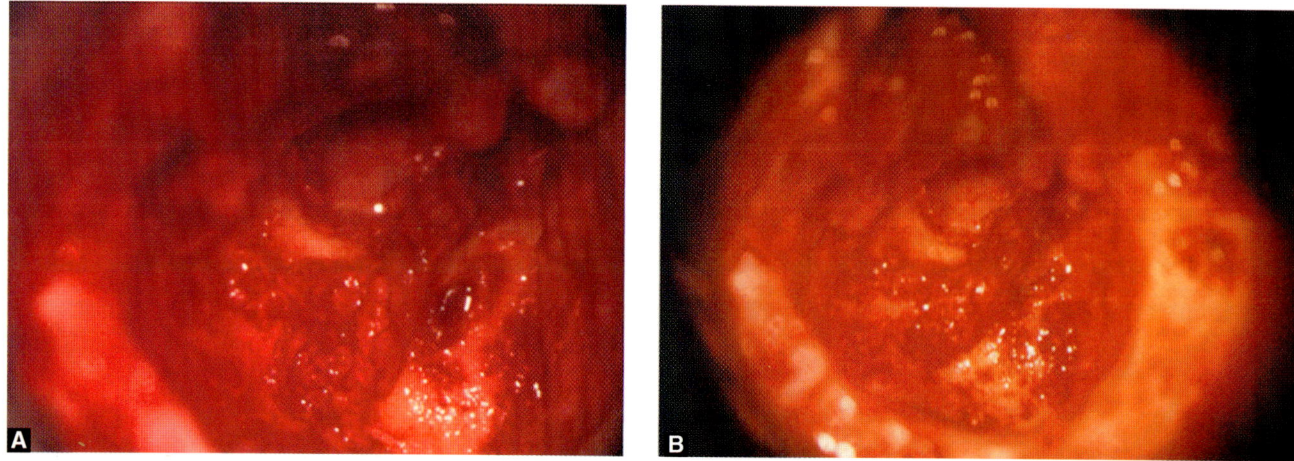

Figs 9.19A and B: (A) Bifid facial nerve in the mastoid with both its branches damaged during previous surgery and lateral semicircular canal fistula; (B) Cut ends of the facial nerve are approximated and were also supported by temporalis fascia. The fistula was closed using double layered temporalis fascia graft

Making the Surgeon Competent

- Temporal bone dissection: This helps in knowing the exact course, size, shape and appearance of facial nerve under microscope.

- To watch visual aids preferably videos: To know and learn the exact method of handling facial nerve during surgery, its variations and pathological conditions leading to its palsy. Also videos can be seen repeatedly and at leisure. Various surgical conditions can be reviewed within a specific time period.

- To see facial nerve surgery intraoperatively so as to become familiar with depth perception, instrumentation, operative set-up and management of patient and surgical expertise.

To Identify Important Landmarks

Tympanic part does not as such require any landmarks as it is seen easily. But, it can still be located by noting the stapes and processes cochleariformis and above it the nerve continues up to the cog.

In the mastoid segment and second genu, the pyramidal process, lateral semicircular canal, short process of incus and the diagastric ridge give the exact level of the facial nerve. While performing mastoid exenteration, the warning signals indicating that the facial nerve is being approached are:

- Mastoid cells become smaller
- Bone becomes whiter and denser
- Bleeding from vessels over the nerve sheath.

However, one has to realize that in case of an iatrogenic palsy, all anatomical landmarks are destroyed and hence the above-mentioned indi-cations/warning signals are usually absent. Hence, the surgeon has to largely depend on his surgical expertise and experience.

CONCLUSION

The facial nerve being the longest and thickest structure to run through the mastoid and middle ear should be easily identified as a thick white cord. Avoidance of iatrogenic trauma to the facial nerve mainly includes the surgeon's thorough knowledge and familiarity with the normal anatomical landmarks, anomalous course of the facial nerve and the skill in handling the nerve when required to do a timely exploration and to decompress or repair the damaged facial nerve. Even after surgery, medical line of treatment is important which includes steroids, antibiotics and physiotherapy under supervision.

In my experience, nerve conduction studies and EMG are important prognostic investigations and help to detect the stability, presence and conductivity of the nerve graft or the sutured nerve ends. Hence, I perform these tests at regular intervals to monitor the response of impulses being conducted through the repaired nerve.

The outcome of the surgery depends on the process of regeneration. The timing of surgery should be such that maximum ability of nerve regeneration is achieved before degenerative changes occur. There are various factors which influence regeneration like age, nutrition, type and duration of injury, infection, hematoma formation, fibrosis of cut ends of the nerve and hormonal.

In our view, I feel, type of injury to the facial nerve, choice of surgery and expected regeneration are interlinked and they along with the factor mentioned above are important in recovery of facial nerve function.

BIBLIOGRAPHY

1. Green ID Jr, Shelton C, Brackman DE. Iatrogenic facial nerve injury during otologic surgery. Laryngoscope. 1994;104:922-6.
2. Green ID Jr, Shelton C, Brackman DE. Surgical management of iatrogenic facial nerve injuries. Otolaryngology and Head and Neck Surgery. 1994;111:606-10.
3. Grewal DS, Hathiram BT. Facial nerve repair after iatrogenic injury following tympanomastoidectomy surgery—Our technique. Indian Journal of Otology. 1999;5:131-3.
4. Grewal DS. Iatrogenic facial palsy following surgery of chronic suppurative otitis media. Indian Journal of Otology. 1996;2:161-5.
5. Mayer TG, Crabtree JA. Archives of Otolaryngology. 1976;102:744-6.
6. Shambaugh, Glasscock. Surgery of the Ear (4th edn). Facial nerve surgery, WB Saunders and Co. 1990. pp. 435-65.

10

Traumatic Facial Nerve Paralysis

O Nuri Özgirgin

TEMPORAL BONE TRAUMAS

Blunt Traumas

The prognosis of incomplete facial paralysis that occurs following the blunt traumas of the temporal bone is good. In such cases, corticosteroids should be delivered as early as possible. Additionally, antiviral treatment should be accompanied by considering the trauma could also trigger the activation of herpes virus genomes that to induce facial paralysis. The facial paralysis that develops following blunt temporal bone traumas should be regarded similar to Bell's palsies. During this period the prognostic tests should be performed to monitor the progress of the paralysis. In case of having total denervation of the nerve within two weeks, the decompression of the nerve could be considered.

Temporal Bone Fractures

The temporal bone fractures should be classified in two groups in regard to the relation of the fracture line with the pyramids. If the fracture line is parallel to the pyramidal surface of the temporal bone, the fracture should be regarded as longitudinal, however, if it crosses the pyramis then transverse fractures should be the case. The blunt traumas mainly injure the pre-geniculate area and give damage to the superficial petrosal nerve (Ishman et al. 2004).

Besides the axis of the fracture line, temporal bone fractures are also classified as whether the otic capsule is involved within the fracture line or not. The fracture lines involving the otic capsule affects the inner ear by resulting with sensorineural hearing loss, cerebrospinal fluid (CSF) otorrhea and facial nerve paralysis. In cases with otic capsule injuries, the intracranial involvement with epidural and subdural hematoma development is not rare (Brodie et al. 1997).

All the structures within temporal bone will inevitably be affected by the fractures. The demonstration of air by the X-rays of intracranial compartments, temporo-mandibular joint and the soft tissue surrounding the temporal bone is the evidence of fracture even if the fracture line cannot be visualized clearly. So, the computerized tomography (CT) X-rays should initially be obtained.

Both right and left sides are similarly affected. In 10% of cases, the paralysis is bilaterally developed. Among 24 to 81% of cases, the hearing is affected.

The hearing loss is in conductive type, it generally resolves spontaneously. If the conductive hearing loss becomes permanent, this will be the sign of disrupted ossicular chain. Facial nerve paralysis occurs in 7 to 50% of cases with temporal bone trauma. The swelling of the nerve and its compression within the fallopian canal are the main causes of the nerve lesion. The nerve can be enhanced in T1 magnetic resonance images (MRI) with gadolinium. The vessels feeding the nerve can be affected, or regeneration, fibrosis or scar tissue formation may be the cause of this enhancement. (Sartoretti-Schefer S, et al. 1997).The facial paralysis is partial and delayed in most of the cases. The prognosis is not good in immediate facial paralysis and surgery should be considered earlier in these cases. In traumas, the nerve is involved less in children as compared with the adults.

EVALUATION OF THE INJURY

The temporal bone and the facial nerve should be evaluated within the first opportunity that the general conditions permit. The degree of facial nerve dysfunction should be the first to be evaluated, followed by a thorough examination of the external auditory canal and the functions of the middle and inner ear. The presence of hematoma or lacerations over the external auditory canal and even on the tympanic membrane should be regarded. Any kind of dizziness and vertigo should be noted. Cerebrospinal fluid (CSF) rhinorrhea or otorrhea should be checked. Tuning fork tests and audiological evaluation of the patient should be performed. High resolution CT X-rays should be obtained to evaluate if fracture line is present and where it is located.

TYPES OF FACIAL NERVE INJURIES IN TEMPORAL BONE FRACTURES

In case of having facial nerve paralysis that is simultaneously developed with the time of the trauma either complete laceration of the nerve or contusion should be regarded.

In delayed paralysis, arterial spasm or thrombus formation or either the external compression of the nerve by the soft tissue edema may be the cause of the facial nerve dysfunction. The most frequent finding is the bleeding within the nerve tissue and the swelling of the nerve due to edema. This is the cause of the delayed paralysis. The prognosis is complete resolution in most cases.

The sharp ends of the bony fragments may interfere with the nerve to create an avulsion or defect on the nerve fibers. Its incidence is less frequent. The integrity of the nerve may be interrupted in such cases. The axonoplasmic process is disrupted and ischemia of the distal part of the nerve develops. This lesion will be the cause of either complete or partial paralysis of the facial nerves that develops simultaneously with the trauma. In such a case, the bony fragments and spicules should be removed otherwise the fibrosis that replaces the nerve lesion will be the cause of permanent dysfunction of the nerve. Rarely, the total transection of the nerve may be present. In such cases, complete facial paralysis develop, immediately. The transection of the nerve may be complete or partial.

If the contributing effect is compression, the lesion that develops on the nerve is known as neuropraxia. In such cases, injury is located on the myelin sheath of the nerve but the axons are intact. Most of the cases completely resolve. In cases where the axons are injured but the nerve sheath is intact the lesion is known as axonotmesis and Wallerian degeneration develops in these cases within a week. Additionally, total nerve transection is called as neurotmesis. (Baumann BM, et al. 2008).

Longitudinal Temporal Bone Fractures

The fracture line progresses in parallel to the superior wall of the external auditory canal (EAC), crosses the middle ear, eustachian tube and the carotid canal. The tympanic membrane is frequently lacerated and the ossicular chain is disrupted. Conductive type of hearing loss is present. Bleeding through the external auditory canal can be observed. Sometimes CSF otorrhea can be added. The involvement of the geniculate ganglion is frequently the cause of the facial paralysis. The incus when dislocated because of the trauma can also compress the facial nerve. Temporal bone traumas result mostly with longitudinal fractures in 80% of cases. However, because of the axis of the fracture line being in parallel to the facial nerve, paralysis develops in only 20% of these cases. Clinically, the cases with longitudinal fractures and total paralysis can have the best facial function HB Grade 3 (Danner CJ 2008) (Fig. 10.1).

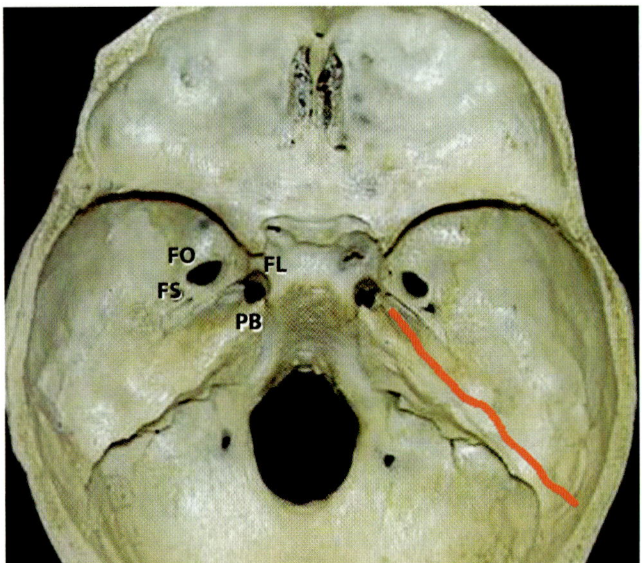

Fig. 10.1: Longitudinal temporal bone fracture (FO: Foramen ovale, FS: Foramen spinosum; FL: Foramen lacerum; PB: Petrose bone)

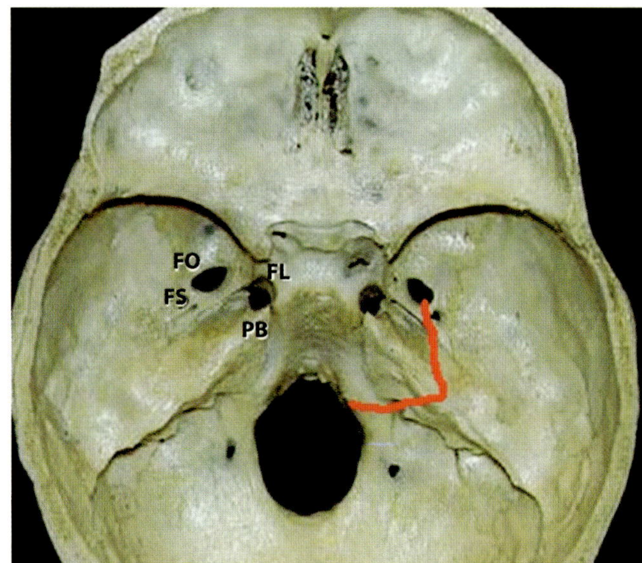

Fig. 10.2: CT X-ray of a patient with gun-injury. Note that the penetrating injury of the bullet is parallel to the long axis of the temporal bone

Transverse Temporal Bone Fractures

Transverse fractures develop as a result of blunt traumas directed to occipital region. The transverse fracture line crosses the posterior petrosal bone and passes between the foramen magnum and foramen ovale. It frequently crosses the otic capsule and the fallopian canal. So the development of facial paralysis is frequent with the transverse fractures. These fractures develop in 20% of cases but facial paralysis appears in half of these cases. As crossing the temporal bone axis, the transverse fractures frequently involves the labyrinth. Sensorineural hearing loss with rotatory vertigo is frequent in such cases. Vertigo subsides by the development of compensation by central nervous system. The tympanic membrane is generally intact with these fractures (Fig. 10.2).

Penetrating Traumas (Gunshot Injuries)

The higher rate of crime and terrorism has also increased the injuries directed to the temporal bone. The penetrating traumas directed to the temporal bone affect the other cranial nerves also; the glossopharyngeal, vagus, accessorius and hypoglossal nerves are also involved. CSF otorrhea frequently accompanies the lesion. The bullet injuries lead to develop multiple bone fragments. These bony fragments will be the focus of infection and osteitis in long term. The skin burn and secondary drainage should also be regarded. Because of these reasons for facial nerve decompression and repair, open cavity techniques should be preferred to prevent the infection and osteitis following the surgery. Some surgeons propose obliterating the cavity with fat tissues at the end of the operation (Fig. 10.3).

It is difficult to maintain the stability of the repaired nerve within the open cavity when a cable graft is used. In such a case, the cavity is more prone to the infections. This coincides with the success rate of graft. It may be advisable to leave the cavity for epithelization before the nerve repair by marking the endings of the lacerated nerve to easily find it.

It is possible to evaluate the nerve and its projection by a high resolution computed tomography (HRCT). It is also possible to detect the location of the bullet and the bony fragments. Especially in penetrating traumas by guns it is advisable not to limit the decompression around the bullet and injury but the nerve completely. As the labyrinth (petrous bone) has a compact bone structure, the bullet generally stops when reaches to the bone and stays within the cellular part of the bone. The best facial nerve function that can be achieved in cases with penetrating traumas made by gun injuries is HB grade 4 or worse. This is

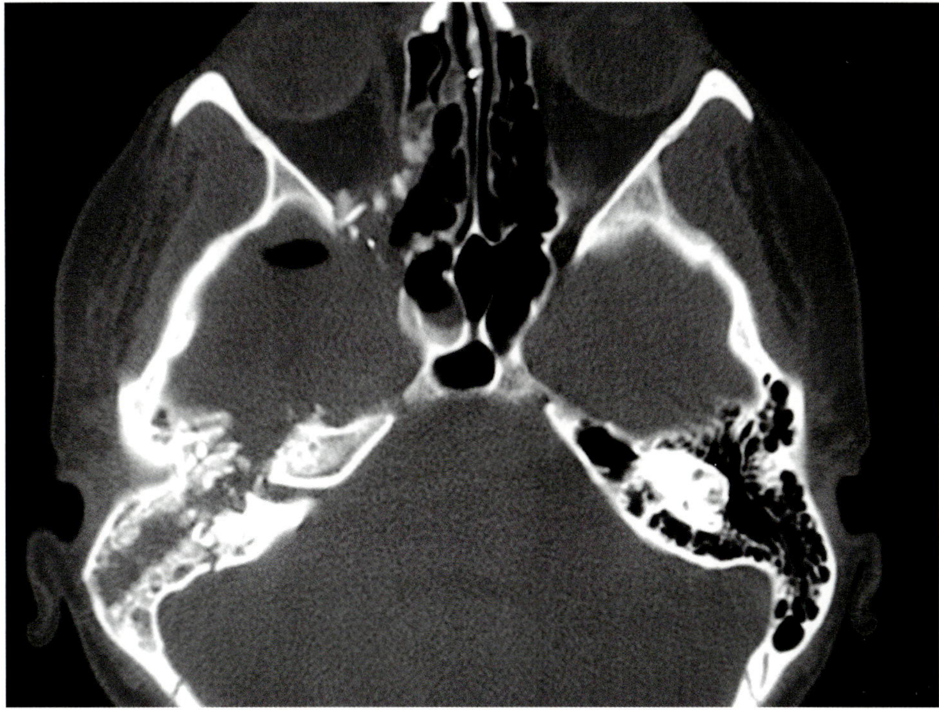

Fig. 10.3: CT X-ray of a patient with gun-injury. Note that the penetrating injury of the bullet is parallel to the long axis of the temporal bone

not better than the facial paralysis cases that happens by other causes (Bento RF et al. 2004).

Iatrogenic Traumas

The iatrogenic facial paralysis is a deep trauma either for the patient or also for the physician, as they develop unintentionally. In such a case, the surgeon should not behave emotionally and assistance should be requested from someone else who has the capability of evaluating the patient objectively and propose the optimal conditions for managing the situation.

It is a good luck if the facial nerve palsy is related with the effect of the local anesthetic material. The anesthetic medication when diffuses into the fallopian canal through the stylomastoid suture, a conduction block on the nerve may develop. In case of unexpected facial paralysis, it is better to wait for a couple of hours before having a new decision. The nerve conduction blocks due to lidocaine will resolve in one hour, however, marcaine will block the nerve for a longer time. If the facial functions do not improve during this period, exploration of the nerve will be necessary.

Delayed type facial paralysis following the ear surgery develops due to nerve compression. This results because of the blunt trauma. The lesion is generally situated at the level of the tympanic segment. Additionally, the heat created by the drill may injure the nerve. In such cases, the nerve heals completely without needing any further treatment. In cases with severe dysfunction, corticosteroids can be administered. The activation of the herpes virus genomes because of the nonspecific surgical trauma has been accused of developing facial paralysis. So, it is reasonable to administer acyclovir or valacyclovir in such cases (Safdar A et al. 2006).

The level of the lesion affecting the nerve is important. In case of having a nerve lesion in less than 1/3rd of the nerve section, it is possible to leave the nerve for secondary healing. However, if the lesion affects the nerve for more than 1/3rd of its section, then the nerve should be transected completely and sutured.

In case of having iatrogenic facial paralysis following the middle ear surgery, it may be necessary to invite an otologic surgeon. The efforts of the primary surgeon alone to decompress the nerve or even delaying the treatment may give more damage to the nerve. Delayed operations may have lower success rate and makes the surgery harder because of the fibrosis and granulation tissue formation.

THE OTOLOGIC AND NEUROTOLOGIC PROCEDURES THAT CREATES RISK OF INJURY ON THE FACIAL NERVE

Stapedectomy

The risk of the facial nerve injury during stapes surgery is low. We should consider the possibility of facial nerve canal bony dehiscence. Facial nerve injury may develop because of the mechanical trauma or laser injury during the stapedectomy. There appears a charcoal on the tip of the laser probe and the heat accumulated on this charcoal may give harm to the dehiscent nerve during the surgery. If laser is being used during the stapes surgery and the nerve is dehiscent wet gel-foam should be placed on the nerve to protect it from the laser beams.

Mastoidectomy and Middle Ear Surgery

During middle ear and mastoid surgery, one of the anatomical landmarks for the facial nerve is the proximal part of the tympanic segment of the facial nerve. This is the area between the geniculate ganglion and the cochleariform process. Once the mentioned area is identified, it is easier to track the nerve toward the pyramidal process. Additionally, the close relation of the nerve with the oval window can be another landmark for the nerve. Especially, the cases where granulation tissue covers and fills the middle ear are more prone to the facial nerve injury if there appears an additional dehiscence on the nerve.

The common pitfalls that cause iatrogenic injury to the facial nerve during middle ear and the mastoid surgery are narrow mastoidectomy openings, insufficient exploration of the tegmen plate and drilling far below the tegmen with the fear of injuring the dura. While performing posterior tympanotomy, the shaft of the drill may be in contact with the second genu of the facial nerve and injures by the heat effect. It is important to identify the projection of the facial nerve during performing mastoidectomy. The easiest landmark for identifying the nerve is the lateral semicircular canal. In the vicinity of lateral semicircular canal, the nerve makes its second genu. If this area is filled with granulation tissue and cannot be accessible, then the digastric ridge should be referred to find out the facial nerve in its proximity to stylomastoid foramen (Fig. 10.4).

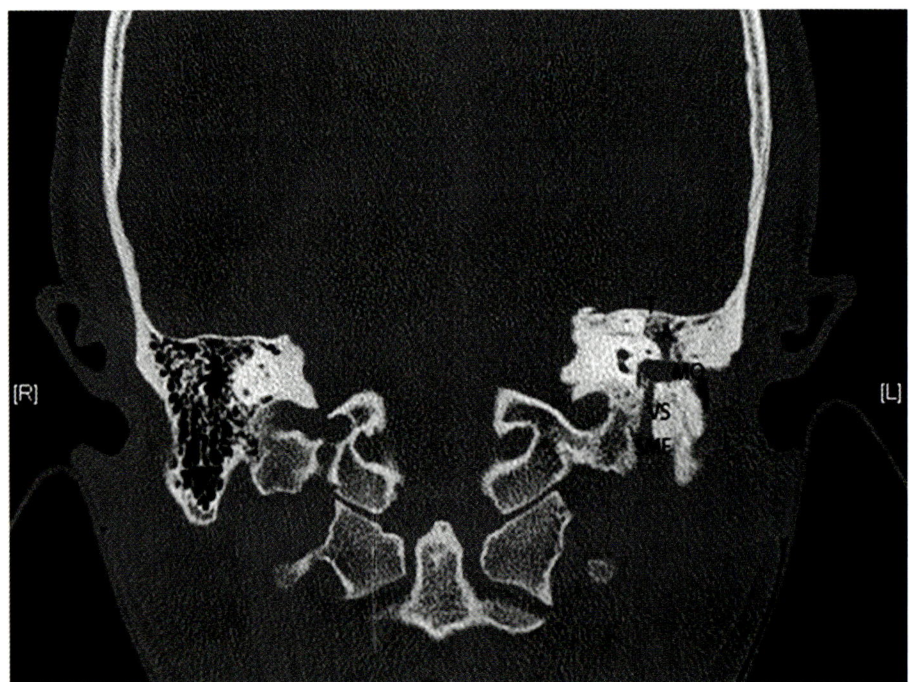

Fig. 10.4: CT X-ray of a patient with iatrogenic facial paralysis. Note that the mastoidectomy (mastoidotomy) opening has been made far below the tegmen level and crossed the facial nerve through the proximal part of its vertical segment; (T: Tegmen, A: Antrum, MO: Mastoidotomy opening, VS: Vertical segment, SMF: Stylomastoid foramen)

While removing the cholesteatoma and its matrix from the epitympanum and the supratubal recess, the geniculate ganglion and the proximal part of the tympanic segment is under risk. In this location, the cochleariform process where the tensor tympani tendon emerges, is a very important landmark for the facial nerve. Facial nerve lies just superior to the cochleariform process. On the other side, the pyramidal genu (the distal part of the tympanic segment and the second genu) is also the place where the nerve is prone to the injury. It is located just below the horizontal semicircular canal. The feeding vessels of the nerve should also be a remark for identifying the nerve in this location (Nilssen EL et al. 1997).

The descending portion of the nerve (mastoid segment) is prone to injury also. The nerve projects laterally to the tympanic ring as it descends toward the stylomastoid foramen. While making canalo-plasty this should be considered (Kartush JM et al. 1994).

Aural Atresia Surgery

During atresia surgery the risk of facial nerve injury is less than expected. The surgeon prepares himself for meeting with the abnormally located facial nerve. On the other side, the atresia surgery is generally performed by the experienced surgeons. The facial nerve anatomy is stable at least within the second genu location.

Endolymphatic Sac Surgery

To find out the endolymphatic sac and to be able to explore the endolymphatic duct completely, it is necessary to drill retro-facial cells. During drilling, the lateral end of the drill may injure the facial nerve (Fig. 10.5).

Transmastoid Labyrinthectomy

The facial nerve is under risk especially when drilling the ampullary ends of the semicircular canals. During opening the vestibule the surgeon have to care on the shaft of the drill. The shaft may be in contact with the nerve while drilling the vestibule and the effect of heat the nerve may be injured.

Translabyrinthine Approach

The facial nerve lies superficial in the level of fundus of the internal auditory meatus. So, it is important not

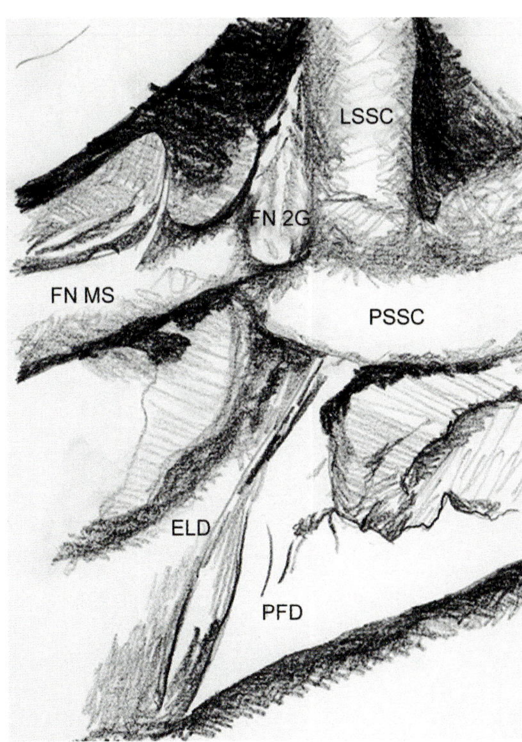

Fig. 10.5: The relation with endolymphatic sac (LSSC: Lateral semi-circular canal; PSSC: Posterior semi-circular canal, ELD: Endolymphatic duct; FN MS: Facial nerve mastoid segment; PFD: Posterior fossa dura)

injure the nerve in this position which is also the narrowest part of the nerve. The diameter of the nerve here is less than one millimeter. The hint for keeping intact the nerve in this position is to keep the dura intact until the drilling completely finishes.

Middle Fossa Approach

The pre-geniculate area is the area which the nerve is mostly susceptible for injury. Within the meatal level, the nerve lies tightly between the basal turn of the cochlea and the ampulla of the superior semicircular canal. All these structures locate within a 4-mm area. It is also very easy to injure the inner ear structures while dealing with the facial nerve. The important landmarks for the facial nerve during the middle fossa approaches are eminentia arcuata and the major superficial petrosal nerve (Fig. 10.6).

Retrosigmoid Approach

While retracting the cerebellum, dissecting the tumor and during the micro-vascular decompression, the

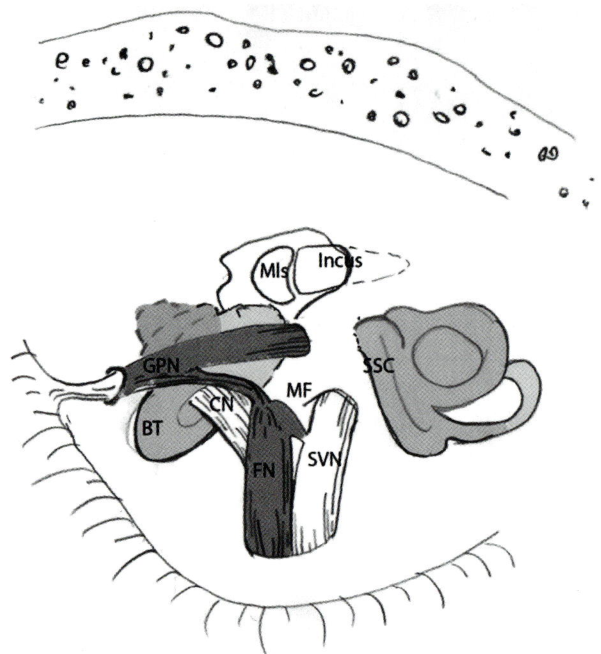

Fig. 10.6: Facial nerve (shown in dark gray) in proximity to the meatal fundus in middle cranial fossa (Mls: Malleus; GPN: Greater petrosal nerve; FN: Facial nerve; SVN: Superior vestibular nerve; MF: Meatal fundus; BT: Basal turn of the cochlea: CN: Cochlear nerve; SSC: Superior semi-circular canal)

facial nerve is under threat. The location of the facial nerve at the level of the internal auditory canal fundus and its porus, are not identical. The nerve rotates antero-inferiorly as it approaches the brainstem.

The cerebellopontine angle should be kept clear while drilling the porus of the internal auditory meatus to preserve the acoustico-facial nerve bundle (Kartush JM et al. 1994).

FACIAL NERVE ABNORMALITIES

The abnormal anatomical projection of the facial nerve in the temporal bone makes it prone to the injuries.

The most frequent abnormality is the dehiscence of the bony fallopian canal. The dehiscence of the tympanic segment generally locates in proximity to the oval window. This part is located lateral, inferior or medial part of the canal. The nerve may even protrude and mask the oval window in some cases.

The nerve may lie superior to the horizontal semicircular canal or pass through the stapes between the crura. It may even lie between the oval and round windows. Persistent stapedial artery and the vein may accompany.

Within its mastoid segment, the nerve may be displaced posterolaterally; it may show bifurcation and trifurcation (LaRouere MJ et al. 1994).

MONITORING THE FACIAL NERVE FUNCTION DURING THE SURGERY

Monitoring the facial nerve functions during ear surgery helps the surgeon to keep the nerve safe. Motorization can remind the surgeon when the nerve is stimulated either mechanically or electrically. The surgical applications made on the nerve such as removal of tumor or cholesteatoma matrix stimulates the nerve mechanically. In such cases, the monitor helps the surgeon to keep the nerve safe.

Two different monitoring systems are described and established. The electrical activity created by the facial muscle contractions are captured by the superficial electrodes as designed by Silverstein (Silverstein H et al. 1991) is one of the systems widely used in the previous decades. A sensor is placed on the cheek to pick up the muscle responses.

The other system is based on receiving the EMG activities. The needle EMG electrodes that are inserted into the orbicularis oculi and oris muscles perceive the electric potentials within the neuromuscular junction and it alerts the surgeon either by sound or EMG waves. These EMG based monitoring systems are more reliable.

The nerve can also be electrically stimulated during the surgery to check its integrity. This can be done either directly contacting the stimulator probe on the nerve itself or also by coupling the stimulator with the surgical instruments to be warned when getting closer to the nerve.

There is a controversy whether the monitoring system should be used in every kind of ear surgery. In many centers, it is not being used during the primary surgery for chronic otitis media, cholesteatoma or stapes surgery. It is advised to set up the system and monitor the nerve especially during neurotologic surgery, skull base surgery and even during revision middle ear surgery. It may be advised to use it during the residency training period.

In normal conditions, the nerve should be stimulated by 0.1 milliamp or lower current values. During stimulation, the electric current should be applied in pulsed modes otherwise the constant stimulation can give rise to paresis of the nerve by creating fatigue on the nerve (Ozgirgin et al. 1993).

The phase of anesthesia is an important issue to deal with. During the induction of general anesthesia and when needed, the neuromuscular blocking agents are administered. During the time interval, when these agents are active, it is not possible to receive responses to electrical stimulation of the nerves. Even the nerve is stimulated mechanically, the responses will be absent during this period and if the surgeon relies only on the monitor the injury applied to the nerve will not remind the surgeon. So it is important to be sure that the muscle relaxing agents should be completely eliminated and there is no block on the neuromuscular junction. For this purpose, it is advised to be in communication with the anesthetist and it may be useful to ask them to stimulate the ulnar nerve to be sure that there is no block on the nerve.

It is not advised to make surgery only by relying on the nerve monitoring systems. Facial nerve monitoring never replaces the anatomy knowledge of the surgeon. It is essential knowing the 3-D anatomy of the temporal bone to able to perform a successful surgery without any complication. Facial nerve monitor is a good servant but a bad master.

Extratemporal Facial Nerve Injuries

The facial nerve can be injured either by blunt or penetrating traumas. The degree of the lesion on the nerve is not more serious than the lesions that occur in the temporal bone. The resolution of the nerve lesions within the temporal bone takes longer than the extratemporal locations (Sharma N et al. 2009).

Additionally complications such as synkinesis develop more frequently in intra-temporal lesions and also the prognosis is better in extra-temporal lesions. The presence of compression on the nerve when located in the temporal bone will be the evidence of unfavorable prognosis. It is important to detect the level of the injury during evaluation process. Stimulating the nerve proximal to the injury can give information about the degree of the injury. The management should be directed to the nerve repair.

MANAGEMENT OF FACIAL NERVE INJURIES

The timing for the surgery is important. In cases with the immediate and complete paralysis the nerve should be explored as soon as possible. However, for the cases with unfavorable improvement or delayed paralysis, it may be possible to explore later within 6 to 12 months.

The most narrow part of the fallopian canal is the proximal end of the labyrinthine segment. Because of this reason, it is important to decompress this portion. In cases with normal hearing, only middle fossa approach can give access to this portion of the nerve. In case of severely or totally impaired hearing, it is possible to use the translabyrinthine approach (Myckatyn TM et al. 2003).

It is necessary to repair the nerve when there appears a defect on the nerve. The purpose should be uniting the nerve endings. The technique should be adopted due to the amount of tissue loss on the nerve. If the nerve damage comprises less than 30% of the nerve section, it is possible to preserve the nerve. However, the lesions more than 30% require totally sectioning the nerve and anastomosing either end-to-end or by inserting a nerve graft between the ends (Green JD Jr et al. 1994).

SURGICAL APPROACHES

The most important issue on deciding the surgical technique is the hearing level of the patient. It is already very well known that the blunt traumas primarily affect the pregeniculate portion of the nerve. Exploration of this area is important in regard to the hearing. Accessing to this location through the mastoid can only be possible by performing labyrinthectomy. This is only possible if the patient's hearing is absent. Otherwise middle fossa approach should be used to keep the patient's hearing levels intact.

If the hearing is absent, transcochlear or translabyrinthine approach can be used. By using this technique, the semicircular canals (lateral and superior), vestibule and a part of cochlea (translabyrinthine approach) or the cochlea completely (transcochlear approach) are drilled. The facial nerve is completely explored from fundus of the internal auditory meatus until the stylomastoid foramen. By using transmastoid approach, the most proximal part of the facial nerve that can be reached will be the cochleariform process level without making labyrinthectomy in case of incus is present. If incus is absent or extracted it may be possible to reach the proximal part of the geniculate ganglion (Figs 10.7 and 10.8).

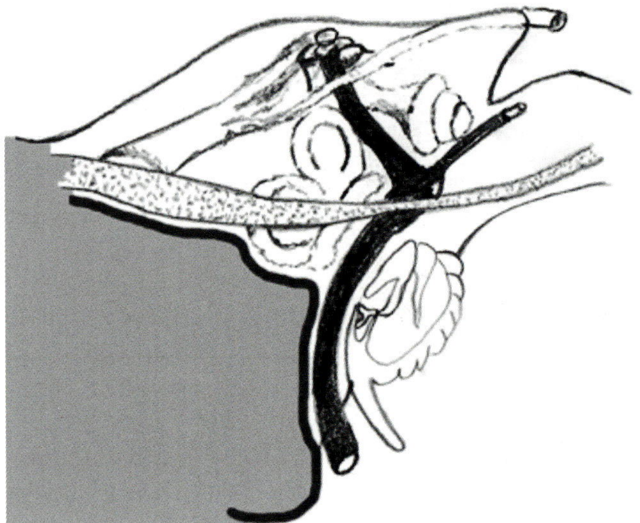

Fig. 10.7: Surgical approach for facial nerve-transmastoid (note that the approach is performed through the mastoid aircells. The labyrinth is preserved. It is only possible to reach until the mid-portion of the horizontal segment of the facial nerve through this approach) *Note:* This figure has been regenerated with permission from the illustration created by Yanagihara et al. Temporal bone fractures including facial nerve paralysis: A new classification and its clinical significance. ENT. 1997;76:79-86

If the hearing is serviceable the middle fossa approach is used. Following craniotomy through the temporal bone the temporal bone is retracted. The surgical field is prepared by defining the anterior border with the middle meningeal artery anteriorly, eminentia arcuata and mastoid tegmen posteriorly. If the internal auditory meatus has to be explored then the medial border should be the superior petrosal sinus (Fig. 10.9).

Following the surgical exploration, the surgeon should consider the nature of the injury on the nerve. If bony fragments are present which interfere with the nerve trunk, only removal of this bony spicule(s) by leaving the nerve for secondary healing will be sufficient. The exploration of the nerve will also serve for decompression in such a case. Whether incising the nerve sheath or not in such conditions is still controversial. In my opinion, the nerve sheath should not be incised unless there is hematoma under the epineurium.

If there is a partial transection on the nerve and if it is more than 1/3rd of its diameter, then the nerve should be completely transected and sutured.

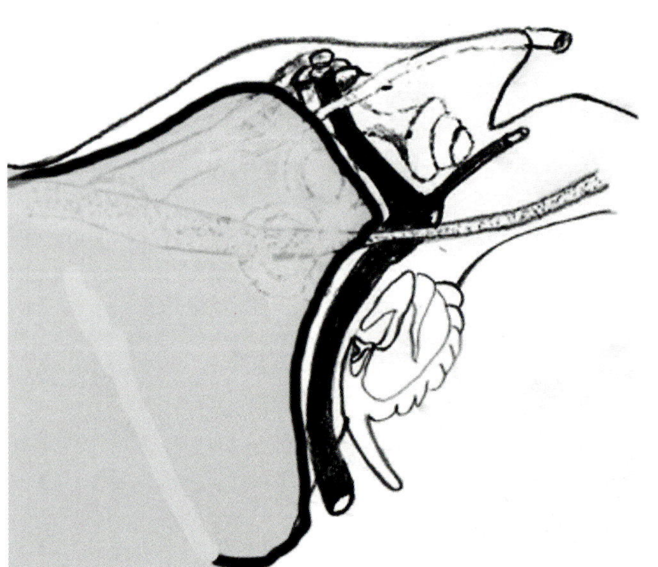

Fig. 10.8: Surgical approach for facial nerve-translabyrinthine (note that the approach is performed through the labyrinth by removing the semicircular canals and partly the vestibule). *Note:* This figure has been regenarated with permission from the illustration created by Yanagihara et al. Temporal bone fractures including facial nerve paralysis: A new classification and its clinical significance. ENT. 1997;76:79-86

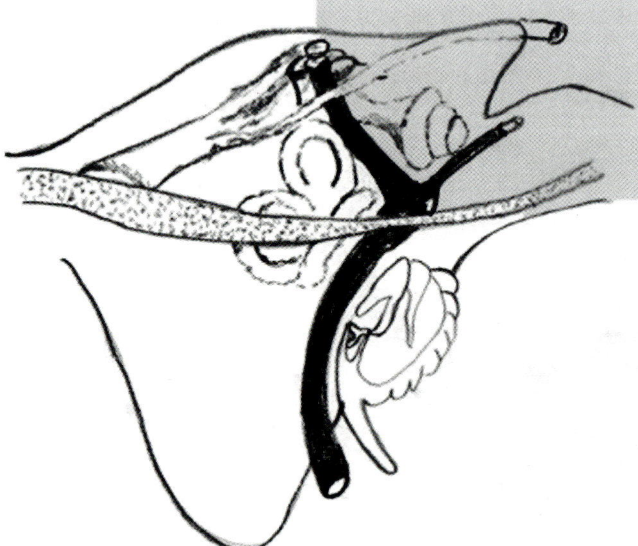

Fig. 10.9: Surgical approach for facial nerve—middle fossa (note that the approach is performed through middle cranial fossa between the cochlea and the superior semicircular canal by preserving these structures). *Note:* This figure has been regenarated with permission from the illustration created by Yanagihara et al. Temporal bone fractures including facial nerve paralysis: A new classification and its clinical significance. ENT. 1997;76:79-86

Techniques for Anastomosing the Nerve

Either suture techniques of fibrin glue can be used to fix the nerve. Monofilament suture materials 8.0 or finer should be preferred. The fibrin glue can only be used either in temporal bone or in the cerebellopontine angle. It is not possible to make sutures within the internal auditory meatus and in its intracranial segment because of the nerve lacking the epineurium. In this location, the fibrin glue should be preferred. Adversely, following the nerve exits from the temporal bone, it should be stabilized by putting sutures (Fig. 10.10). A fascia can be used following the anastomosis is accomplished. In cases with the penetrating injuries, we must rely on obtaining the bacteriologic clearance and for this purpose, it may be necessary to delay the anastomose techniques. In such a case, the nerve endings should be marked by putting mini sutures on it to be identified later on when anastomosing techniques will be used. It may be even necessary to keep the wound open for this purpose. Following eliminating the possibility of residual contamination the nerve can be grafted. In the same stage, the granulation tissue has to be removed and the cut nerve endings should be refreshed.

End-to-end anastomosis can be performed in transected nerve with no defect. The procedure should be performed without creating any tension to the nerve. If there appears tension on the nerve, because of the fibrosis, the number of innervated nerve fibers will be decreased. If a tension should occur the nerve has to be decompressed completely and it has to be relieved by making re-routing. It is possible to gain one centimeter length by rerouting the nerve (Dew LA, et al. 1996).

To be able to perform rerouting it will be necessary to remove the posterior canal wall. In such a case, it will be possible to visualize the whole field and keep the nerve safe. Re-routing should begin with the proximal part of the nerve. Just before making the anastomosis the nerve endings should be refreshed by transecting it with a very sharp surgical knife. The author is using the cornea knives for this purpose. Afterwards the anastomosis should be secured either by using sutures of fibrin glue (Gardetto A, et al. 2002) (Fig. 10.11).

If the defect on the nerve is longer than one centimeter, the cable graft should be preferred.

Literally, it is controversial to make rerouting or cable grafting even for smaller defects. It is believed

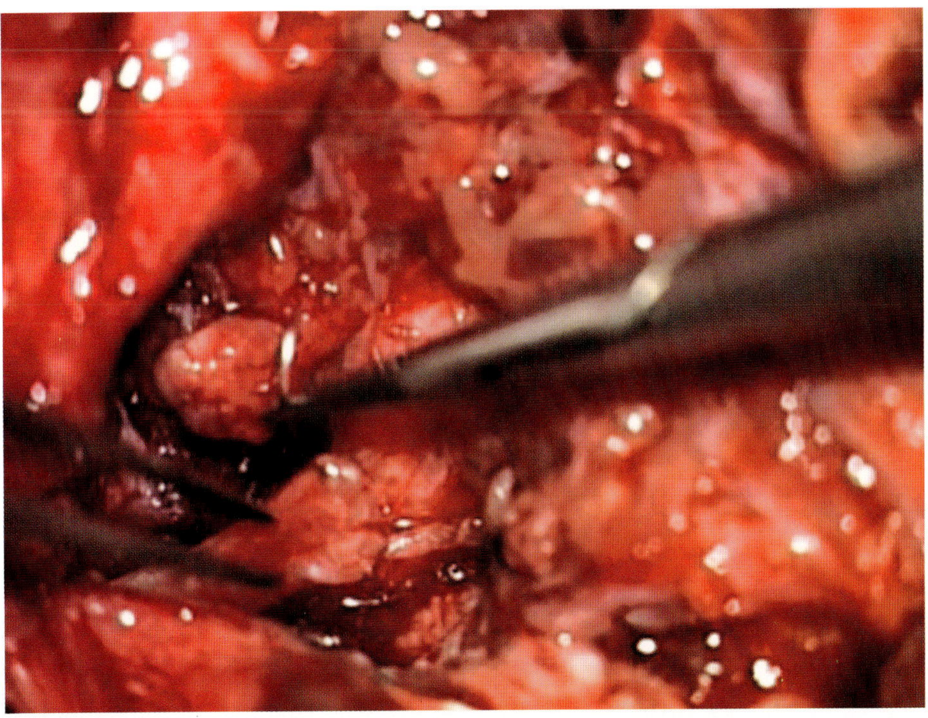

Fig. 10.10: Nerve suture with 9-0 mono-filament material

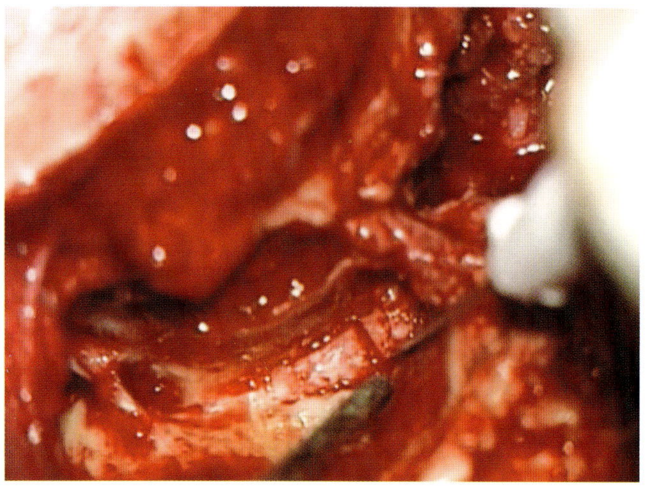

Fig. 10.11: Sectioning the facial nerve for precise anastomosis

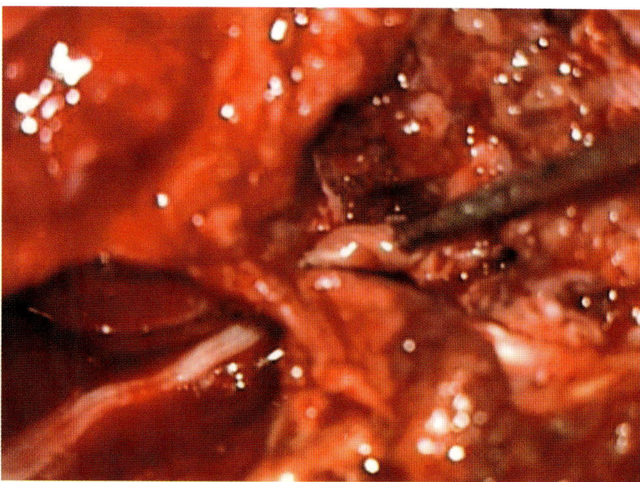

Fig. 10.12: Cable graft received from the sural nerve

that rerouting will conflict with the blood supply of the nerve and many of its fibers will be replaced by fibrosis in long-term. Instead, the cable grafting is believed to have better functional results as compared with rerouting.

Cable grafts should be preferred in cases with nerve defects. In cases where the cable grafts has to be used the proximal end of the nerve should be prepared precisely. The grafts can either be obtained from the greater auricular nerve or from the sural nerve (Humphrey CD et al. 2008).

The greater auricular nerve bisects the virtual line drawn between the mandibular angle and the apex of the mastoid. The nerve gets superficial on the midpart of the sternocleidomastoid muscle posterior to it. It is possible to obtain nerve graft until 4-5 cm from this nerve by using the defined landmarks.

For longer defects the sural nerve should be preferred. The diameter of the sural nerve is completely adaptable to the facial nerve. But as being located far away from the head and neck region it is preferred secondarily. It is easy to locate the sural nerve also. It lies laterally just posterior to the lateral malleolus. Its projection is parallel to the minor saphenous vein. It can be identified easily by making an incision just posterior to the lateral malleolus. It is possible to receive nerve grafts from the sural nerve until 35 cm. The proximal end of the sural nerve should be sutured or anastomosed to the distal end of the facial nerve. This will facilitate the nerve fibers to regenerate properly (Choi D et al. 2001) (Fig. 10.12).

Hypoglossal Facial Anastomosis

The anastomosis of facial nerve with the other cranial nerves has been using for a long time for facial muscles to be innervated and gain function. If it is not possible to reach to the proximal end of the facial nerve (such as having defects at the level of the brainstem), it is reasonable to make anastomosis with the other cranial nerves. The hypoglossal nerve is preferred because it has a strong electrical activity and it may be possible to gain the facial functions easily (Yoleri L et al. 2001).

The cortical projection of the hypoglossal nerve is similar to the facial nerve. Anastomosis can either be performed by end-to-end anastomosis of both nerve endings or by side-to-end anastomosis as suturing the facial nerve onto the trunk of the hypoglossal nerve without transecting it (Rebol J, et al. 2006).

In case of making end-to-end anastomosis there may develop atrophy of the ipsilateral tongue partially. But the electrical stimulation made to the facial nerve will be much stronger in this condition (Atlas MD et al. 1997).

The atrophy of the ipsilateral tongue can be tolerated easily. However in case of multiple cranial nerve pathologies this technique should not be used. Conley and Baker (1972) in their description of the technique reported that there appears a mild atrophy within 53% of cases whereas it is minimal in 22%.

The fibers superior to the hypoglossal nerve do not reach to cervical ansa but maintain mainly the tongue movements. These fibers create strong contraction of the tongue muscles so it is also a strong enough support for the denervated facial nerve. For this reason using only 40% of nerve fibers superior to the hypoglossal nerve can be accepted as a good option to innervate the facial nerve. When using only this portion of the nerve there will be no atrophy of the tongue. With this concept Terzis, described the partial hypoglossal nerve transfer in 1984 (Terzis JK et al. 1990). The purpose is to get benefit of the effects of strong contraction of the motor nerve and on the other side by keeping intact the remaining fibers to prevent any deficit.

It is possible to access to the hypoglossal nerve through the posterior belly of the digastric muscle. The nerve crosses the superior neck after passing slightly superior to the posterior cornu of the hyoid bone. Its projection is lateral to the external carotid artery (Asaoka K et al. 1999). Following identification of the nerve, it should be relieved to be able to get closer until the mastoid apex. The facial nerve is transected at the level of the stylomastoid foramen and the distal end is rotated inferiorly to get contact with the hypoglossal nerve.

Anastomosis with Nervus Accessorius

The accessorius nerve can also be used for anastomosis with the facial nerve. The 12th nerve has an oligofascicular structure. It is possible to divide the nerve longitudinally into colons by using a microscope (Terzis JK et al. 1990). By using this property, it may be possible to spare the 40% of its leaves innervating the sternocleidomastoid muscle and making the anastomosis of the remaining fibers with the facial nerve. So there will not be atrophy and limitations in the shoulder movements.

The accessory nerve bifurcates and gives its internal and lateral branches. The lateral branch innervates the sternocleidomastoid muscle. The nerve is identified lateral to the sternocleidomastoid muscle at the level of fourth cervical vertebra. There are 1500-1700 myelinated axons in this nerve (Chuang DC et al. 2005).

Anastomosis with the accessorius nerve should preferably be performed in cases with Mobius syndrome.

Alternative Surgeries

Following Wallerian degeneration the facial innervation can be completed within 12-18 months.

However, in cases with severe lesions or where the nerve tissue is completely lost there will not be any expectation of reinnervation. Reconstruction techniques should be considered in such cases. The atrophy of the facial muscles will be the major concern in this situation. Whenever, the muscles cannot be innervated or fed with the electrical activity by the nerves, atrophy will develop. For cases having facial paralysis, lasting more than two years, the expectations for the nerve regeneration subsides and the patient will be the candidate for application of the static operations.

Gaining motor innervation to the facial nerve can only be possible by implanting a nerve on it. If the weak innervation can be preserved, a new implantation makes it stronger (Brunelli GA et al. 1993).

One of the major sequels of the facial paralysis is the loss of the cornea reflex. This will create serious functional problems related with the clear vision as well as the esthetic appearance. The cornea reflex can be partially repaired by innervating it through the symmetrical fibers of the orbicularis oculi muscle. Even if the ocular functions can be regained by using other motor nerves, this cannot contribute to the re-establishment of cornea reflex (Terzis JK et al. 2008).

In cases where the muscle atrophy is limited and there is no possibility of further healing of the facial nerve but where the re-innervation potential exists, it is possible to gain movement to the facial muscles by using nerve transfer techniques.

It is possible to deliver electrical activity from the contralateral side of the face inserting the cross nerve grafts. It was Scaramella (Scaramella LF et al. 1973) and Smith (Smith JW et al. 1971) who first used the cross anastomosis techniques. The grafts can be obtained from sural or peroneal nerves. The tunnels already used for facelifting can be created to line the grafts and carry them to the other side. The site of grafting in the paralysis side is important. To re-establish the emotional facial mimics, it is important to patch it to the nerve innervating the greater zygomatic and levator muscles. In long-term paralysis, if the muscle atrophy is apparent, then the cross-grafting should not be used.

To re-establish the symmetry of the facial muscles, it is proposed to combine the crossfacial anastomosis techniques with the partial hypoglossus-facial anastomosis technique. This combined technique has been known as Babysitter method (Mersa B et al. 2000).

In cases having paralysis for less than a year this technique can be used (Thanos PK et al. 1996). For the paralysis manifesting 1-2 years, free muscle graft techniques should be added to the Babysitter method.

Laughing function necessitates a synchronized and coordinated restoration. In cases with less than 6 months of denervation, it is possible to restore the function by grafting the zygomatic branch from the contralateral side.

Additionally, microneurovascular muscle grafts can also be used. Muscle transfers were first performed in dogs by Tamai et al. in 1976 (Harii K et al. 1976). In cases with long-term denervation and muscle atrophy this technique can be used. The purpose is to protect the eye and create the symmetry in resting position as well as oral commissures and facial movements (Rosson GD et al. 2008). The gracilis, latissimus dorsi and pectoralis minor muscles are used for this purpose, but, gracilis is the mostly preferred (Harii K et al. 1998). Pectoralis minor muscle was first used by Terzis (Terzis JK, 1989) and satisfactory results were achieved.

Additionally to restore the facial symmetry, the reposition of the facial muscles, blepharoplasty techniques, eyebrow lifting operations and selective denervation by using Botox and myotomy incisions can be used.

In cases with Mobius disease beyond facial - accessorius anastomosis, Terzis described using the motor fibers of trigeminal nerve in 1980's. In 1989, Zuker et al. (1989) proposed using the masseter muscle. The transfer of the motor branch of the cervical plexus has also been proposed. However, the number of motor fibers is limited in this nerve, so it is not preferred.

In long-term paralysis (patient's general conditions, co-morbid diseases, patient's attitude) and also if there is no expectation of nerve regeneration static operations can be used. The correction of the ptosis of the eyebrows, oculoplastic surgery of the paralytic eye, modification of the nasolabial fold, static facial suspension surgeries and external nasal valve repair techniques can be used in these patients (Mehta RP, 2009).

Traction techniques are the mostly used among static operations (Ozaki M et al. 2008). The purpose is to regain symmetry to the paralytic face. However, it is not possible to contribute to the facial function during this process. The traction materials are fixed to the skin by using face lifting incisions. Frequently labial commissure and superior labia are tracked and the nasolabial fold is recreated (Alam D, 2007). The temporalis muscle is used for traction. The superior and posterior parts of the temporalis muscle have their angles 45° to the oral commissure. Within this angle, it is possible to elevate the oral commissure and also remove the flaccidity. The surgical technique limits itself in the face and does not require tissue transfers from remote areas (Byrne PJ et al. 2007).

BIBLIOGRAPHY

1. Alam D. Rehabilitation of long-standing facial nerve paralysis with percutaneous suture-based slings. Arch Facial Plast Surg. 2007;9:205-9.
2. Asaoka K, Sawamura Y, Nagashima M, et al. Surgical anatomy for direct hypoglossal-facial nerve side-to-end "anastomosis". J Neurosurg. 1999;91(2):268-75.
3. Atlas MD, Lowinger DS. A new technique for hypoglossal-facial nerve repair. Laryngoscope. 1997;107:984-91
4. Baumann BM, Jarecki J. Posttraumatic delayed facial nerve palsy. Am Jo Em Med. 2008; 26,115.e1-115.e2
5. Bento RF, de Brito RV. Gunshot wounds to the facial nerve. Otol Neurotol. 2004;25:1009-13.
6. Brodie HA, Thompson TC. Management of complications from 820 temporal bone fractures. Am J Otol. 1997;18:188-97.
7. Brunelli GA, Brunelli GR. Direct muscle neurotization. J Reconstr Microsurg. 1993;9:81-90; discussion 89-90.
8. Byrne PJ, Kim M, Boahene K, et al. Temporalis tendon transfer as part of a comprehensive approach to facial reanimation. Arch Fac Plast Surg. 2007;9:234-41.
9. Choi D, Dunn LT. Facial nerve repair and regeneration: an overview of basic principles for neurosurgeons. Acta Neurochir (Wien). 2001;143:107-14.
10. Chuang DC. Nerve transfers in adult brachial plexus injuries: my methods. Hand Clin. 2005;21:71-82.
11. Conley J, Baker DC. Hypoglossal-facial nerve anastomosis for reinnervation of the paralyzed face. Plast Reconstr Surg. 1979;63:63-72.
12. Danner CJ. Facial Nerve Paralysis. Otolaryngol Clin N Am. 2008;41:619-32.
13. Dew LA, Shelton C. Iatrogenic facial nerve injury: prevalence and predisposing factors. Ear Nose Throat J. 1996;75:724-9.
14. Gardetto A, Kovacs P, Piegger J, et al. Direct coaptation of extensive facial nerve defects after removal of the superficial part of the parotid gland: an anatomic study. Head Neck. 2002; 24:1047-53.

15. Green JD Jr, Shelton C, Brackmann DE. Surgical management of iatrogenic facial nerve injuries. Otolaryngol Head Neck Surg. 1994;111:606-10.

16. Harii K, Asato H, Yoshimura K, et al. One-stage transfer of the latissimus dorsi muscle for reanimation of a paralyzed face: a new alternative. Plast Reconstr Surg. 1998;102:941-51.

17. Harii K, Ohmori K, Torii S. Free gracilis muscle transplantation, with microneurovascular anastomoses for the treatment of facial paralysis: a preliminary report. Plast Reconstr Surg. 1976;57:133-43.

18. Humphrey CD, Kriet JD. Nerve repair and cable grafting for facial paralysis. Facial Plast Surg. 2008;24:170-6.

19. Ishman SL, Friedland DR. Temporal bone fractures: traditional classification and clinical relevance. Laryngoscope. 2004;114:1734-41.

20. Kartush JM. Overview of the facial nerve surgery. In: Neurotology (Ed): RK Jackler, DE Brackmann. Mosby: St Louis; 1994. pp. 1257-69.

21. LaRouere MJ, Lundy LB. Anatomy and physiology of the facial nerve. In: Neurotology. Eds. Ed RK Jackler, DE Brackmann. Mosby:St Louis; 1994. pp. 1271-81.

22. Mehta RP. Surgical Treatment of Facial Paralysis. Clin Exp. ORL. 2009;2:1-5.

23. Mersa B, Tiangco DA, Terzis JK. Efficacy of the "baby-sitter" procedure after prolonged denervation. J Reconstr Microsurg. 2000;16:27-35.

24. Myckatyn TM, Mackinnon SE. The surgical management of facial nerve injury. Clin Plast Surg. 2003;30:307-18.

25. Nilssen EL, Wormald PJ. Facial nerve palsy in mastoid surgery. J Laryngol Otol. 1997; 111:113-6.

26. Ozaki M, Takushima A, Momosawa A, et al. Temporary suspension of acute facial paralysis using the S-S Cable Suture (Medical U&A, Tokyo, Japan). Ann Plast Surg. 2008; 61:61-7.

27. Özgirgin N, Özçelik T, Aksoy S, et al. Fasial sinir monitorizasyonu. Kulak BurunBogaz ve Bas Boyun Cerrahisi Dergisi. 1993;1:205-9.

28. Rebol J, Milojkovic V, Didanovic V. Side-to-end hypoglossal-facial anastomosis via transposition of the intratemporal facial nerve. Acta Neurochir (Wien). 2006;148:653-7.

29. Rosson GD, Redett RJ. Facial Palsy: Anatomy, Etiology, Grading, and Surgical Treatment. J Reconstr Microsurg. 2008;24:379-89.

30. Safdar A, Gendy S, Hilal A, Walshe P, Burns H. Delayed facial nerve palsy following tympano-mastoid surgery: incidence, aetiology and prognosis. J Laryngol Otol. 2006; 120:745-8.

31. Sartoretti-ScheferS, Scherler M, Wichmann W, et al. Contrast-enhanced MR of the facial nerve in patients with post-traumatic peripheral facial nerve palsy. AJNR. 1997;18:1115-25.

32. Scaramella LF, Tobias E. Facial nerve anastomosis. Laryngoscope. 1973;83:1834-40.

33. Sharma N, Cunningham K, Porter RG, et al. Comparison of Extratemporal and Intratemporal Facial Nerve Injury Models. Laryngoscope. 2009;119:2324-30.

34. Silverstein H, Rosenberg S. Intraoperative facial nerve monitoring. Otolaryngol Clin North Am. 1991;24:709-25.

35. Smith JW. A new technique of facial animation. In: Huston JT (Ed): Transactions of the 5th International Congress of Plastic Surgery. London, England: Butterworth;1971. p:83.

36. Terzis JK, Konofaos P. Nerve Transfers in Facial Palsy. Facial Plastic Surgery. 2008; 241771-93.

37. Terzis JK. Babysitters. An exciting new concept in facial reanimation. In: Castro D (Ed): Proceedings of the 6th International Symposium on the Facial Nerve. Amsterdam, Berkeley, Milano: Kugler and Ghendini Publications;1990.

38. Terzis JK. Pectoralis minor: a unique muscle for correction of facial palsy. Plast Reconstr Surg. 1989; 83:767-76.

39. Thanos PK, Terzis JK. A histomorphometric analysis of the cross-facial nerve graft in the treatment of facial paralysis. J Reconstr Microsurg. 1996;12:375-82.

40. Yoleri L, Songur E, Mavioglu H, et al. Cross-facial nerve grafting as an adjunct to hypoglossal-facial nerve crossover in reanimation of early facial paralysis: clinical and electrophysiological evaluation. Ann Plast Surg. 2001;46:301-7.

41. Zuker RM, Manktelow RT. A smile for the Mobius' syndrome patient. Ann Plast Surg. 1989;22:188-94.

11

Facial Nerve in the Parotid Gland

DS Grewal

SURGICAL ANATOMY OF THE PAROTID GLAND

The parotid gland is a unilobular, flat and triangularly shaped salivary gland, lying mainly in the retro-mandibular sulcus. It is enclosed within a fibrous capsule, which sends septae into the glandular substance dividing it into lobes.

The facial nerve emerges from the stylomastoid foramen (3-4 mm deep to the outer edge of the bony EAC), runs anteriorly, inferiorly and laterally to enter the posteromedial aspect of the parotid gland. The nerve bisects it unequally into a large part, which lies lateral to the nerve, called the superficial lobe and a smaller part, which lies medial to it, called the deep lobe. Most parotid tumors are found superficial to the facial nerve since they affect the superficial lobe. In between the two lobes is the facial venous plane (of Patey) containing the facial nerve along with the retromandibular vein and the branches of the external carotid artery.

LANDMARKS OF THE FACIAL NERVE IN PAROTID

Different methods to locate the nerve in the parotid gland are:

- *Tragal pointer (of Conley)*: The nerve is located medial and about 1 cm inferior to the tragal cartilage
- *Tympanomastoid suture*: This is located at the apex of the vaginomastoid angle or valley of the nerve. It is the angle where the vaginal process of the tympanic portion of the temporal bone meets the mastoid process. The facial nerve runs just deep to this suture
- *Styloid process*: The nerve passes lateral to the styloid process at the skull base
- By tracing the terminal branches of the facial nerve backwards:
  - The ramus frontalis is located by a line from the tragus to lateral canthus
  - The ramus buccalis is located by a line from the tragus towards the alae of the nose parallel to the zygoma but 1 cm below
  - Ramus mandibularis is near the angle of the mandible at a point 4-4.5 cm from the attachment of the lobule of the pinna
- Tendon of the posterior belly of digastric muscle
- Posterior auricular vein or the retromandibular vein.

FACIAL NERVE DIVISION AND BRANCHES IN THE PAROTID AND FACE

The nerve divides into two main divisions, one cm beyond its entry into the parotid gland at the pes anserinus:

1. Upper division is stouter and consists of the temporal, zygomatic and upper and lower buccal branches.
2. Lower division is thinner and consists of mandibular and cervical branches.

Sometimes, the buccal branch may arise from the bifurcation.

Lower zygomatic branch lies just superior to the parotid duct. Damage to the mandibular branch results in paralysis of depressor anguli oris during surgery of the upper neck such as parotidectomy, submandibular gland excision, etc (Figs 11.1 to 11. 4).

ANATOMIC VARIATIONS OF FACIAL NERVE

Following are the anatomic variations of the facial nerve which can occur in the face or parotid region:

- Variations in branching pattern of the main branch or its branches
- Formation of a loop due to anastomosis between the branches of the facial nerve can be a short, long or multiple (Fig. 11.2A and B).
- Plexiform communications between the various branches of the facial nerve
- Variations of the facial nerve in relation to the superficial veins. This can be either branches of the facial nerve passing through the clefts in the superficial veins or formation of the nerve loops through which superficial veins pass.

INVOLVEMENT OF THE FACIAL NERVE IN RELATION TO PAROTID

The facial nerve may be damaged in the following lesions involving the parotid gland:

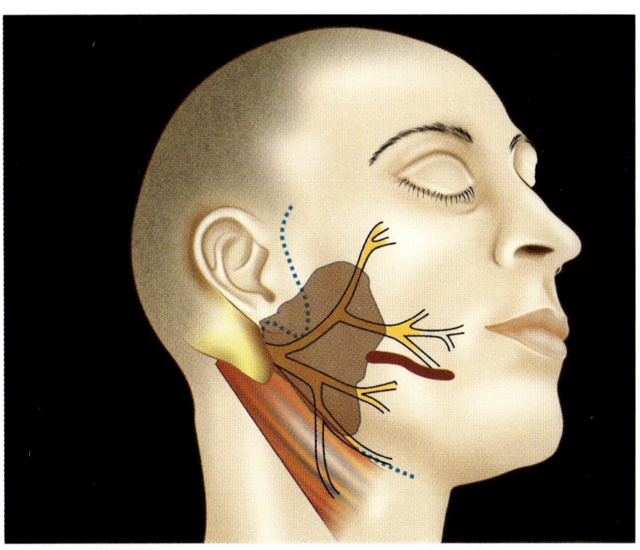

Fig. 11.1: Facial Nerve and its branches in face

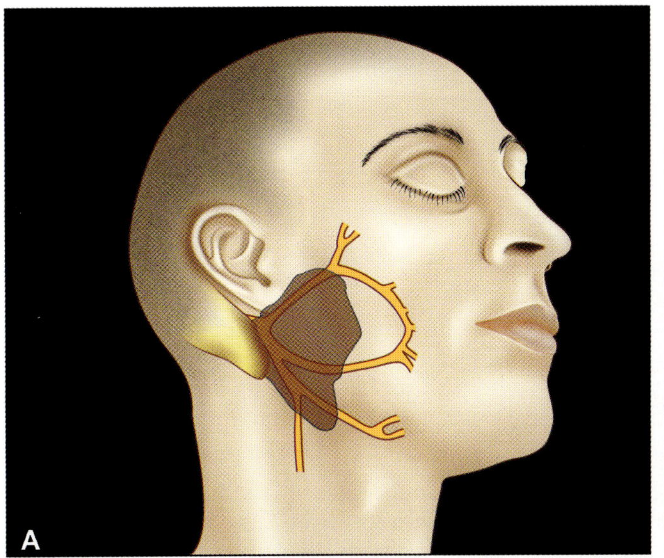

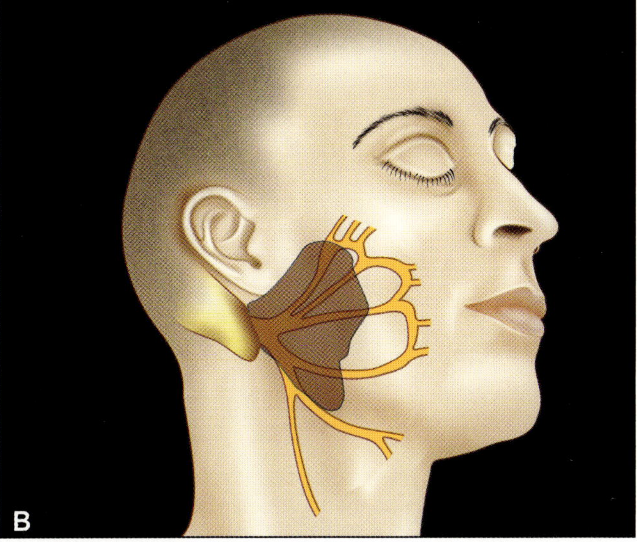

Figs 11.2A and B: (A) Diagrammatic representation of single large loop formation due to anastomosis between the branches of facial nerve; (B) Multiple loop formation

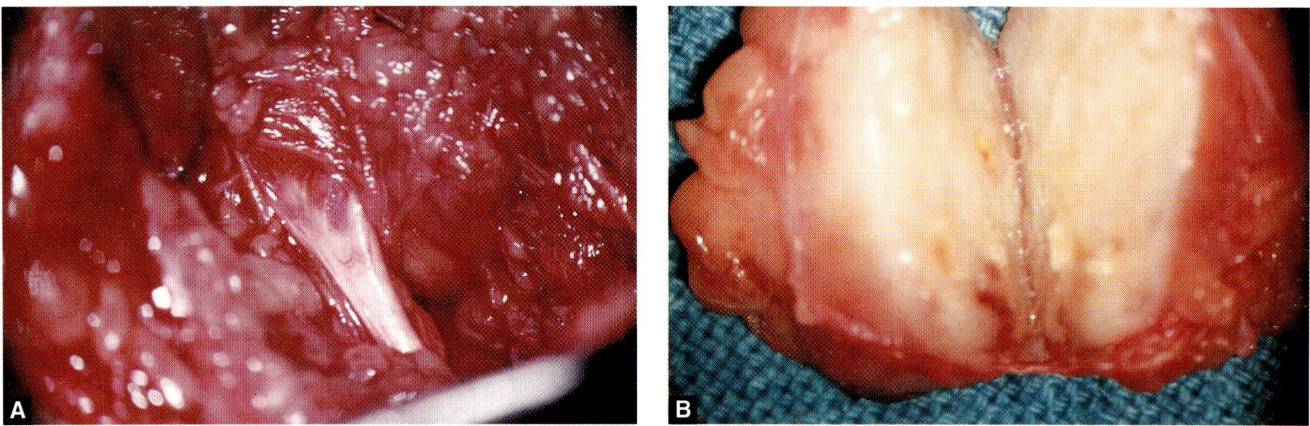

Figs 11.3A and B: (A) Intraoperative photograph of superficial parotidectomy being performed for parotid adenoma showing facial nerve; (B) Pleomorphic adenoma

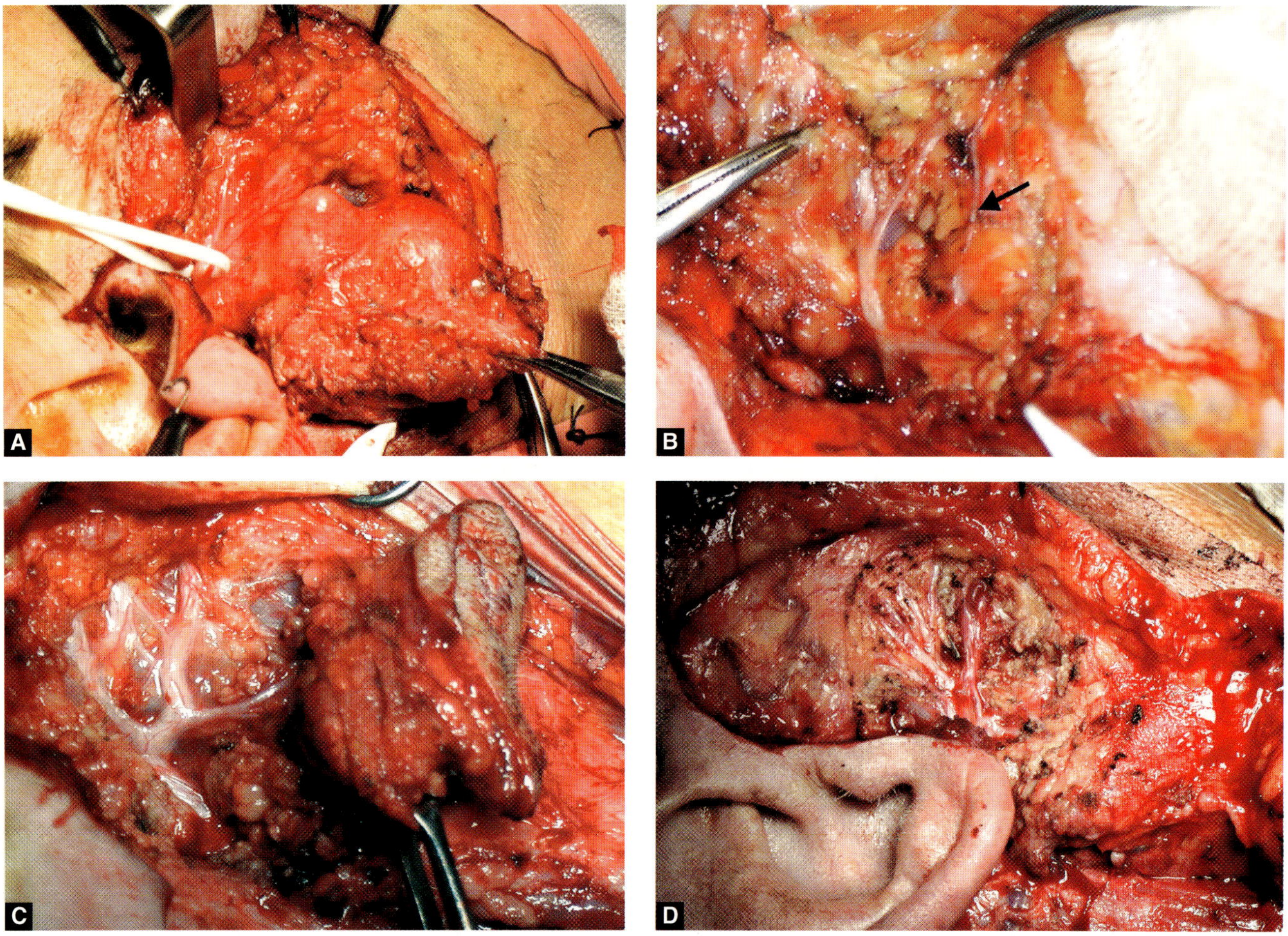

Figs 11.4A to D: (A) Removal of pleomorphic adenoma from deep lobe of parotid, note its relation to the facial nerve; (B) Superficial parotidectomy being performed for Pleomorphic adenoma, note the big loop like communication between the branches of the facial nerve; (C) Superficial parotidectomy being performed for pleomorphic adenoma, note the anastomosis between the branches of facial nerve forming small loop; (D) Branches of the facial nerve after resection of basal cell carcinoma infiltrating the parotid, clip marks the deep margin (images contributed by Dinaz Irani and Brandon Hitchcock, BOPDHB, Tauranga Hospital, Tauranga, New Zealand)

- Congenital lesions
- Inflammatory lesions
- Traumatic, which may be iatrogenic or accidental trauma
- Neoplastic lesions.

Facial Nerve Injury due to Trauma

Penetrating trauma, lacerations and injury to the facial nerve are the most common causes of extratemporal facial nerve paralysis.

Facial nerve injuries are classified as:
- Compression
- *Pulsion*: Pulling/tearing of the nerve as in severe injury to the nerve during birth
- Crushing
- *Transection*: Clear-cut injury with or without missing segment.

Facial Nerve in Parotid Neoplasms

1. Lymphangiomas of the parotid gland surround the facial nerve and then spread downwards into the submandibular gland.
2. Facial nerve should be dissected out from beyond the periphery of the neoplasm.
3. Pleomorphic adenomas may lie in intimate contact with the undersurface of facial nerve or may involve the facial nerve sheath.

Trauma to the Facial Nerve during Surgery

- Part of the parotid, which lies superficial to the facial nerve, is peeled off the nerve together with the tumor in partial parotidectomy
- In total conservative parotidectomy, the nerve may be injured when the tumor is being delivered through a gap between the branches of the facial nerve or being scooped out inferiorly from under the facial nerve.

Facial Nerve Weakness after Parotidectomy

It is usually temporary and commonly affects the mandibular and frontal branches of the facial nerve. It is more prone to occur in elderly patients, in those with slender rather than stout branches where an unusual degree of trauma occurs in the vicinity of nerve, due to pressure or traction on the nerve or constant suction on its surface. It may also occur due to excessive drying of its sheath or heat from diathermy.

Facial Nerve in Malignancy of the Parotid

Adequate resection of tumor is performed and the branches or even the main trunk of facial nerve may be resected, if involved.

Facial nerve involvement (extratemporal) in congenital lesions is seen in the following conditions:
- Malformations of ear
- Excessive growth of styloid process which leads to hypoplasia of the nerve.

Injury to Facial Nerve in Parotid and its Repair (Fig. 11.5)

Facial nerve divisions in parotid have various connections and form a webbed network called Pes anserinus.

Injury to the main trunk or temporozygomatic or cervicofacial divisions is always repaired.

In clear facial lacerations, with immediate onset of facial nerve palsy, repair is undertaken in the first three days, or if not possible, then three weeks later.

In case of gross contamination, proximal and distal segments should be identified and tagged.

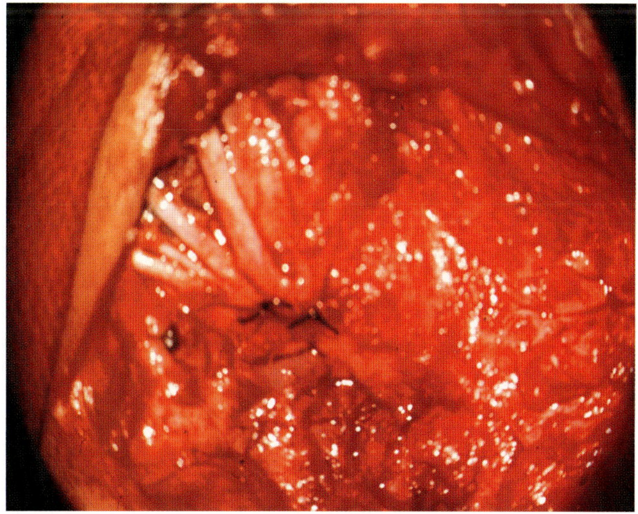

Fig. 11.5: Intraoperative photograph showing sutured branches of the facial nerve in the parotid following cut injury due to a stab wound

Primary end-to-end an astomosis results in greater functional return than interposition grafting with multiple anastomosis.

In gunshot wounds or blasts, extensive soft tissue injury occurs and if nerve loss is extensive then interposition graft is used.

In parotid surgery when facial nerve is to be preserved, it is stimulated near the stylomastoid foramen before wound closure if there is no movement then careful inspection under microscope is carried out for evidence of injury like accidental ligature on nerve or crush injury.

When facial nerve injury occurs posterior to the anterior margin of masseter muscle concomitant injury to parotid duct is looked for.

BIBLIOGRAPHY

1. Johns M, Kaplan M. Neoplasms-Salivary Glands. Cummings CW. 2:1039-41.
2. May M. Disorders of facial nerve. Scott-Brown's Otolaryngology, 6th Edn. 3:24/10-12.
3. Miehlke J. Parotid tumors and Facial nerve. Surgery of facial nerve. 125-28.
4. Proctor B. Anatomy of the facial nerve. Otolaryngologic Clinics of North America. 1991;24(3): 499-503.
5. Shaheen OH. Benign salivary tumours. Scott-Brown's Otolaryngology. 6th Edn. 352-5.
6. Warren AJ, Osguthorpe D. Management of trauma of the facial nerve: Otolaryngologic Clinics of North America. 1991;24(3):587-92.

12

Hemifacial Spasm

DS Grewal

Hemifacial spasm is the symptom complex of unilateral facial nerve hyperactive dysfunction characterized by the onset of mild and intermittent spasms in the orbicularis oculi muscle that gradually progress in severity and frequency. It spreads gradually to include all the muscles of facial expression. A mild muscular weakness may also be seen over a period of months or years (Janetta et al. 1977).

The facial spasm may be primary or secondary. Primary spasm is the idiopathic hemifacial spasm while secondary spasm is usually secondary to a recovering facial paralysis and are often combined with contractures. It may be occasionally confused with a facial tic. However, a facial tic is psychogenic. It is the habit of shutting the eyelids or blinking, distorting the mouth and wrinkling the nose. Patients suffering from facial tics usually require psychiatric help.

The idiopathic hemifacial spasm of one side of the face are agitated by paroxysmal, clonic, voluntary and episodic muscular contractions. The spasms are more noticeable in the lower eyelid and the oral commissure. This unpleasant grimace is aggravated under emotional tension, which makes the patient irritable especially in the presence of a third person.

ETIOLOGY

The etiology of idiopathic hemifacial spasm is unknown. There are several theories proposed to explain it:

- *Otologic theory*: In this, the causative lesion is an edema of the facial nerve or a fibrous constriction of its sheath (Woltman, et al. 1951; Pulec, 1972). Those who accepted this etiological thesis postulated the existence of an irritable focus in any segment of the facial nerve, which causes a short-circuiting of impulses.
- *Neurosurgical theory*: The lesion could be caused by a continuous and prolonged pressure upon the seventh nerve by a vascular structure in the posterior cranial fossa (Janetta, 1972).
- *Neurological theory*: The pathological condition could be located in the motor nucleus of the facial nerve in the brainstem (Wartenberg, 1952; Crue et al. 1968). Supporters of this theory believe that these impulses originate in the ganglion cells of the facial nerve in brainstem.

The lack of a consensus on the causes of idiopathic hemifacial spasms suggests that the exact cause is still not known and in different cases, it may have different etiologies. Clinically, it is very difficult but not impossible to determine in a patient with this disease, whether the lesion is in the nucleus, the cerebellopontine angle or in the fallopian canal.

TREATMENT

Generally, medical measures fail to control the symptom and surgery is the only available therapeutic or palliative option. Operative treatment depends largely on the various etiological theories. The medical line of treatment includes drug treatment and also treatment with botulinum toxin.

Drug Treatment

Various drugs have been tried for the treatment of hemifacial spasms. They reduce the severity and the frequency of spasms but the results are disappointing. Carbamazepine may be used in doses from 100 mg once daily to 12 hourly to a maximum of 200-400 mg given 8 hourly. The drug dosage is increased over a period of 2-3 weeks to get an optimum therapeutic concentration of 30-50 mol/lt and to prevent sedative side effects. Phenytoin may be used in a range of 150-500 mg (average 300 mg) depending upon the tolerance of the patient; to achieve a plasma level of about 40-80 mol/lt. Clonazepam 0.5-2.0 mg 8 hourly is effective at times (Cull and Will, 1995).

Botulinum Toxin Injection

Injection of Botulinum toxin type A is another effective method of temporary relief from hemifacial spasm. Botulinum toxin is produced by the bacteria *Clostridium botulinum*. It has a molecular weight of 150 kDa and is capable of neuromuscular blockage due to its single polypeptide chain to dichain molecules held by disulphide bonds. The heavy chain portion of the molecules binds irreversibly to the presynaptic cholinergic nerve terminals at specific receptor sites causing a reversible neuromuscular junction blockade. It has shown good results in 90% of the patients treated for hemifacial spasm.

0.1-0.2 ml of a diluted form of toxin may be injected around the eye in the orbicularis oculi muscle and in the zygomaticus major muscle for periorbital and perioral twitches (Fig. 12.1). The effects of the toxin become apparent within 2-7 days and maximum effects are seen by the 10th day. The effects of the treatment last for about 10 weeks.

The disadvantages include:
- Local pain at the injection site
- Periorbital bruising
- Diplopia
- Ptosis
- Ectropion with misting of vision
- Drooping of the angle of the mouth.

Operative Procedures

The procedures to relieve the spasms can be divided into a number of categories based on the theoretical factors implicated.

Facial Nerve Needling

This treatment is based on the theory originally proposed by Fergusson (1978) that the deafferentiation of the central pontine nucleus secondary to peripheral nerve injury results in abnormal discharges that are manifested as hemifacial spasms. McCabe and Boles (1972) and Karnik and Jain (1973) have proposed that the motor fibres that supply the facial musculature originate in the suppressor area of the motor cortex and any damage to this leads to the overactivity of the facial nerve causing hemifacial spasms.

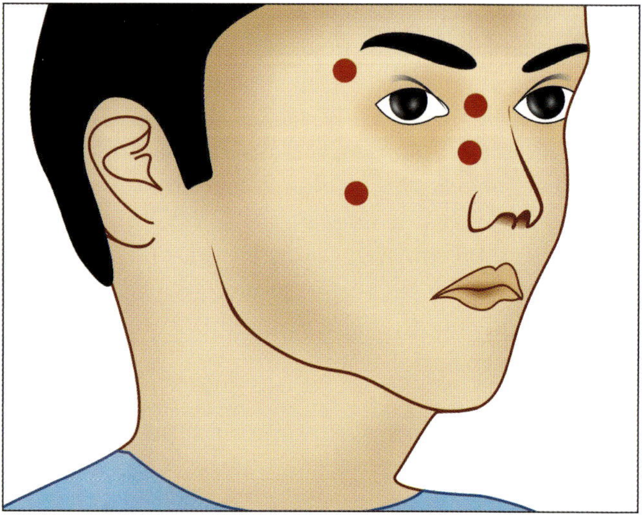

Fig. 12.1: Diagrammatic representation showing sites of injection to treat periorbital and perioral twitching

Facial nerve needling cuts down peripheral motor units and causes muscle weakness. However, it gives relief from the spasms. The sites include the mastoid segment (Celis et al. 1974), the stylomastoid foramen (Wakasugi, 1972) or the branches within the parotid gland (Fisch and Esslen, 1972). Ludman and Choa (1985) in their study of 62 patients have described the operation of transtympanic facial nerve needling. Out of the 54 patients that followed up 22 patients showed complete or almost complete relief of spasm in the first operation itself. A few of the patients had to undergo the operation again. Ogale et al. (1995) in their study of 10 patients who underwent transtympanic facial nerve needling in the horizontal segment have reported six patients completely relieved of their symptoms.

The operative procedure for transtympanic facial nerve needling entails an endomeatal approach with exposure of the tympanic segment of the facial nerve. The fallopian canal of the facial nerve is thinned and removed. The facial nerve is then punctured with a fine microsurgical pick making 4-6 punctures. This technique was based on cutting down the number of motor units in the peripheral musculature by inducing lesions in the peripheral course of the facial nerve. Here, minimal facial weakness is traded for relief of spasms.

The advantage of transtympanic facial nerve needling is the ease of the procedure but the chances of recurrence are higher than with microsurgical decompression technique.

Partial Neurectomy

This treatment is based on the same principle as facial nerve needling. Hemi-section of the facial nerve can be done in the mastoid segment (Ludman and Choa, 1985) or longitudinally splitting at the cerebello-pontine angle (Fan, 1993). Of the 33 cases Fan (1993) treated, none of the 20 cases that followed up for one year showed recurrence. The failure rate in this series was 10%.

Vascular Decompression of Facial Nerve

This treatment is based on the belief that this disorder is peripheral in origin due to decompression of the nerve trunk. The compression of the nerve could be due to an aberrant blood vessel loop at the Root exit zone (REZ) at the cerebellopontine angle or the porous

of the internal auditory meatus (Gardner and Sava 1962, Janetta et al. 1977).

Janetta et al. (1977) in their study of 45 patients with classical hemifacial spasms have described the decompression of the facial nerve at the cerebello-pontine angle. The cause of hemifacial spasm was found to be a vascular cross-compression usually by an arterial loop. The facial root exit zone is decompressed by changing the axis of the arterial loop through interposition of a small prosthesis of a non-reabsorbable spongy material, e.g. a piece of muscle or a ivalon sponge or teflon between the artery and the facial nerve and the vestibule-cochlear nerve. The artery may be large such as a vertebral or the basilar artery or small such as the posteroinferior cerebellar artery or the anteroinferior cerebellar artery. They have reported excellent results in 38 of the 45 patients on which the surgery was performed.

Any posterior fossa neurosurgical operation, no matter how skillfully performed, is more hazardous than an operation in which the nerve is approached extracranially, with the risk of cochlear nerve damage, aseptic meningitis or a small chance of mortality. Nowadays, with the use of an endoscope for this procedure, the morbidity and the complication rate have significantly decreased.

The treatment of hemifacial spasm has undergone evolution and it is now possible to do vascular decompression of facial nerve with the help of endoscope which is step forward in its safe and effective treatment.

Other Procedures

Some of the other procedures that can be done for hemifacial spasms include:
- Facio-hypoglossal anastomosis (Andrew, 1981)
- Total decompression of the intratemporal course of the facial nerve (Pulec, 1972)
- Orbicularis oculi stripping (Elston, 1988).

However, the results have not been very encouraging.

BIBLIOGRAPHY

1. Andrew J. Surgery for involuntary movements. Br J Hosp Med. 1981;26(5):522-4,526-8.
2. Blaubach AC, Castillo AH. Idiopathic Hemifacial Spasm-New Method of Surgical Treatment. Acta Otolaryngologica. 1974;77:221-7.

3. Celis-Blaubach and A. Higuera Castillo Idiopathic hemifacial spasm,Acta-otolaryngologica. 1974;77:221-7.

4. Crue BL, Todd EM, Carregal EJ. Compression of Intracranial portion of the facial nerve and section of 114 Atlas of Surgery of the Facial Nerve nervus intermedius for hemifacial spasm. Bull Los Angeles Neurology Soc. 1969;33:70.

5. Cull RE, Will RG. Diseases of the nervous system. Davidson's Principles and Practice of Medicine. 1995;17:1021-3.

6. Elston JS. The clinical use of botulinum toxin. Seminars in Ophthalmology III. 1988;249-60.

7. Fan Zhong. Intracranial longitudinal splitting of the facial nerve—a new approach for hemifacial spasm. Annals of Otology, Rhinology and Laryngology. 1993;102(2):108-9.

8. Ferguson J. Hemifacial spasm and the facial nucleus. Annals of Neurology. 1978;4:97.

9. Fisch U, Esslen E. The surgical treatment of hemifacial spasm. Archives of Otolaryngology. 1972;95:402-5.

10. Gardner WJ, Sava GA. Hemifacial spasm—a reversible pathophysiologic state. Neurosurgery. 1962;19:240.

11. Hawthorne MR, White K. Practical use of botulinum toxin in head and neck dystonia. Recent Advances in Otolaryngology. 1995;7:253-70.

12. Janetta PJ, Abbssay A, Maroon JC, et al. Etiology and definite microsurgical treatment of hemifacial spasm. Journal of Neurosurgery. 1977;47:321-8.

13. Janetta PJ ,Taking pressure off facial nerves Medical world 1972:13-55.

14. Karnik PP, Jain JC: Hemifacial spasms. Indian Journal of Otolaryngology. 1973;25:31-4.

15. Ludman H, Choa DL. Hemifacial spasm. Operative treatment. Journal of Laryngology and Otology. 1985;99:239-45.

16. McCabe BF, Boles R. Surgical treatment of essential blepharospasm. Archives of Otolaryngology. 1972;81:611-8.

17. Ogale SB, Chopra S, Thakkar S. Transtympanic facial nerve needling. Acta Otolaryngologica. 1995;115:405-7.

18. Pulec JL. Idiopathic facial spasm—pathogenesis of segmental decompression. Presented to the American Otological Society on April 24th 1972, Palm beach, Florida.

19. Wakasugi B. Facial nerve block in the treatment of facial spasm. Archives of Otolaryngology. 1972;95:356.

20. Wartenberg R. Facial nerve block in the treatment of facial spasm. New York: Oxford University press. 1952;80.

21. Woltman HW, Williams HL, Lambert EM. An attempt to relieve hemifacial spasm by neurolysis of the facial nerve. A report of two cases of hemifacial spasm with reflections on the nature of the spasm, the contracture and mass movement. Proceedings of Staff Meeting of Mayo Clinics. 1951;26:36.

13

Syndromes Associated with Facial Palsy

DS Grewal

MELKERSSON-ROSENTHAL SYNDROME

Melkersson-Rosenthal syndrome is a rare neuromyocutaneous disorder characterized by a triad of recurrent facial paralysis, recurrent facial and labial edema (cheilitis granulomatosa) and fissured tongue (lingua plicata). In 1928, Melkersson was the first to describe a symptom complex of facial edema and recurring facial palsy. In 1931, Rosenthal added a fissured tongue or "Lingua plicata" to this symptom complex, thus completing the triad of recurrent swelling of the lips or the face, alternating facial nerve palsy and fissured tongue. In the past, Hubschmann (1894) and Rossolimo (1901) had described a similar syndrome of relapsing facial paralysis and facial edema. However, Hubschmann did not document the tongue involvement and Rossolimo included migraine headache. In 1945, Miescher described several patients with "cheilitis granulomatosa". However, Dhar and Kanwar (1995) failed to find any granuloma from lip biopsy in 5 out of 6 reported cases (Figs 13.1 and 13.2).

Although the Melkersson-Rosenthal syndrome frequently begins in childhood, it was not reported in pediatric literature until Ehmann and Stickl (1962) described the syndrome in two children aged 22 months and 8 years respectively. It is more common in females than in males (Mistry et al. 1995). The exact etiology is unknown and theories of the etiology of this syndrome include infection, allergy and hereditary along with familial causes (Alexander and James, 1972). Carr (1966) has proposed that Melkersson-Rosenthal syndrome is an autosomal dominant trait, while Lygidakis et al. (1979) suggest that "Melkersson-Rosenthal Syndrome gene" is situated at 9p11 locus.

The diagnosis of this syndrome is essentially a clinical one. It can be differentiated from Heerfordt's syndrome by the absence of fever, uveitis and parotitis and it is differentiated from the Aschner's syndrome or "Double lip syndrome" by the absence of thyroid enlargement, blepharochalasis and presence of facial palsy (Mistry et al. 1995). It is often associated with migraine, megacolon, facial swelling and stress, which suggest vasomotor instability fundamental to autonomic dysfunction. Rarely, other cranial nerves are involved.

However, this syndrome may manifest with two instead of three symptoms (atypical cases) and can thus be divided into three clinical forms:

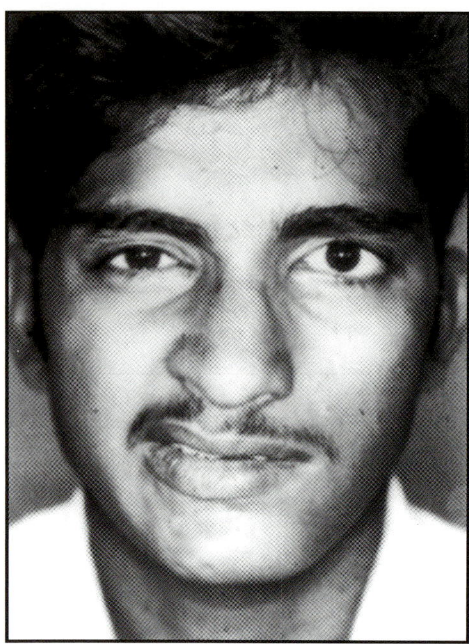

Fig. 13.1: A patient of Melkersson-Rosenthal syndrome with facial palsy

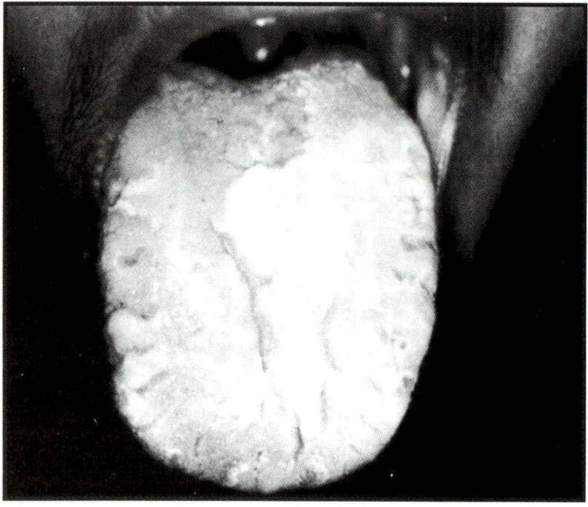

Fig. 13.2: Fissured tongue in the same patient (Fig. 13.1)

1. Complete
2. Oligosymptomatic
3. Monosymptomatic.

The syndrome can occur in the following combinations:

- Facial paralysis and edema, without lingua plicata
- Facial edema and lingua plicata without facial paralysis
- Facial paralysis and lingua plicata without edema (Klaus and Brunsting, 1959).

The facial paralysis is most commonly recurrent, but may be unilateral or bilateral; simultaneous or alternating and occurs only in 1/3rd of the cases (Zimmer et al. 1992). The first episode is commonly seen before the 20th year of life. It is usually complete and of the lower motor neuron type. Facial edema affecting the lips and adjacent areas of the face is the most common feature. The eyelids, nose, tongue, upper alveolar process and chin may also be affected. Clinically, the edema is similar to Quincke's edema. Lingua plicata or fissured tongue is seen in only 25% of cases (Auckland,1958).

Histological findings of sarcoid-like granulomas from skin or oral mucosa are helpful in the diagnosis. The biopsy of the tongue and the mucosa shows hyperplastic rete pegs, dilated lymphatic channels, fibrosis and perivascular infiltrates of lymphocytes, plasma cells and histiocytes. Granulomatous inflammation is typical of Melkersson-Rosenthal syndrome, but is not mandatory as Melkersson-Rosenthal syndrome is essentially a clinical diagnosis and not a histopathological one.

Therapy for this syndrome is mainly directed to the treatment of facial palsy and correction of the facial disfigurement due to edema. Initially, facial palsy is managed by warm compresses, analgesics, oral corticosteroids, antibiotic eyedrops and ointment, eye shields and active and passive physiotherapy. The facial palsy usually recovers completely, however recurrences are known to occur. Various therapeutic agents have been tried including vitamin D, anti-tuberculous drugs, penicillin, ultrasound, surgical excision along with plastic reconstruction of the facial edema and facial nerve decompression. However, the results are far from encouraging. Rarely, facial nerve decompression can be considered if the symptoms last for a longer duration or if the facial palsy fails to resolve in untreated cases. Facial nerve decompression may be done with the hope of preventing the disfiguring facial synkinesis and increasing facial paresis with each episode. If the lip swelling is cosmetically disfiguring, a plastic surgical repair can be performed, whereas the lingua plicata does not merit any therapy.

Recent advances in management include the use of oral clofazimine or laser beam acupuncture according to traditional Chinese medicine that have proved to be helpful in recovery (Hornstein, 1997; Dhar and Kanwar, 1995).

BIBLIOGRAPHY

1. Alexander RW, James RB. Melkersson-Rosenthal syndrome- review of literature and report of a case. J Oral Surg. 1972;30(8):599-604.
2. Auckland G. Melkersson's syndrome. Br J Dermatol. 1958;70(12):458-9.
3. Carr RD. Is Melkersson-Rosenthal syndrome hereditary? Arch Dermatol. 1966;93(4):426-7.
4. Dhar S, Kanwar AJ. Melkersson-Rosenthal syndrome in India: Experience with six cases. J Dermatol. 1995;22(2):129-33.
5. Ehmann B, Stickl H. Recurring facial paralysis and swelling—a pediatric contribution to the Melkersson-Rosenthal syndrome. Z. Kinderheilk. 1962;110:541-3.
6. Hornstein OP. Melkersson-Rosenthal syndrome: a challenge for dermatologists to participate in the field of oral medicine. J Dermatol. 1997;24(5):281-96.
7. Hubschmann Von P. Ueber recidive und diplegie bie der sogenannten rheumatischen facialislahmung. Zbl Neurochir. 1894;13:815.
8. Klaus SN, Brunsting LA. Melkersson-Rosenthal syndrome (persistent swelling of the face, recurrent facial paralysis, and lingua plicata): report of case. Proc Staff Meet Mayo Clin. 1959;34:365-70.
9. Lygidakis C, Tsankanis C, Ilias A, et al. Melkersson-Rosenthal syndrome in four generations. Clin Genet. 1979;15(2):189-92.
10. Melkersson E. Ett fall av recidiverande facialispares i samband med angioneurotisk oedem. Hygiea. 1928;20:737-41.
11. Miescher G. Uber essentielle granulomatoze Makrocheilie. Dermatologica. 1945;91:57-85.
12. Mistry B, Khan S, Gaikwad N, et al. The Melkersson-Rosenthal syndrome. The Bombay Hospital Journal. 1995;37:399-401.
13. Rosenthal C. Klinisch-erbbiologischer Beitrag zur Konstitutionspatiologie. Gemeinsames Auftreten von (rezidivierender familiarer) Facialislahmung, angioneurotischem Gesichtsodem und Lingua plicata in Arthritismus-Familien. Z Gesamte Neurol Psychiatry. 1931;131:475-501.
14. Rossolimo GJ. Recidiverende facialislahmung bei migrane. Zbl Neurochir. 1901;20:744.
15. Smeets E, Fryns JP, Van Der Berghe H. Melkersson-Rosenthal syndrome and de novo t (9:21) (p11:p11) translocation. Clinical Genetics. 1994;45:323-4.
16. Zimmer WM, Rogers III, RS, et al. Orofacial manifestations of Melkersson-Rosenthal syndrome. Oral Surgery, Oral Medicine and Oral Pathology. 1992;74:610-9.

RAMSAY HUNT SYNDROME

Ramsay Hunt syndrome is also known as herpes zoster oticus or herpes zoster cephalicus. This syndrome is associated with facial palsy, hearing loss, dizziness and herpetic eruptions and is caused by a neurotrophic virus, the herpes zoster virus. Hunt (1907) first described it as a viral prodrome associated with severe pain in and around the ear and vesicles involving the pinna. In its severe form, it may be associated with vesicles on the tongue and buccal mucosa, lower motor neuron facial palsy, sensorineural hearing loss, disturbance of vestibular function or involvement of several cranial nerves (trigeminal, vestibulocochlear, vagus and glossopharyngeal nerves). It is more commonly seen to affect elderly males.

It is caused by a specific neurotropic virus but the mode of transmission is yet not well known. However, it causes facial palsy due to a severe lymphocytic infiltration of the geniculate ganglion or the intratemporal segment of the facial nerve.

The characteristics which differentiate Herpes zoster oticus from Bell's palsy include absence of complete recovery in approximately 40% patients and failure of recurrence (Bell's palsy is known to recur in 12% cases). Ramsay in his original description proposed that herpes zoster virus causes affection of the geniculate ganglion resulting in ganglionitis and herpetic eruption of the "geniculate zone". This "zone" is supplied by the sensory portion of the seventh cranial nerve and is situated within the auricle and the external auditory canal (Figs 13.3A and B).

Depending on the clinical presentation, Hunt (1907) classified the Ramsay Hunt syndrome into:
- Herpes auricularis (without neurological signs)
- Herpes auricularis with facial palsy
- Herpes auricularis with facial palsy and auditory symptoms.

This classification can also be divided as:
- Herpes auricularis (geniculate herpes)
- Herpes facialias (gasserian herpes)
- Herpes occipitofrontalis (cervical herpes).

Treatment of this syndrome is essentially conservative with the use of:
- *Antiviral agents (Acyclovir)*: Requires a virus specific enzyme for conversion to active metabolite that inhibits DNA synthesis and viral replication

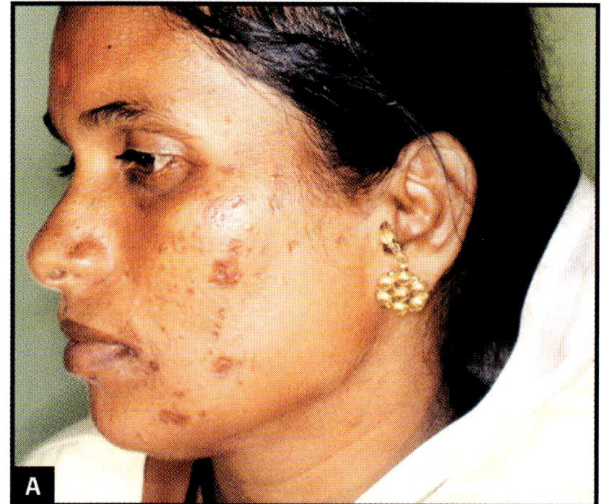

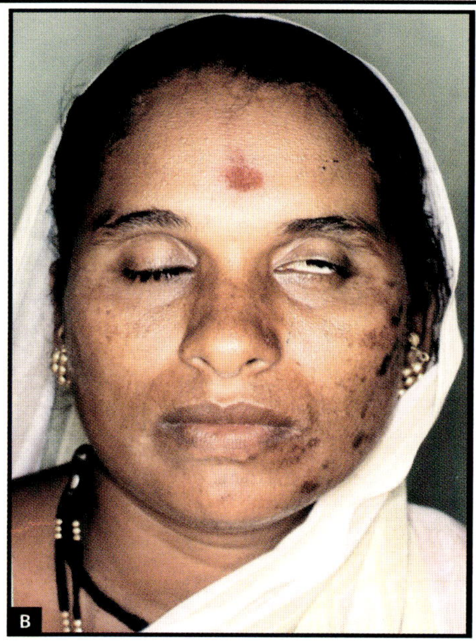

Figs 13.3A and B: A patient of Ramsay Hunt syndrome showing presence of facial plasy and healed vesicles around the pinna

- Dose: 800 mg 5 times/day for five days or 5-10 mg/kg/8 hr IV for seven days, Valacyclovir 1 gm tds and Famcyclovir 500 mg tds are also recommended
- Analgesics
- Local application of soothing anesthetic ointment
- Eye care
- Active and passive physiotherapy.

Various researchers like Ballance and Duel (1932), Findlay (1949) and Cawthorne (1965) have advocated facial nerve decompression in cases of Ramsay Hunt syndrome to prevent residual facial palsy and for a speedier recovery. However, the recovery is rarely complete.

BIBLIOGRAPHY

1. Ballance C, Duel AB. Operative treatment of facial palsy. Archives of Otolaryngology. 1932;15:1-70.
2. Cawthorne T. Bell's palsies. Archives of Otolaryngology. 1965;81:502.
3. Findlay JP. Herpes zoster of the nervus chorda tympani with facial paralysis. Med J Aust. 1949;2(11):380-2.
4. Hunt JR. On herpetic inflammations of the geniculate ganglion: a new syndrome and its complications. J Nervous and Mental Diseases. 1907;34:73-96.
5. Hunt JR. A further contribution to herpetic inflammations of the geniculate ganglion. Am J Med Sci. 1908;136:226-41.

MOEBIUS SYNDROME

It is a rare congenital disorder usually characterized by bilateral facial palsy, unilateral or bilateral Abducens palsy, anomalies of the extremities and involvement of the other cranial nerves especially the hypoglossal with absence of various muscle groups particularly the pectoral group of muscles.

The etiology is unknown but four modes of developmental pathologies are known. These are:
- Hypoplasia or absence of central brain nuclei
- Destructive degeneration of central brain nuclei
- Peripheral nerve involvement
- Myopathies.

Treatment includes reconstructive surgery such as orthognathic and static sling surgery.

HEERFORDT SYNDROME

It is a peculiar symptom complex commonly seen in sarcoidosis. It is also known as uveoparotid fever and is characterized by acute onset uveitis, iritis, parotid enlargement and fever.

This symptom complex is also associated with Bell's palsy and Sjögren's syndrome. The disease is usually benign and resolves without any specific treatment.

FREY'S SYNDROME

Synonyms

- Auriculotemporal syndrome
- Gustatory hyperhydrosis

History

It was described by Duphenix in 1757.

Lucy Frey, a French neurologist, implicated the auriculotemporal nerve in her account of a Polish cavalry officer with an infected parotid wound.

Definition

It is a symptom complex that includes localized facial sweating and flushing during mastication of food and cutaneous hyperesthesia in front of and above the ear.

Etiology

Injury to auriculotemporal nerve gives rise to this syndrome. This nerve can be injured during:

- *Parotidectomy*: 35-60% of post-parotidectomy patients within 6 weeks to 3 months of operation present with this
- Parotid abscess drainage
- Accidental injury.

Pathology

The auriculotemporal nerve provides both, parasympathetic innervation to the parotid gland and sympathetic innervation to the sweat glands and subcutaneous blood vessels. The neurotransmitter for both fibers is acetylcholine. Following injury to the auriculotemporal, regrowth of the secretomotor parasympathetic fibers into the distal cut ends of the sympathetic fibres in the skin causes gustatory sweating.

Treatment

- Most patients require only reassurance as it resolves spontaneously in a vast majority
- Conservative therapy:
    - *Anti-perspirant*: Aluminium chloride hexahydrate
    - *Topical anticholinergics*: Glycopyrrolate
    - *Botulinum toxin A*: Interferes with exocytosis of synaptic vesicles at cholinergic nerve endings.
- Surgical treatment
    - *Tympanic neurectomy*: Transection of Jacobsons nerve running on promontory
    - Interposition of fascia lata or fat between secretomotor fibers and the skin
    - Stellate ganglion block
    - Intracranial neurolysis of the glossopharyngeal nerve.

To reduce the incidence of Frey's syndrome-modifications of parotidectomy have been developed-elevation of a superficial musculoaponeurotic flap or a sternomastoid flap as interposition to prevent autonomic re-innervation of the skin.

MONDINI'S DEFECT

This is a congenital defect that includes:

- Cochlea with one and a half turns and the apical coil replaced by a distal sac
- Dilated vestibular aqueducts
- The organ of corti may be absent or reduced to a mound of undifferentiated cells
- The patient is partially or completely deaf.

14

Tumors Causing Facial Palsy

David Moffat

INTRODUCTION

The surgeon with good clinical acumen (Moffat et al. 1998) will be aware of the importance of excluding pathology throughout the whole anatomical length of the facial nerve and its central connections before making a definitive diagnosis of idiopathic facial palsy or Bell's palsy (Fig. 14.1).

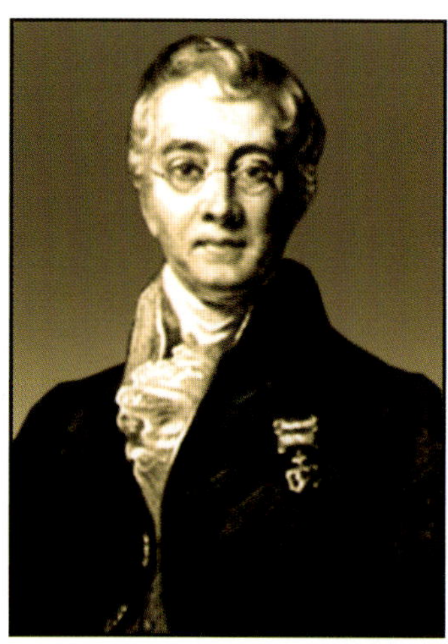

Fig. 14.1: Sir Charles Bell

Tumors affecting the facial nerve represent one of the greatest challenges facing both the neurotologist and the neuroradiologist. The nerve transgresses the traditional domains of the head and neck surgeon, otologist and neurosurgeon. Mastery of the facial nerve, therefore, represents the cornerstone of the discipline of skull base surgery.

The surgeon depends on accurate imaging by his radiologist at all stages of the management of tumors affecting the facial nerve. Imaging is cardinal in the diagnosis, the determination of treatment and the follow-up of these patients (Moffat et al. 1993). Furthermore, the role of the interventional radiologist in skull base surgery has become invaluable.

This chapter represents the author's experience of tumors causing facial palsy over a 30-year period in the University Department of Otoneurological and Skull Base Surgery at Addenbrooke's Hospital in Cambridge.

CLASSIFICATION

Tumors manifesting with facial nerve palsy have been classified into those that are intrinsic to its nerve fibers

(Fig. 14.2), and those extrinsic (Fig. 14.3) and adjacent to its course.

The extrinsic tumoral causes arise in the anatomical regions of the:

- Facial nucleus and supranuclear connections
- Cerebellopontine angle
- Temporal bone
- Parotid.

Tumors of the facial nucleus and supranuclear connections are mentioned for completeness but excluded from review in this chapter.

CLINICAL PRESENTATION

A complete facial palsy is easily recognizable (Fig. 14.4) but an early partial palsy is a subtle sign (Figs 14.5 and 14.6) (Moffat, 2001). The earliest sign of a facial palsy is a delay in blinking and the physician should

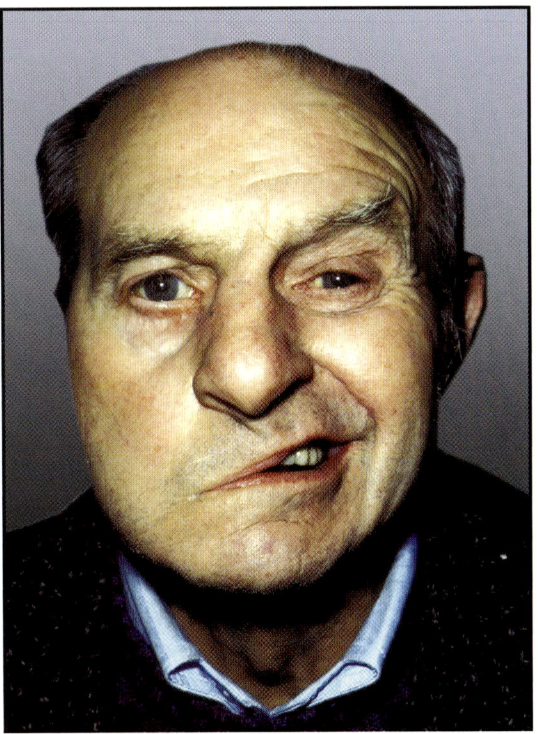

Fig. 14.4: House-Brackmann grade VI facial palsy

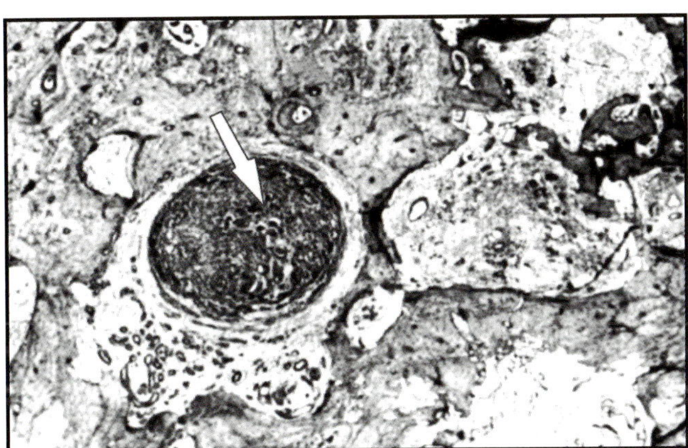

Fig. 14.2: Histopathology of tumor infiltration of the facial nerve (white arrow)

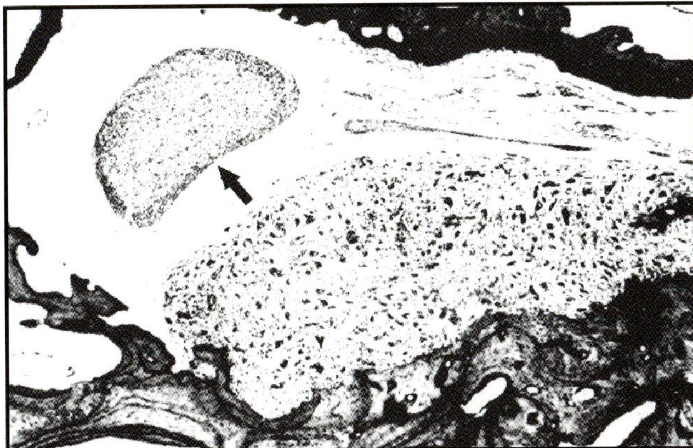

Fig. 14.3: Histopathology of neoplastic tissue causing facial nerve compression (black arrow)

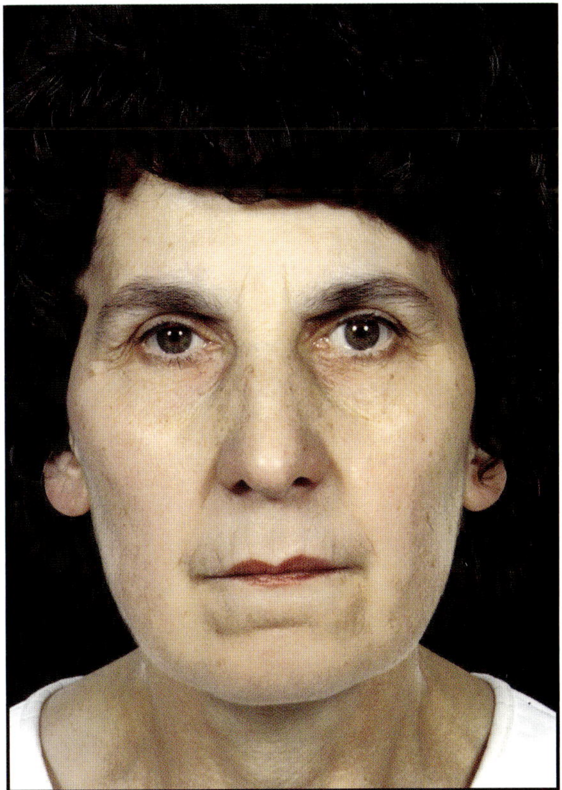

Fig. 14.5: Normal face at rest

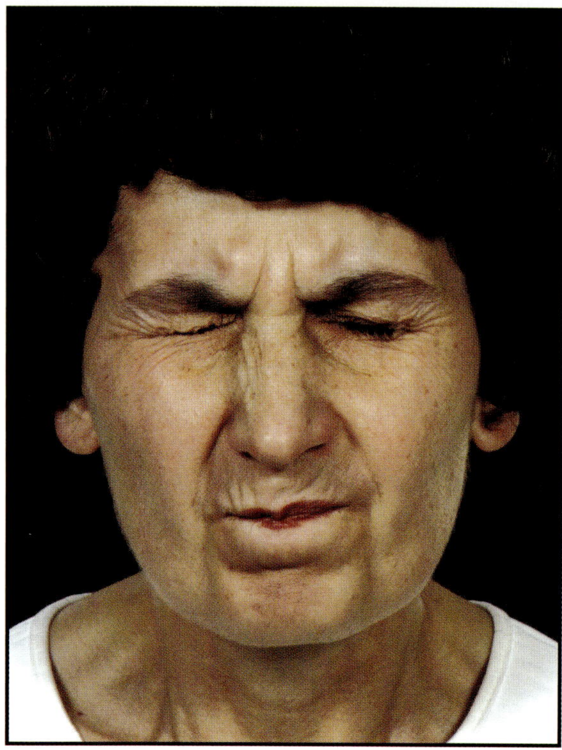

Fig. 14.6: House-Brackmann grade II manifest on screwing up the face

always elicit a blink reflex by asking the patient to look straight ahead and then rapidly tapping the glabellar region with the tester's finger initially hidden from view.

Diagnosis can be a challenge and the symptoms may be slow and insidious (Moffat et al. 1993) and thus the diagnosis may be delayed. The diagnosis of "Bell's palsy" is one of exclusion and a neoplastic cause must be excluded by high resolution imaging of the entire course of the facial nerve.

INTRINSIC LESIONS OF THE FACIAL NERVE

Intrinsic lesions of the facial nerve are:
- Schwannoma (neuroma)
- Hemangioma.

Facial Nerve Schwannomas (Neuroma)

Schwannoma is synonymous with neurilemmoma. These tumors arise from the Schwann cells of the nerve sheath and are often multicentric in origin. They are commonly intratemporal but may occur anywhere along the course of the nerve (Fig. 14.7). Tumors of

the chorda tympani (Huoh et al. 2010) and the greater superficial petrosal nerve (Amirjamshidi et al. 2010) have recently been described. The posterior fossa and/or internal auditory canal (IAC) segment is involved in 50% of cases and they comprise 1% of all cerebello-pontine angle (CPA) tumors (Moffat et al. 1993). Eighty percent involve two adjacent segments and are dumb-bell in shape and may have an intratemporal component, normal nerve in the IAC and tumor in the CPA. They may erode the otic capsule. There have been occasional reports of malignancy.

The anatomical location in order of frequency is as follows:
- Geniculate ganglion
- Horizontal portion
- Vertical portion
- Internal auditory canal
- Labyrinthine segment
- Extra-temporal portion.

Facial nerve shwannoma can be asymptomatic or can present with progressive or acute total facial nerve palsy. Interestingly, only 32% of facial neuromas in the CPA present with facial weakness (Moffat and Ballagh, 1995). Associated otological symptoms such as conductive and/or sensorineural hearing loss, tinnitus or vertigo can also occur (Marzo et al. 2009).

Auditory brainstem evoked responses (ABR) are abnormal in 83% of IAC and CPA facial neuromas. Electroneuronography (ENOG) may show diminished amplitude of the nerve action potential.

Computed tomography (CT) may show a widened fallopian canal (Fig. 14.8) and on both CT and magnetic resonance imaging (MRI) the appearances in the IAC and CPA are identical to acoustic neuroma.

Masses may be present in the posterior and middle cranial fossae. MRI is useful for showing the facial nerve within the temporal bone. T1 weighted images are isointense or hypointense (Fig. 14.9). T2 weighted images are hyperintense and tumors enhance with gadolinium DTPA (Moffat and Ballagh, 1995).

The surgical approach depends on the anatomical location and extent of the tumor (Gunther et al. 2010). The surgeon should be prepared to operate on the entire length of the facial nerve from the CPA to the parotid. Rerouting of the facial nerve with direct anastomosis is sometimes possible but cable grafting with greater auricular or sural nerve is usually necessary.

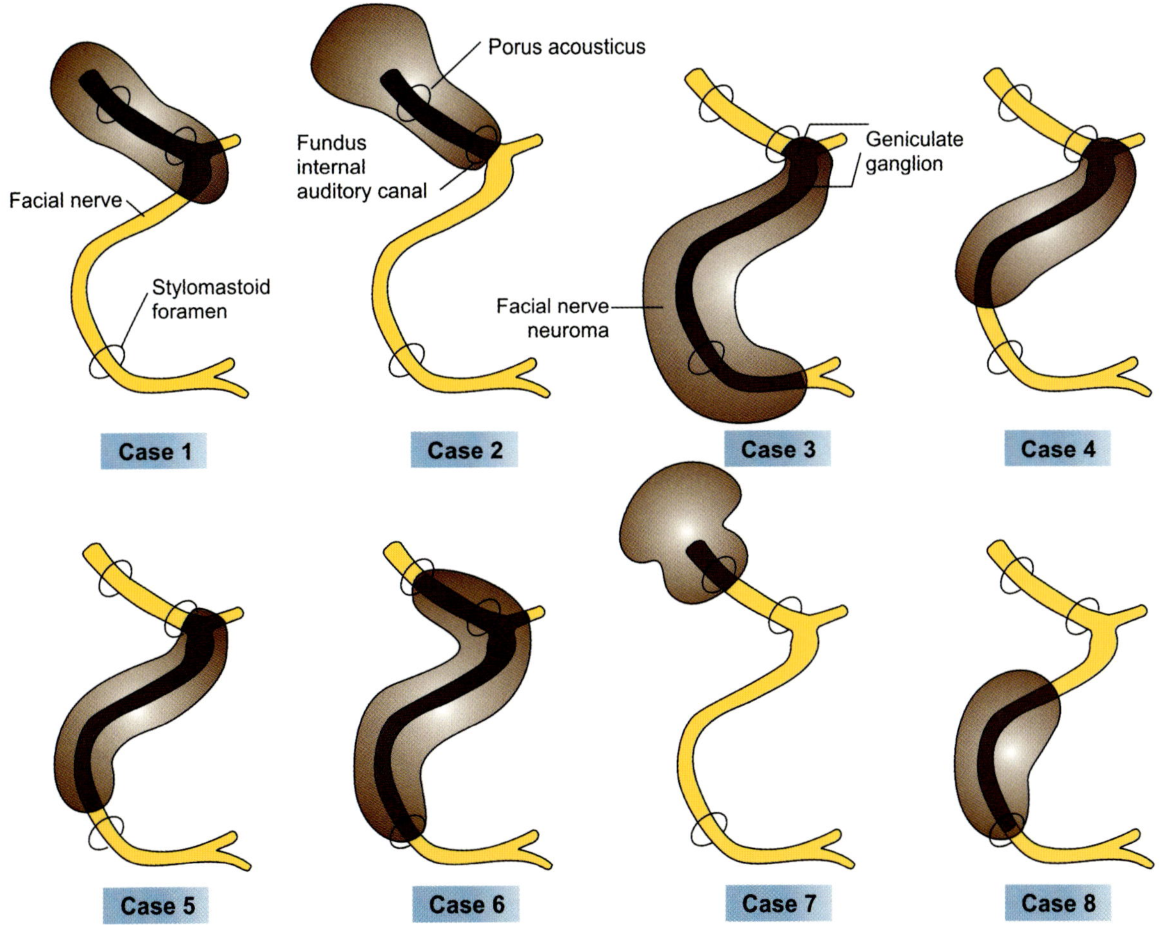

Fig. 14.7: Diagrammatic representation of the facial nerve in Cases 1 to 8, shaded area represents involvement by facial nerve neuroma. Segments of the facial nerve which may be involved in facial neuroma

Facial Nerve Hemangioma

These are vascular hamartomas and are predominantly capillary or cavernous (Fig. 14.10). They may present in the temporal bone, IAC or the CPA and may mimic acoustic neuromas (Shaida et al. 2000). They occur most commonly at the geniculate ganglion due to the rich vascular network around it and are usually capillary hemangiomas at this site (Semaan et al. 2010). They may occur in association with a facial nerve neuroma (Towfighi et al. 2008). Ossifying hemangiomas are due to dystrophic change and bone remodeling.

High resolution CT scanning demonstrates calcium stippling and IV contrast does not enhance the lesion. MRI reveals hyperintensity of the signal on both T1 and T2 weighted images with no contrast enhancement (Fig. 14.11) (Shaida et al. 2000).

They can produce a facial palsy even when very small. Sensorineural hearing loss may occur.

A venous angioma of the facial nerve producing a progressive facial palsy has been reported by Ray, et al. in 2004.

EXTRINSIC LESIONS OF THE FACIAL NERVE

Lesions of the Facial Nucleus and Supranuclear Connections

Lesions of the CPA

Vestibular schwannoma: This is the most common pathology in the CPA occurring in 80.7% of cases

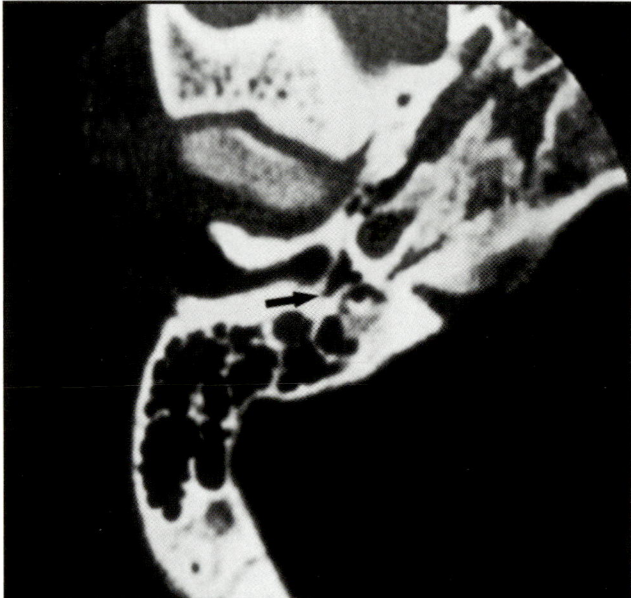

Fig. 14.8: Axial CT scan of the right temporal bone showing bone erosion in the region of the geniculate ganglion (black arrow)

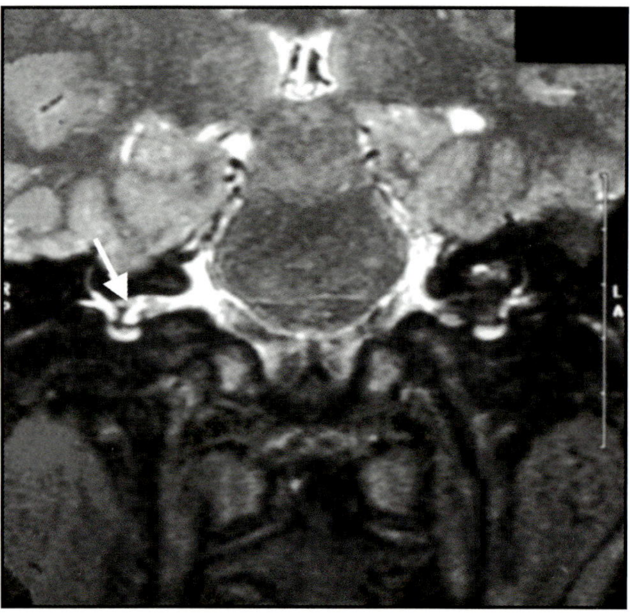

Fig. 14.9: T2W coronal MRI scan showing a facial neuroma on the right side (white arrow)

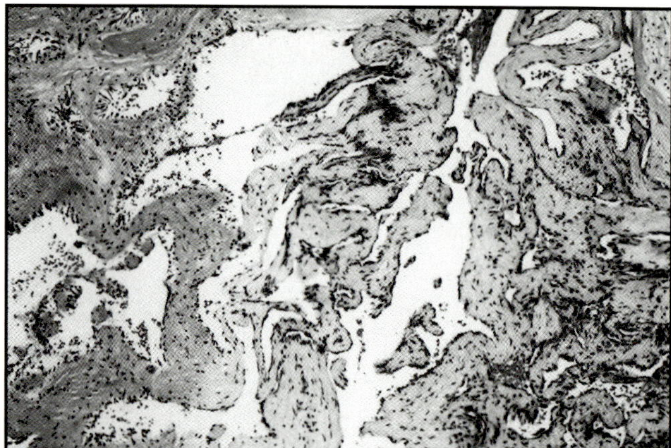

Fig. 14.10: Histopathological features of a cavernous hemangioma

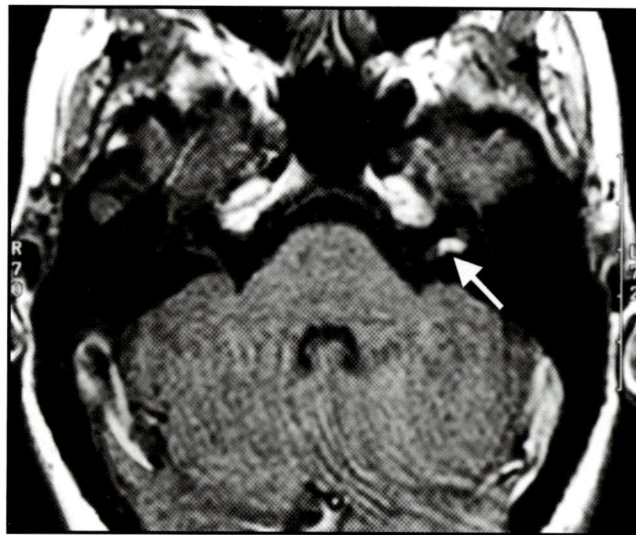

Fig. 14.11: Axial T1W MRI scan showing the hyperintense lesion in the left IAC without contrast enhancement representing a hemangioma of the facial nerve (white arrow)

(Fig. 14.12) (Moffat et al. 1993). It occurs at a frequency of 1 per 100,000 of the population per year (Moffat et al. 1989). These benign schwannomas grow at a variable rate but in the majority of cases they are slowly growing at a rate of 1-2 mm per year. They may go for long periods without growing. In the Cambridge series of patients undergoing a Watch, Wait and Rescan Management Policy 60% of tumors were found not to be growing over the observation period (Quaranta et al, 2003). For a benign tumor, acoustic neuromas bear a remarkably sinister reputation. They are usually silent at first presenting with a little unilateral tinnitus and a progressive sensorineural hearing loss (Baguley et al. 1989). In 10% of cases, the deafness is sudden (Moffat et al. 1994) presumably due to compression of the internal auditory artery by the expanding tumor in the IAC. Distortion for hearing more marked than the pure tone threshold would indicate the hallmark of these tumors. Expansion to touch the trigeminal nerve with its concomitant alteration in sensation on the skin of the face in the distribution of this nerve then occurs and the corneal reflex is depressed. If growth continues, the tumor will begin to indent the brainstem and vestibular disturbance is more likely to occur. Brainstem compression will produce a Brun's nystagmus (Moffat et al. 1988) and increasing unsteadiness on the feet along with obstruction of the cerebrospinal fluid pathways as the tumor completely fills the CPA cistern. Hydrocephalus and raised intracranial pressure will lead to papilledema and a deterioration in visual acuity. Ataxia and dysdiadochokinesis will result. Neural plasticity particularly in young people will allow remarkable compensation to occur but when decompensation occurs it is often rapid and expedient treatment needed. to enable the patient to survive.

CT scanning will only detect vestibular schwannomas when they have grown out into the CPA (Moffat et al. 1993). MRI scanning is the gold standard investigation and often a fast spin echo T2 W image is sufficient to visualize the tumor. If in doubt the patient should be given gadolinium DTPA contrast enhancement.

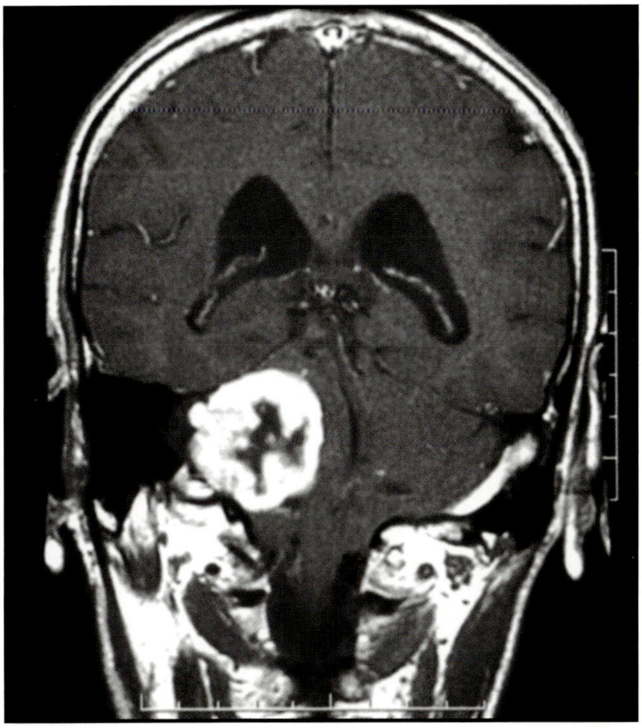

The management options are:
- Watch, Wait and Rescan
- Surgery via a translabyrinthine (Hardy et al. 1989. 1, 2), (Moffat et al. 1996), retrosigmoid or middle fossa approach
- Stereotactic radiotherapy either by single dose or gamma knife therapy or by LINAC in multiple doses.

Rare Tumors

Rare tumors of the CPA account for 19.3% of cases (Fig. 14.13). An analysis of the frequency of these rarer lesions can be seen in the pie diagram in Figure 14.14 (Moffat et al. 1993). Meningioma at 6.5% and primary cholesteatoma at 4.3% together make more than half of these rarer CPA tumors.

Meningioma

Meningiomas account for between 3% and 13% of CPA tumors in the literature and in our series 6.5% (Moffat et al. 1993) (Harada et al. 1994). Ten percent of all meningiomas are in the CPA. Macroscopically, they are globular masses with a thin capsule. They displace but do not invade nerves. They arise on the posterior surface of the temporal bone off-center from the IAC and may be intratemporal.

Fig. 14.12: Coronal T2W MRI scan showing large cystic vestibular schwannoma with marked brainstem compression and shift of the 4th ventricle

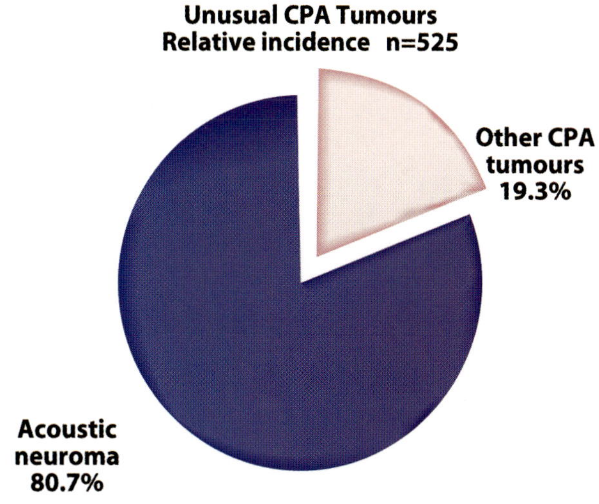

Fig. 14.13: Exploded pie diagram showing percentage of non-acoustic neuroma lesions of the CPA

Unusual Cerebellopontine Angle Tumors

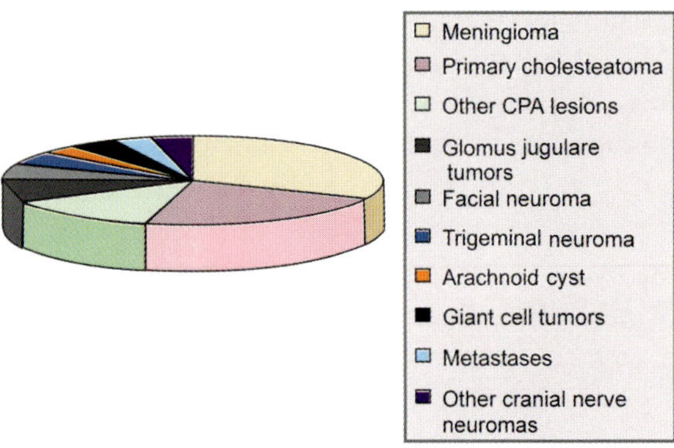

Fig. 14.14: Pie analysis of rare lesions of the CPA

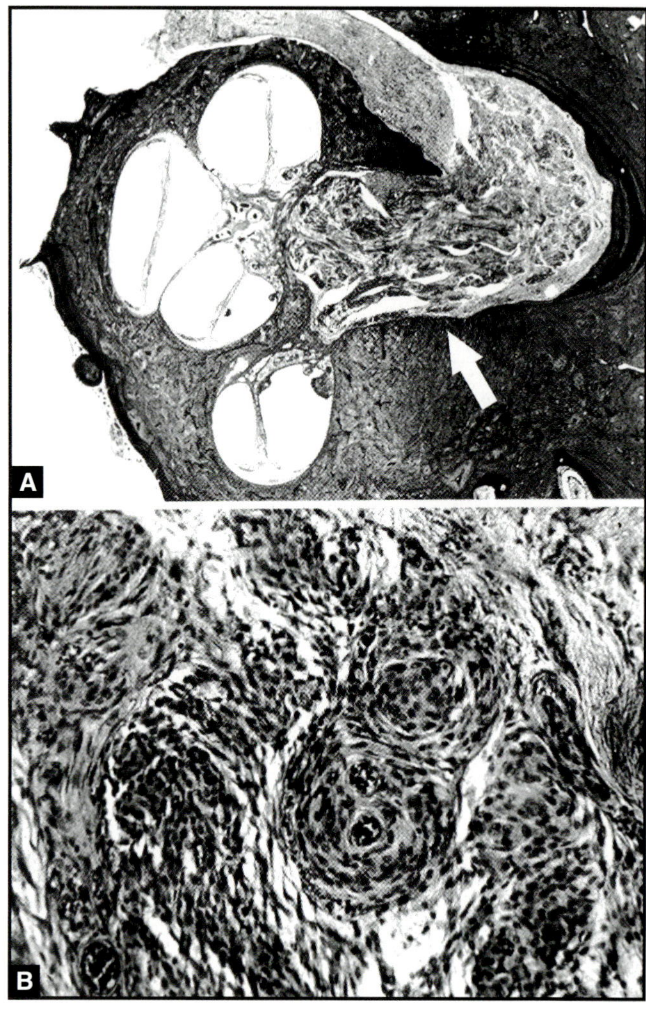

Figs 14.15A and B: Histopathology of a meningioma in the IAC (white arrow)

The characteristic histopathological features can be seen in Figure 14.15.

Clinically, patients present with audiovestibular symptoms often of shorter duration than with acoustic neuroma (Baguley et al. 1995). The hearing loss tends to occur later and other cranial nerves are more frequently involved.

Pure tone hearing thresholds tend to be better than in vestibular Schwannoma. In 75% of cases, the ABR is positive compared with 96% in vestibular schwannoma where a response can be obtained.

In plain X-rays bone destruction or hyperostosis may be seen.

CT scans show the tumor off-center from the IAC. The tumor mass is dense and homogeneous. There is considerable tumor enhancement with contrast. Calcification and bony changes may be seen.

MRI scans show a tumor which is less intense than a vestibular schwannoma due to their greater vascularity. Delineation between the tumor and the cranial nerves may be seen. The tumors have a flat base since they arise from the posterior face of the temporal bone. They are eccentric to the IAC and the angle between the posterior surface of the temporal bone and a tangent drawn to the tumor is greater than 90°. On the T1-W image, the tumor is isointense to hypointense (Fig. 14.16). The T2-W signal is variable but 50% are hypointense (Fig. 14.17). Gadolinium DTPA enhancement is less than with vestibular schwannoma.

These tumors are not very radiosensitive and surgery is the treatment of choice (Grey et al. 1996) (Ramina et al. 200 8) in the fit patient. Recurrences due to incomplete resection are common. Gross and microscopic invasion of the temporal bone occurs frequently and resection of the underlying bone should be undertaken.

Cholesteatoma (CPA Epidermoid)

This pathology comprises 4.3% of CPA tumors. It arises from epithelial rests. The tumor is lined with squamous epithelium and filled with keratin (Fig. 14.18). Cranial nerves are compressed and irritated. The cholesteatoma insinuates between and around nerves rather than displacing them.

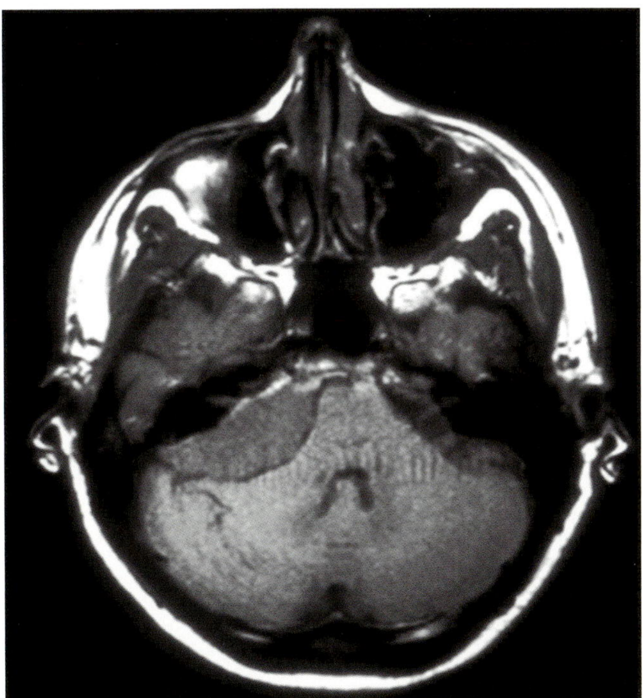

Fig. 14.16: T1W axial MRI scan of large meningioma arising from the posterior face of the temporal bone. The tumor is hypointense when compared with normal brain tissue. Note the flat base and the tumor mass eccentric to the IAC. The angle between a tangent drawn to the tumor and the posterior face of the temporal bone is more than 120 degrees

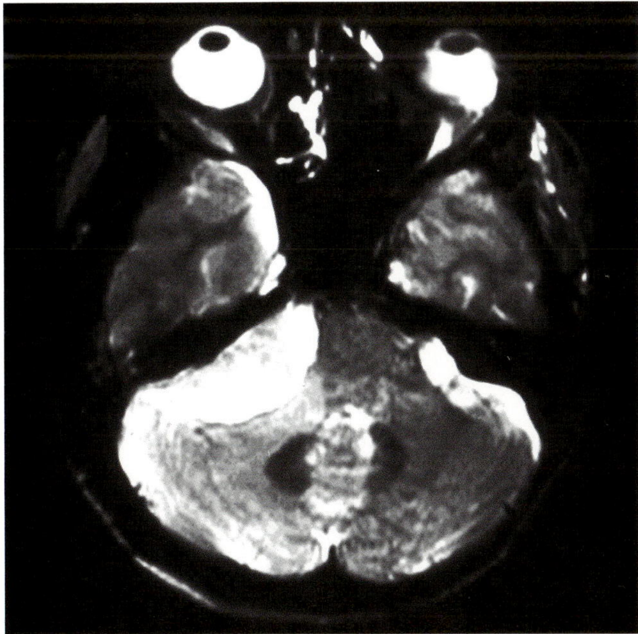

Fig. 14.17: Same tumor on the T2W image. The tumor is hyperintense

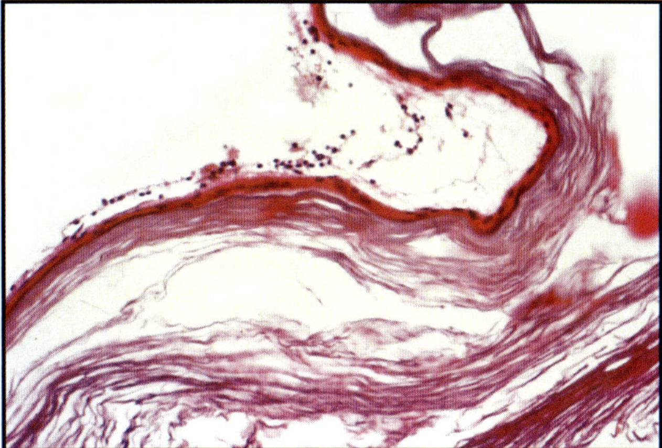

Fig. 14.18: Typical histopathological appearance of a cholesteatoma with squamous epithelium and layers of keratin

The clinical features include facial twitching which may be an early sign. Progressive facial paralysis is more common than with vestibular schwannoma. Pure tone audiometry often reveals well preserved hearing thresholds (Quaranta et al. 2003) but the speech audiogram tends to reveal poor speech discrimination scores. Dysequilibrium and rotatory vertigo, which may be positional (Beynon et al. 2000), can occur.

Plain X-rays show a smooth scalloped destruction of bone.

CT scan shows a lesion less dense than brain with irregular margins and eccentric to the IAC. Intravenous contrast shows no enhancement (Moffat et al. 1993).

MRI demonstrates a heterogeneous mass usually hypointense and of the same intensity as cerebrospinal fluid on the T1-W image (Fig. 14.19). The T2-W image shows an hyperintense tumor (Fig. 14.20). There is no enhancement with gadolinium DTPA. This compares with cholesterol granuloma where the lesion is hyperintense on both the T1-W and T2-W images (Moffat et al. 1993).

A method of staging CPA cholesteatoma has recently been devised based on the anatomical regions involved (Moffat et al. 2002).

Surgical treatment is hampered by the difficulty in excising the cholesteatoma matrix in its entirety. Denaturing the protein matrix with a defocussed laser may prove to reduce the likelihood of recurrence. The patients require follow-up for life and interval imaging. Recurrences may occur and require further surgery.

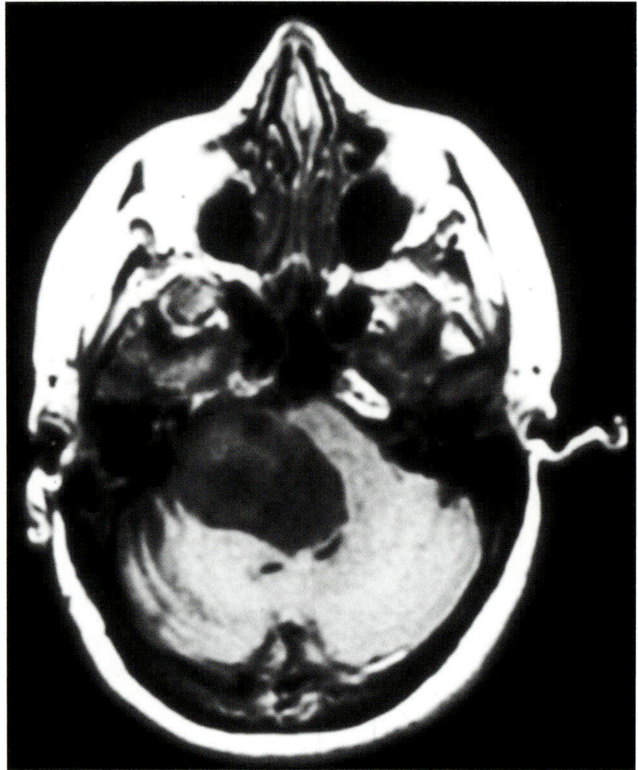

Fig. 14.19: Axial T1W MRI scan of a CPA cholesteatoma showing an hypointense mass (the same intensity as cerebrospinal fluid)

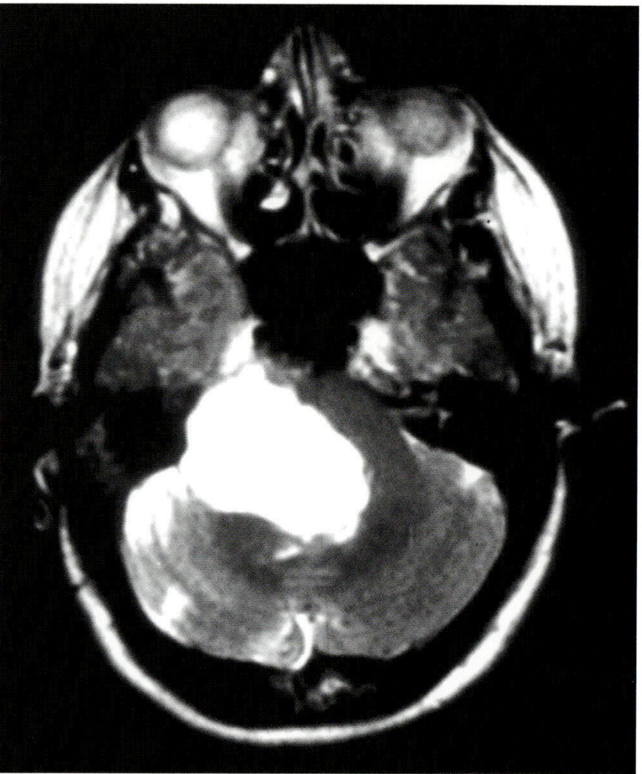

Fig. 14.20: Axial T2-W MRI scan of the same lesion demonstrating the hyperintensity of the mass on the T2

Glomus Jugulare Tumors (Fisch Type D-intracranial)

Fisch type D glomus jugulare tumors account for 1.7% of CPA tumors. The female to male ratio is 2:1 (Moffat et al. 1993).

Classically, patients present with pulsatile tinnitus, hearing loss and dysequilibrium. Pulsatile headaches may be responsible for a considerable deterioration in the patient's quality of life. Dysphonia, dysphagia and shoulder weakness may be present indicating involvement of the nerves around the jugular foramen, namely the glossopharyngeal, vagus and accessory nerves.

These lesions may be multicentric. Very rarely these tumors are malignant and metastasise (Brewis et al. 2000).

Conductive hearing loss and the otoscopic finding of a red pulsatile mass behind the tympanic membrane arising from the hypotympanum (the rising sun sign) are characteristic features (Fig. 14.21). The jugular foramen syndrome with palsies of all or any combination of the last four cranial nerves may be present. Facial and sixth nerve palsies may also occur.

Pure tone audiometry may be normal but typically there is a conductive hearing loss and bone conduction thresholds may reveal some loss of cochlear reserve in large tumors where there is some erosion of the otic capsule.

CT scanning demonstrates a mass of soft tissue density in the middle ear with erosion of the jugular foramen. There is irregular ragged loss of the margin of the bone of the jugular bulb which may be seen on the axial (Fig. 14.22) and coronal views.

Loss of the bony spur between the jugular and carotid canals is clearly seen on the coronal cuts. Marked contrast enhancement occurs in these tumors.

Multiplanar MRI images give accurate information of the extent of the tumor (Moffat et al. 1993). Marked contrast enhancement occurs with gadolinium DTPA (Fig. 14.23). It is essential to use CT and MRI in a complimentary fashion in the investigation of glomus jugulare tumors since CT will delineate the extent of the bony erosion and MRI will delineate the size and precise anatomical location of the tumor.

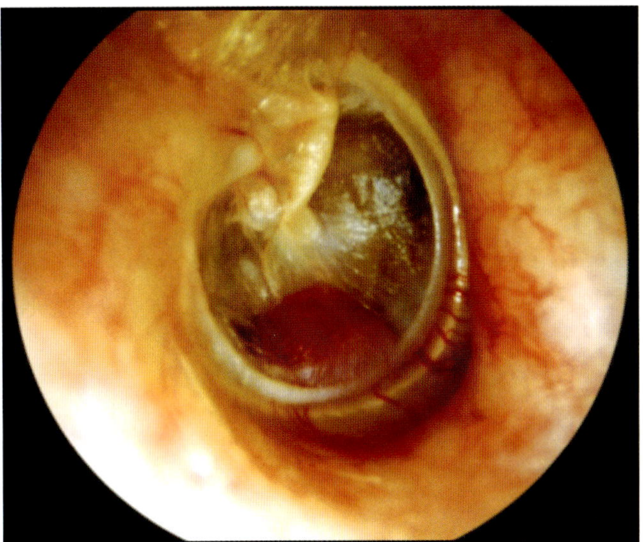

Fig. 14.21: Otoscopic view of the "rising sun sign" produced by a red vascular pulsatile glomus tumor arising from the hypotympanum

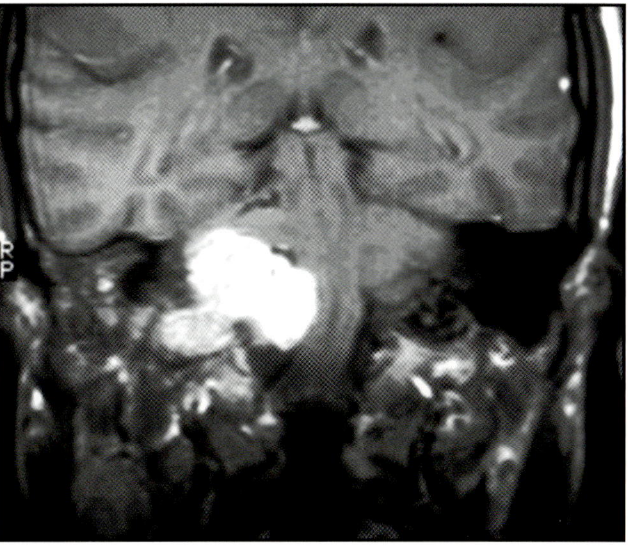

Fig. 14.23: Coronal T1W MRI scan of vast Fisch type D glomus tumor with marked brainstem compression and shift of the 4th ventricle

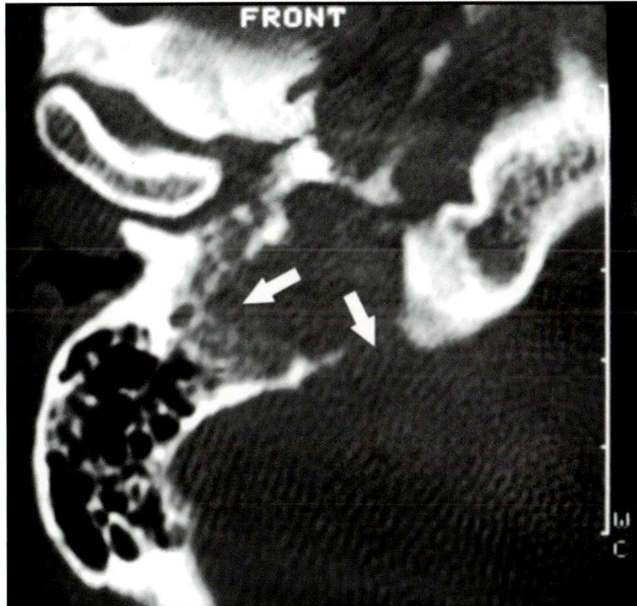

Fig. 14.22: Axial CT scan of skull base showing ragged erosion of the jugular bulb by a large glomus jugulare tumor (white arrows)

MR arteriography may be employed to assess the vascularity and feeding vessels but may not give as much information as conventional carotid ateriography which demonstrates the extent of the tumor and the degree of vascularity. It is important to establish the main feeding vessels not only to assist the surgery but also for preoperative embolization.

These tumors have a complex and incredibly rich blood supply which includes feeding vessels from the external and internal carotid arteries and the vertebral artery. The ascending pharyngeal artery is often the main feeding vessel (Fig. 14.24) and this may arise from the carotid bifurcation. The carotico-tympanic arteries are a challenge for the otoneurosurgeon.

These tumors are not very radiosensitive and surgery is the only curative treatment. However, a recent study of 88 cases of jugular paraganglioma comparing radiotherapy and surgery found that radiotherapy achieved local control in 96% of patients (Huy et al. 2009). This is most commonly performed via trans- and infratemporal approach with blind sac closure of the external auditory canal (Moffat and Hardy, 1989). The defect is obliterated with fat and fascia lata. Large Fisch type D tumors will require fascial grafting of the dura in the middle and/or posterior cranial fossae. Preoperative selective embolization with coils and feathers is helpful in reducing intraoperative blood loss. Recently, surgical approach selection based on tumor relationships with the facial nerve has been proposed by Borba et al (2010). Post-operative conformal or stereotactic radiotherapy may be necessary. This can be given as a single dose in gamma knife therapy. New palsies of the IX, X, XI and XII cranial nerves resulting from surgery can pose a real problem particularly for the elderly patient, who will not compensate, as well as for a younger patient. Dysphagia and aspiration may necessitate percutaneous gastrostomy and possibly tracheostomy; and medialization thyroplasty can improve vocal quality. It is therefore important to consider excisional surgery very carefully, particularly in the elderly patient with a big tumor who is neurologically intact preoperatively. Removal of the transverse process of the atlas will facilitate access to the jugular foramen and hence increase the likelihood of preserving neural function. Opening the jugular foramen and preserving the wall of the vein and bulb will increase the risk of leaving residual tumor but will decrease the risk of neurological deficit in the last four cranial nerves. Transposing the facial nerve is not always necessary, but if it is, it will result in a grade II or III face postoperatively.

Trigeminal Neuroma

These interesting and difficult lesions very rarely cause facial palsy. They present with facial numbness and/or pain and are usually not clinically manifest until they are large.

CT scanning demonstrates smooth enlargement of Meckel's cave or foramen lacerum.

MRI reveals an enhancing iso- or hypointense mass on T1W image (Fig. 14.25). The T2W images are isointense (Moffat et al. 1993). There is an absence of flow related signal void.

Atleast 27% of these tumors extend into the middle and posterior cranial fossae. They usually require a combined posterior and middle cranial fossa surgical approach. Anterior tumors require a Fisch type C inratemporal approach. Total resection may be difficult (Moffat et al. 2006; Sharma et al. 2008).

Arachnoid Cyst

Arachnoid cysts account for 0.7% of CPA tumors (Moffat et al. 1993). They are most commonly situated in the middle cranial fossa. They may occur in the CPA and/or IAC or over the convexity of the cerebellum and can present with a facial palsy (Diwan et al. 2005).

Pathologically, they are formed by splitting and duplication of the arachnoid layer. They are lined by arachnoid or ependyma and filled with cerebrospinal

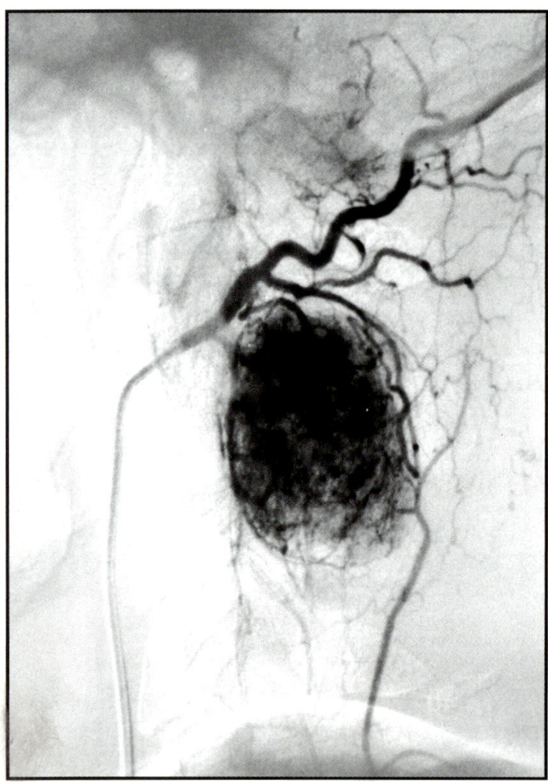

Fig. 14.24: Carotid arteriogram of a glomus jugulare tumor demonstrating that the ascending pharyngeal artery is the main feeding vessel

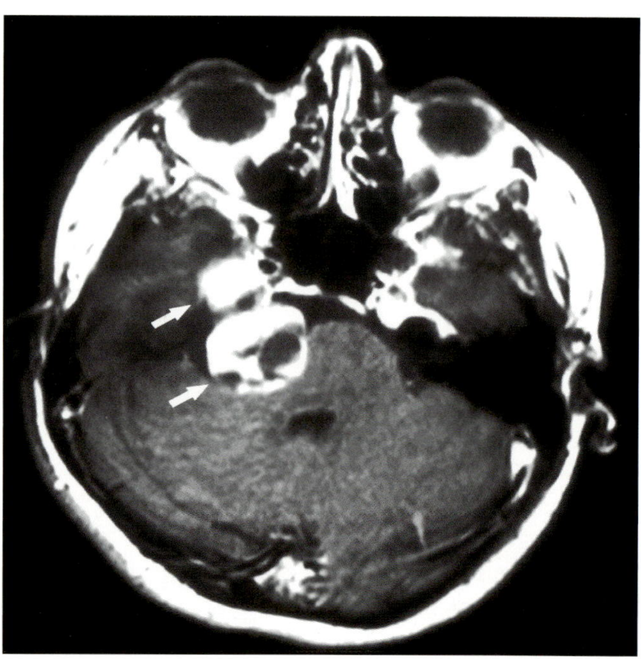

Fig. 14.25: Axial T1-W gadolinium DTPA enhanced MRI scan showing a large right cystic trigeminal neuroma present in the middle and posterior cranial fossae (white arrows)

or xanthochromic fluid (Fig. 14.26). The large pseudotumor variety may fill the CPA and erode bone. They may be congenital or ac quired.

Congenital arachnoid cysts may remain clinically silent.

Acquired cysts arise from trauma or inflammation. They may be associated with intracranial extra-axial tumors.

Imaging reveals an enlarged IAC in more than 50% of cases.

CT scanning may be normal for small cysts. The lesion is hypodense with smooth edges. It does not enhance with intravenous contrast.

MRI reveals a hypointense lesion on T1 W images (Fig. 14.27) and markedly hyperintense image on T2W (Moffat et al. 1993).

Small cysts may never require treatment. In those requiring surgery, complete excision of the cyst is not necessary. Decompression via a retrosigmoid approach is recommended. Smaller cysts may be decompressed via the retrolabyrinthine approach. Small cysts within the IAC can be tackled by a middle fossa approach.

Metastases

Like arachnoid cysts they also comprise 0.7% of CPA lesions (Moffat et al. 1993). The symptoms and signs depend upon the site (Fig. 14.28). Primary tumors are most commonly of the breast (Guilemany et al. 2005)

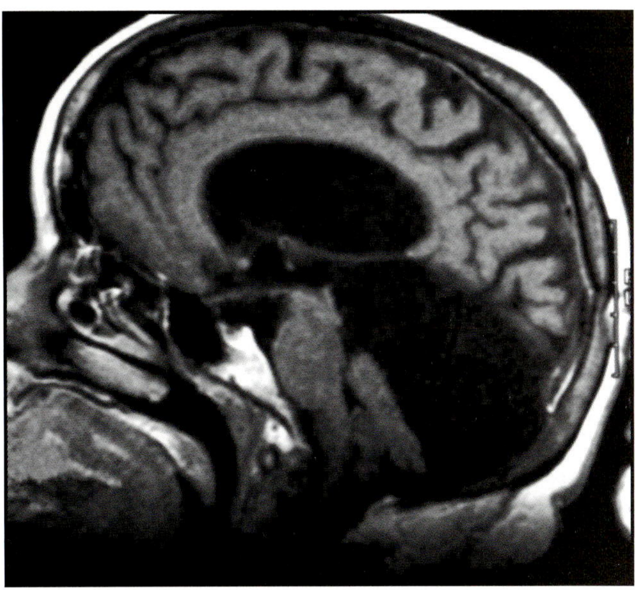

Fig. 14.27: Sagittal T1W MRI scan of an arachnoid cyst. The lesion shows marked hypointensity

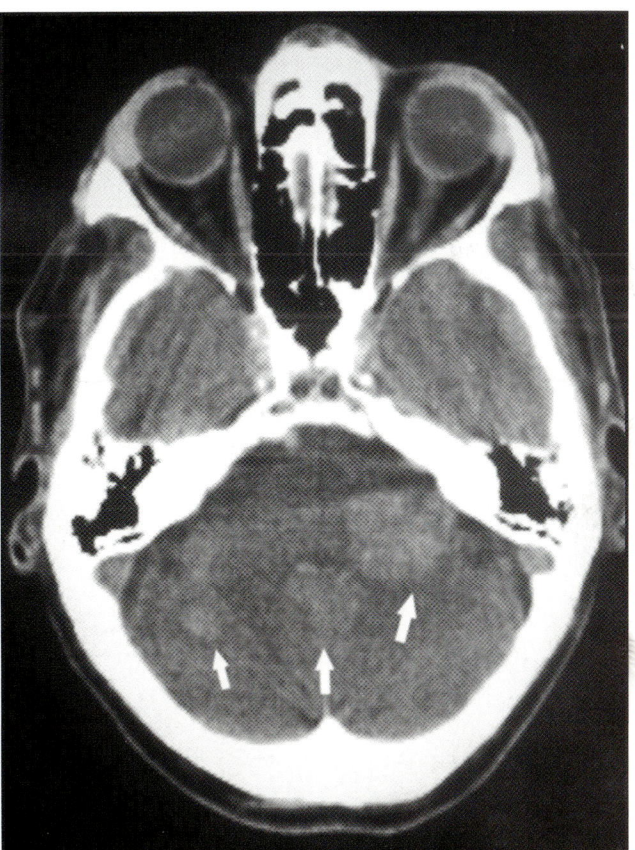

Fig. 14.28: Axial CT revealing three hyperintense metastases secondary to prostatic carcinoma in the posterior cranial fossa (white arrows)

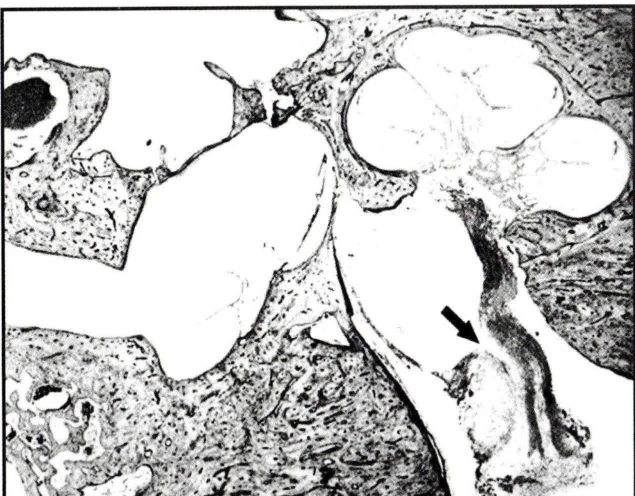

Fig. 14.26: Histopathology of an arachnoid cyst in the IAC formed by splitting and duplication of the arachnoid layer (black arrow)

and lung (Shrock et al. 2006) and also of the gastrointestinal and urinary tracts, or thyroid and sinuses and very rarely malignant melanoma (Brackmann et al. 2007) and deposits from blood dyscrasias such as B-cell non-Hodgkin lymphoma (Knapp et al. 2008).

Treatment is by palliative radiotherapy but local excision of solitary lesions can be remarkably beneficial.

Other Cranial Nerve Neuromas

The incidence of these neuromas is 0.2% (Moffat et al. 1993). These are mainly jugular foramen schwannomas and the clinical features depend upon the nerve of origin (Bakar, 2008). Histopathologically, they are schwannomas and identical to acoustic neuromas.

CT and MRI features are the same as vestibular schwannoma but anatomical localization depends upon the nerve of origin. Glossopharyngeal and vagal neuromas are more inferior in the CPA and eccentric to the IAC (Fig. 14.29).

Surgery may require a combined transtemporal and retrosigmoid approach with resection of tumor in the skull base and neck.

Lipoma

Lipomas comprise 0.14% of CPA tumors (Moffat et al. 1993). Histopathologically, they comprise mature fat cells (Fig. 14.30) and arise from embryological rests in the meninges. They differ from other intracranial lipomas in that they infiltrate cranial nerves and present with focal symptoms. The presenting symptoms and signs are similar to vestibular schwannomas (Monem et al. 1999). Facial weakness is not usually present.

CT scanning shows a homogeneous and very hypodense lesion which does not enhance.

The characteristic feature of a lipoma on MRI is a lesion of very high intensity on the unenhanced T1W image (Fig. 14.31) (Monem et al. 1999). There is no difference between the pre- and post-contrast images (Fig. 14.32). The lesion is also hyperintense on the T2W image. Fat suppressed images will markedly reduce the intensity of the lesion making the diagnosis.

These are usually indolent lesions many of which are not growing. They rarely require surgical resection and attempted surgery runs a high-risk of facial nerve palsy.

Cavernous Hemangioma (Extrinsic to Facial Nerve)

There are only a few reported cases in the CPA and IAC (Samii et al. 2006). Capillary hemangioma occurs

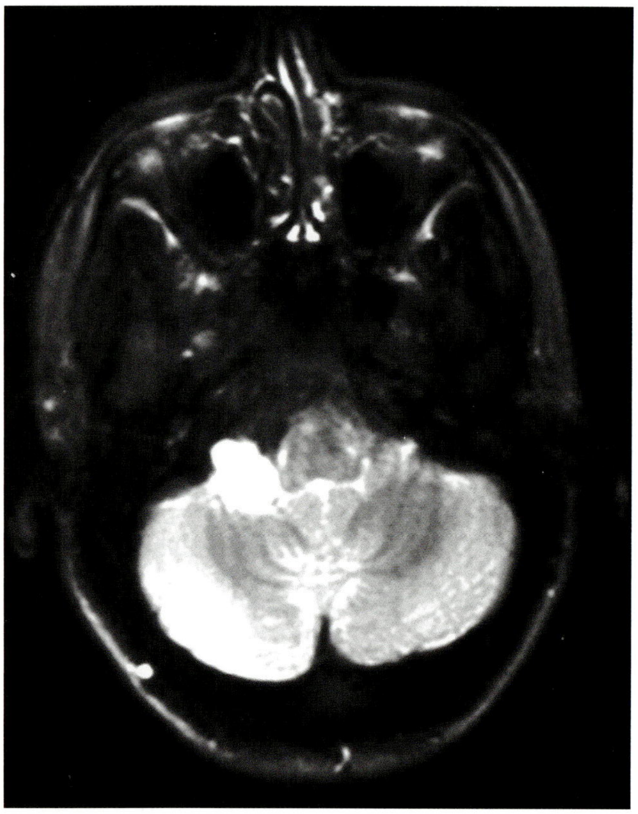

Fig. 14.29: Axial gadolinium DTPA-enhanced T1-W MRI of a glossopharyngeal neuroma eccentric from the IAC and inferior to it

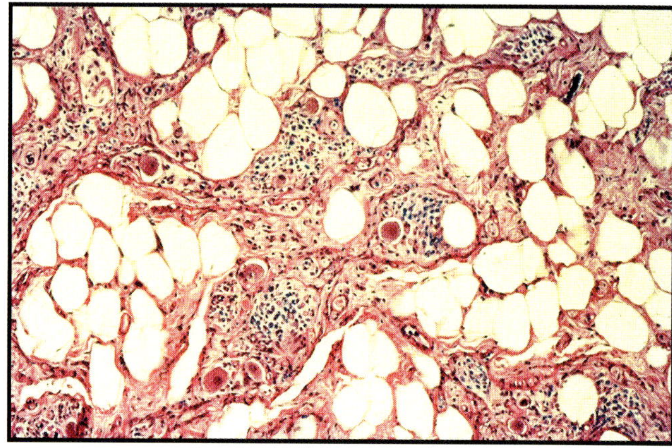

Fig. 14.30: The histopathological features of a lipoma with mature fat cells clearly seen

in the temporal bone and may be an intrinsic facial nerve lesion. Cavernous hemangiomas may occur in the CPA (Fig. 14.33) or the IAC (Shaida et al. 2000) and mimic vestibular schwannoma.

Enlargement of the IAC is common.

CT scanning shows calcium stippling at high resolution. Intravenous contrast does not enhance the lesion.

MRI scanning reveals increased signal intensity on T1W (Fig. 14.34) and T2W images (Moffat et al. 1993).

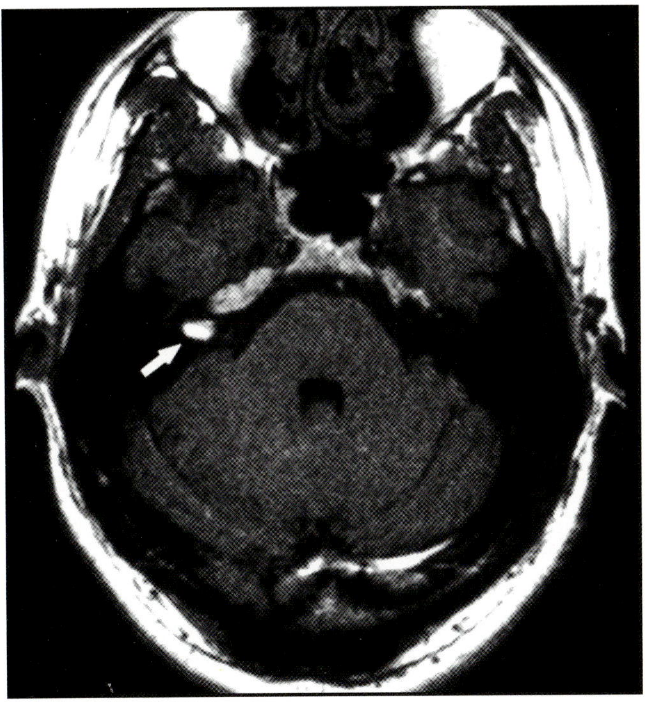

Fig. 14.31: Axial unenhanced T1W MRI scan of a lipoma of the right IAC showing the markedly hyperintense lesion (white arrow)

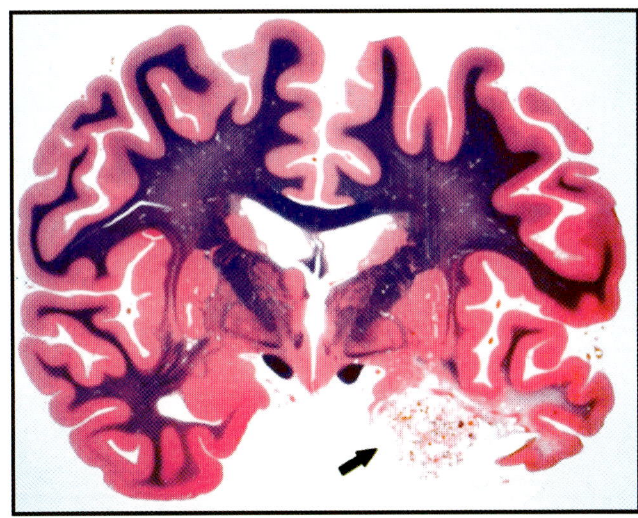

Fig. 14.33: Coronal section through the brain showing the macroscopic features of a cavernous hemangioma

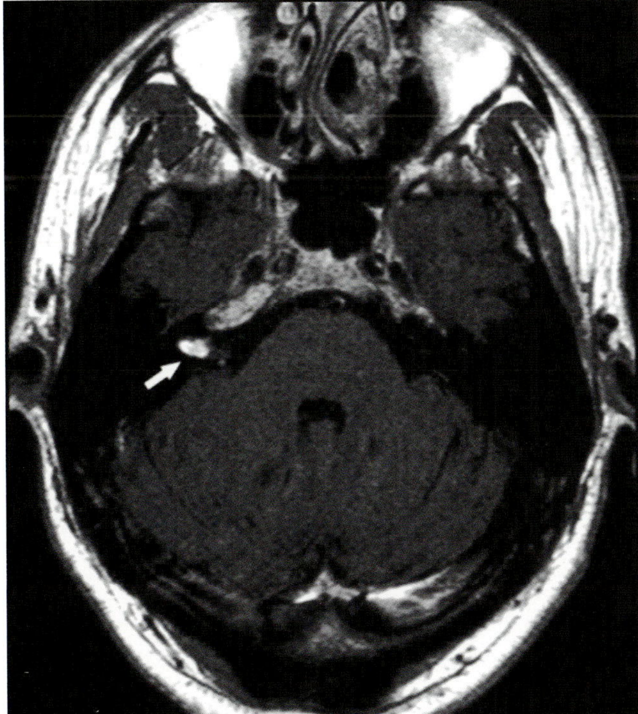

Fig. 14.32: Axial contrast T1W scan of the same patient revealing that there is no difference between this and the unenhanced image (white arrow)

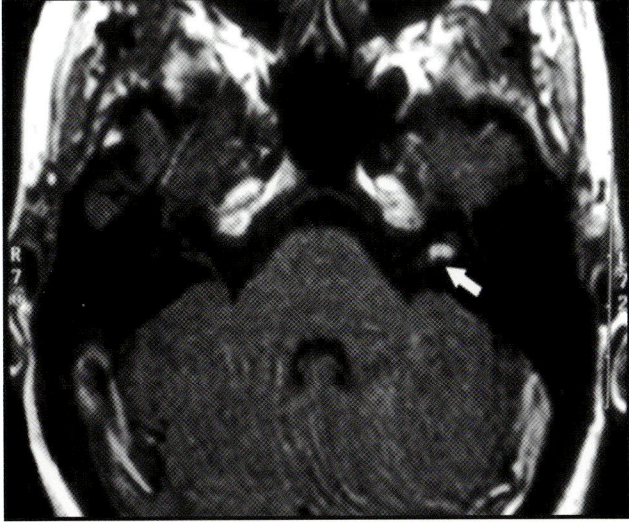

Fig. 14.34: Axial T1W MRI scan of a small intracanalicular left-sided hemangioma. Note the hyperintensity of the lesion on the unenhanced scan (white arrow)

Arteriovenous (AV) Malformation

These congenital lesions may be truly arteriovenous malformations or may arise due to a developmental venous anomaly (Moffat et al. 1993). They may occur in the CPA or on the dura where an audible bruit may be present. They rarely require treatment.

Dural AV malformations can be successfully treated by stereotactic radiotherapy and comprise a substantial proportion of all gamma knife treatments.

AV malformations in the CPA may spontaneously thromboze and largely disappear. They may be responsible for the enigmatic "disappearing CPA tumor"! (Figs 14.35 to 14.37).

Vertebral Artery Aneurysm

These may present as a CPA lesion and cause contralateral mass effect (Monksfield et al. 2005). Three-dimensional imaging reconstruction followed by endovascular coiling of the aneurysm may be possible.

Neurofibromatosis Type 2 (NF 2)

This is an autosomal dominant hereditary condition which may be devastating for the patient in its aggressive early onset Wishart type and still

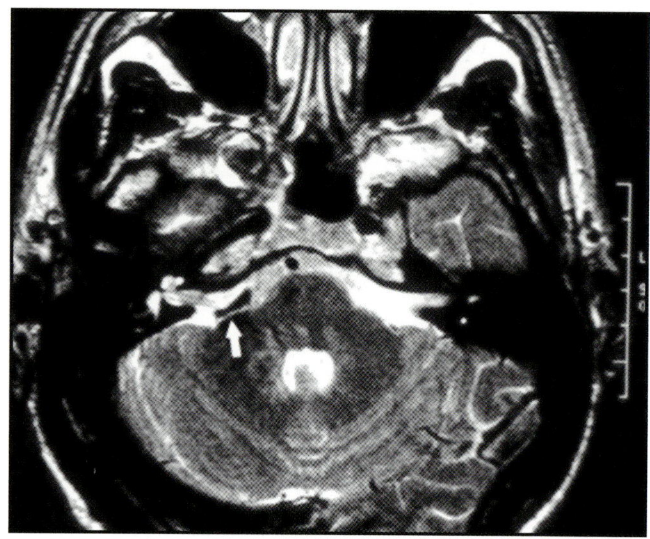

Fig. 14.36: Axial T2W image of same lesion having almost disappeared 6 months later (white arrow)

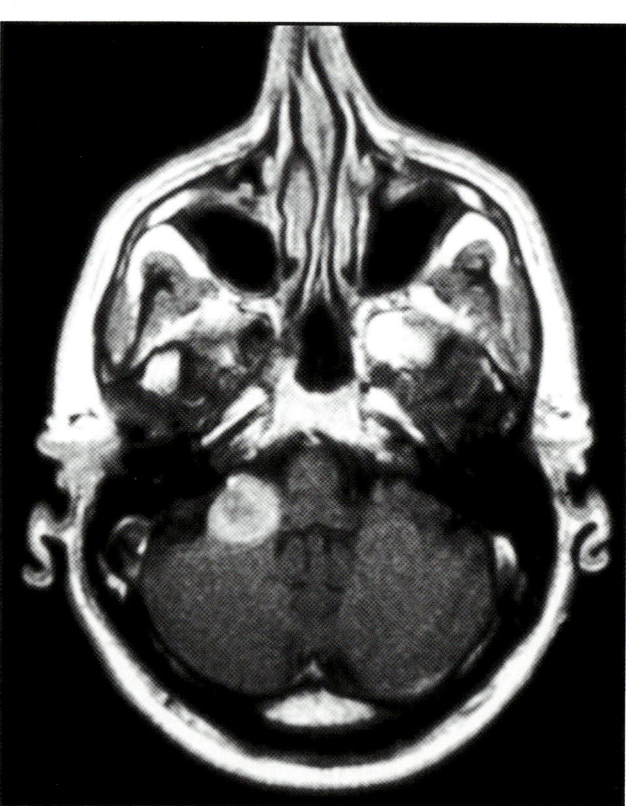

Fig. 14.35: Axial T1W MRI scan of hyperintense thrombosed AV malformation

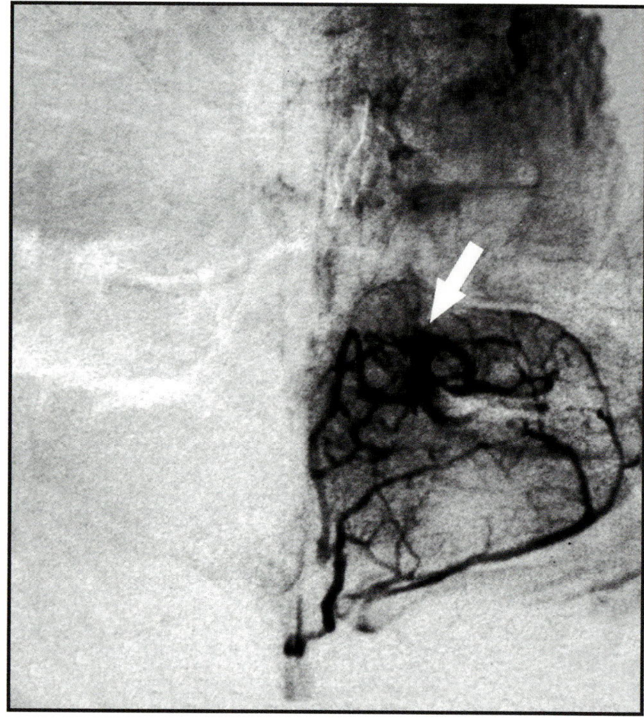

Fig. 14.37: Venous phase of an arteriogram showing a developmental venous anomaly of the posterior cranial fossa (white arrow)

incapacitating in its less aggressive later in onset Gardiner type (Irving, et al. 1997). It has the highest penetrance (95%) for an autosomal dominant. It usually arises from a gene deletion on the long arm of chromosome 22 at the locus of the amino acid sequence producing the protein merlin which is a tumor suppressor (Irving et al. 1994). Spontaneous mutations may be responsible for cases of NF2 without a family history and sporadic mosaics may produce multiple but unilateral tumors. It is characterized by bilateral vestibular schwannomas with central and peripheral nerve tumors (Moffat et al. 1993). The patients often have multiple handicaps which may be bilateral. Its management poses one of the greatest challenges in modern skull base surgery.

The characteristic features of bilateral vestibular schwannomas (Fig. 14.38) are not infrequently associated with multiple meningiomas (Figs 14.39 and 14.40), low grade astrocytomas, ependymomas, gliomas, dermal fibromas, intrinsic (Fig. 14.40) and

extrinsic spinal tumors, other cranial nerve schwannomas and meningiomas as well as posterior subcapsular cataracts.

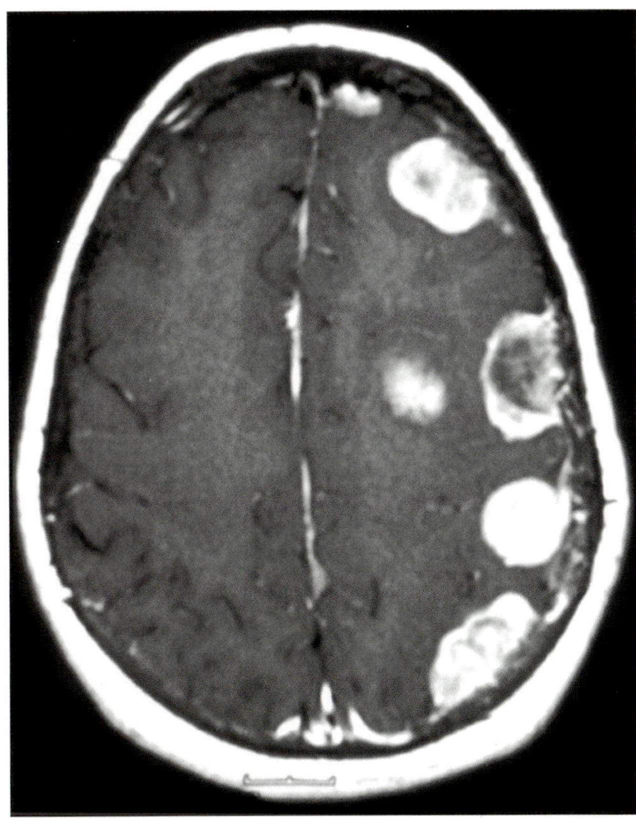

Fig. 14.39: Axial-enhanced MRI scan demonstrating multiple meningiomas in a case of NF2

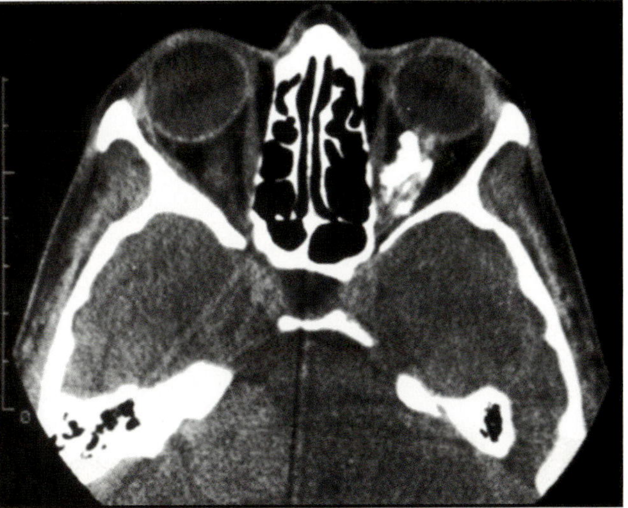

Fig. 14.40: Axial CT of optic meningioma in the left orbit in a case of NF2

Fig. 14.38: Gadolinium DTPA-enhanced axial MRI scan showing bilateral large vestibular schwannomas in a patient with neurofibromatosis type 2 (NF2)

Rarely spectacular abdominal schwannomas are seen (Fig. 14.41).

Intrinsic spinal lesions may be unresectable (Fig. 14.42).

The dilemma in the management of this condition is polarized by the case illustrated in Figure 14.43 (Chang and Moffat, 2000). This 30-year-old female presented with a small meningioma en plaque on the right side where she had no hearing and total seventh nerve palsy. On the left side can be seen a very large cystic vestibular schwannoma, with normal hearing. She had bilateral optic neuromas and was blind in the right eye. Thus, she only had hearing and eyesight on the side of this enormous lesion (Fig. 14.43).

The Cambridge Surveillance Protocol for NF2 consists of an annual MRI head scan and review in a multidisciplinary tertiary referral clinic which includes skull base and neurosurgeons, geneticists and counselors. An initial MRI scan of the whole spine is followed by biannual scans in those patients with spinal tumors and repeat spinal scanning in those without only, if suspicious neurological symptoms and signs emerge. Annual audiometry, both pure tone and

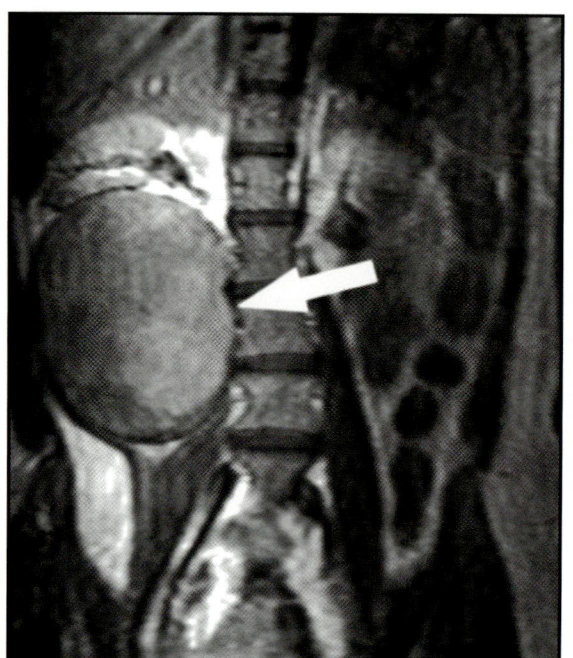

Fig. 14.41: MRI scan of large abdominal neurofibroma in a case of NF2 (white arrow)

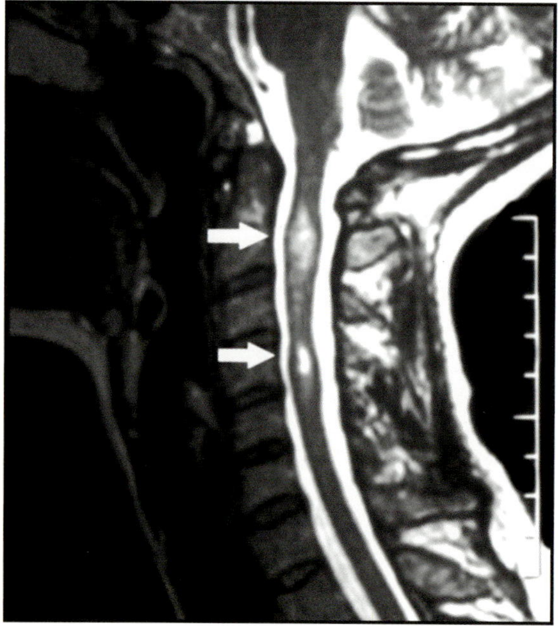

Fig. 14.42: Sagittal T2W MRI scan of spinal cord showing intrinsic spinal lesions in NF2 (white arrows)

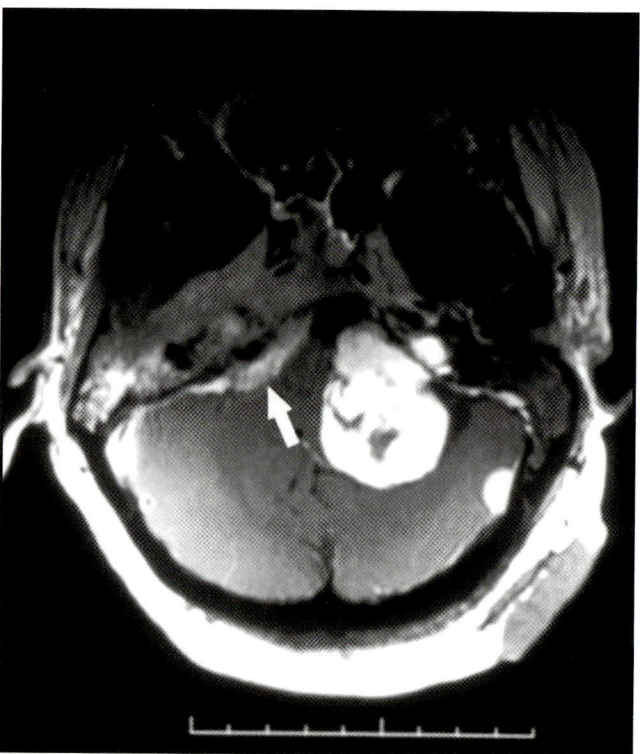

Fig. 14.43: Axial T2W MRI scan of female patient-aged 30 years with the Wishart type of NF2. Note the meningioma en plaque on the right (white arrow) where she had no hearing, a total facial palsy and a blind right eye due to bilateral optic gliomas. On the left side, there is a large vestibular schwannoma where serviceable hearing is present

speech audiograms and regular ophthalmic examinations are necessary (Evans et al. 2004).

Management options (Moffat et al. 2002) include:

- Regular surveillance with interval imaging
- Surgery to lesions causing threatening neurological compromise
- Auditory brainstem implantation as a "sleeper" if inserted at the time of excision of the first vestibular schwannoma and certainly for the second side
- Stereotactic radiotherapy has a limited place in the management of NF2. The results are not as good as in unilateral vestibular schwannoma and there is an increased risk of radiotherapy inducing malignant change in the tumor. Surgical excision of a tumor following stereotactic radiotherapy is associated with poor facial nerve results.

Lesions of the Temporal Bone

Cholesteatoma

Cholesteatoma of the temporal bone may be congenital or acquired.

Congenital Cholesteatoma

Congenital cholesteatomas arise from embryonic undifferentiated cells which differentiate into squamous cells. Historically, the term congenital cholesteatoma was reserved for those lesions of the cerebellopontine angle and petrous apex (Fig. 14.44). Although there is argument about the possible role of such embryonic epidermoid cysts in the genesis of middle ear cholesteatoma, most modern otologists and many pathologists believe this to be the case.

Cholesteatomas erode bone by three mechanisms:
1. Pressure on surrounding structures
2. The secretion of osteolytic enzymes
3. Osteitis due to surrounding granulation tissue.

The latter is likely only to be associated with acquired cholesteatomas.

Acquired Cholesteatoma

Primary acquired cholesteatoma refers to a lesion arising in the attic or posterosuperior part of the middle ear, when there has been no previous history of otitis media. Initially, whatever their mode of origin may be, these may be uninfected, certainly so long as the keratin desquamated within them can be shed to the

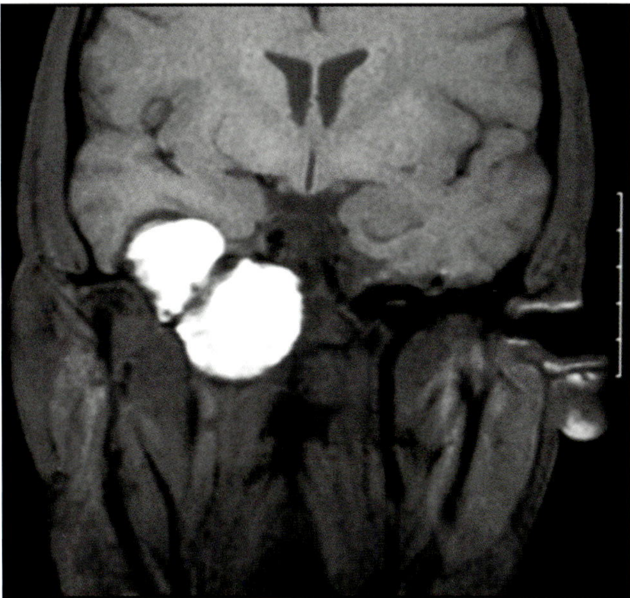

Fig. 14.44: Coronal MRI scan showing a large CPA cholesteatoma

external ear canal. The disease may be silent at this stage but eventually the keratin becomes moist and infected. The effect of surface infection on the skin from which it has been shed is to encourage more desquamation and to impair surface migration, so that yet more infected keratin accumulates. This will actively erode bone.

Secondary acquired cholesteatoma follows active middle ear infection, usually with large postero-marginal defects of the tympanic membrane. Since this type of cholesteatoma is infected from the start it becomes apparent early because of foul smelling often scanty otorrhea.

These cholesteatomas erode bone and may therefore cause facial palsy.

CT scanning reveals a mass of soft tissue density and it is difficult to differentiate this from mucosal thickening or fibrosis. Smooth "scalloped" erosion of bone may make the otologist suspicious. Advances in imaging and higher resolution scanning as well as the utilization of MRI B1000 or diffusion weighted images is helpful in differential diagnosis and the concomitant management of the patient.

The propensity for extension of the cholesteatoma to invade the otic capsule and beyond to the petrous apex (Fig. 14.45) (Atlas et al. 1992) makes imaging invaluable for surgical planning and patient counseling.

Involvement of the IAC may occur (Fig. 14.46) and this has great implications for the facial nerve, hearing and of course the risk of cerebrospinal fluid leakage.

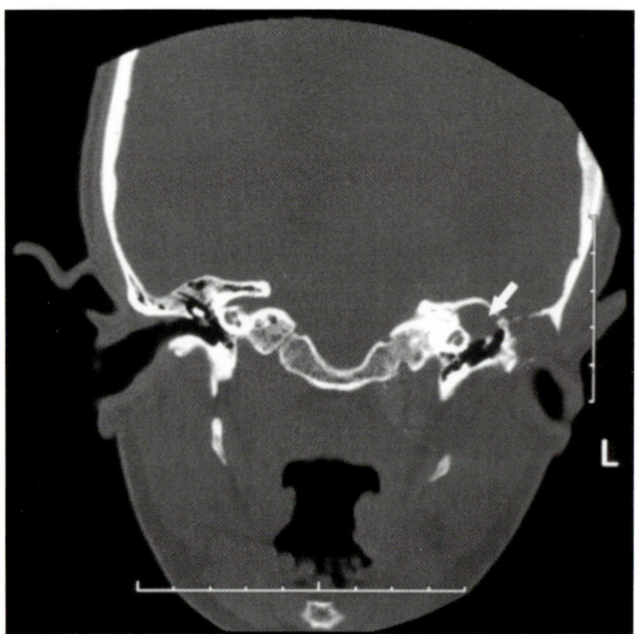

Fig. 14.45: Coronal CT scan showing extensive cholesteatoma in the left temporal bone. It is involving the otic capsule (white arrow)

Cholesterol Granuloma

MRI helps in differentiating cholesteatoma from cholesterol granuloma (Moffat et al, 1993). In cholesteatoma, the lesion is isointense or hypointense on the T1W image and hyperintense on the T2W image. In cholesterol granuloma, the lesion is hyperintense on both the T1W and T2W images (Figs 14.47 and 14.48).

In this patient, there is a bony defect in the middle fossa plate clearly seen on the coronal CT (Fig. 14.49).

The MRI scan shows what we have described as the "billiard pocket sign" (Quaranta et al, 2002). On the coronal T1W image, there is an area of hypointensity at the level of the middle fossa defect and also just superior to it in the middle fossa and above this an area of hyperintensity. Presumably, this represents cholesteatoma extending through the middle fossa defect with an associated cholesterol containing cyst (Figs 14.50 and 14.51).

Malignant Otitis Externa

This rare condition which may occur in diabetics produces a slowly expanding inflammatory granulomatous erosion of the temporal bone which

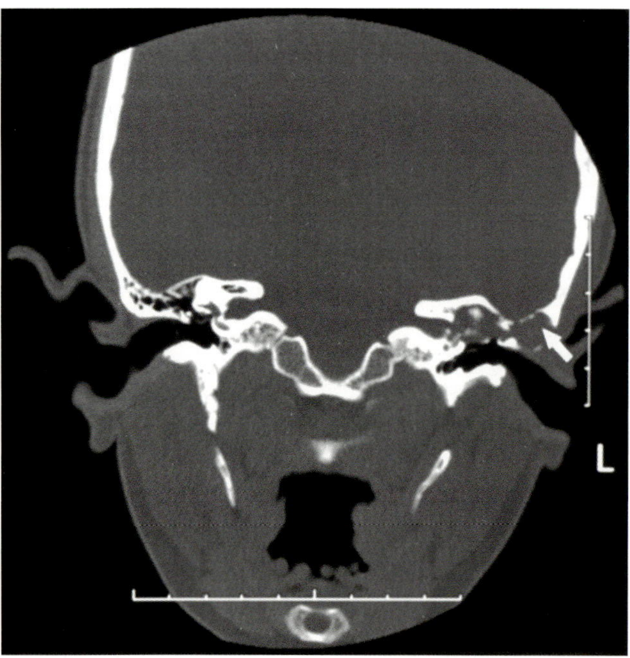

Fig. 14.46: Coronal CT of same patient revealing cholesteatomatous erosion into the IAC

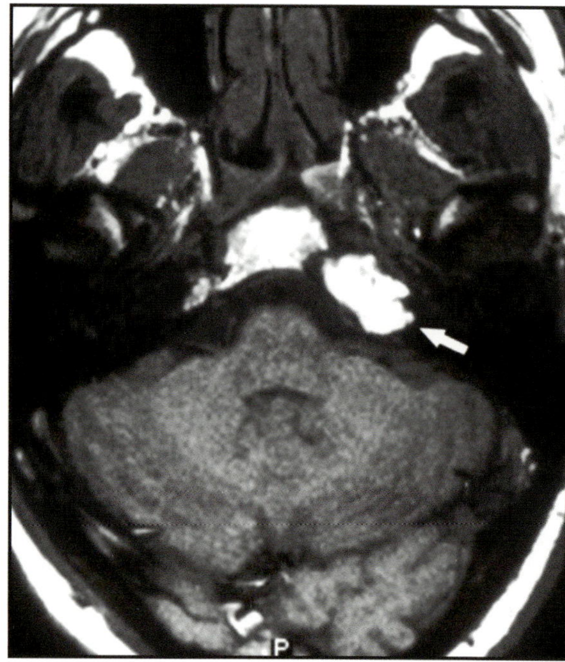

Fig. 14.47: Axial T1W MRI scan showing an hyperintense cholesterol cyst of the petrous apex (white arrow)

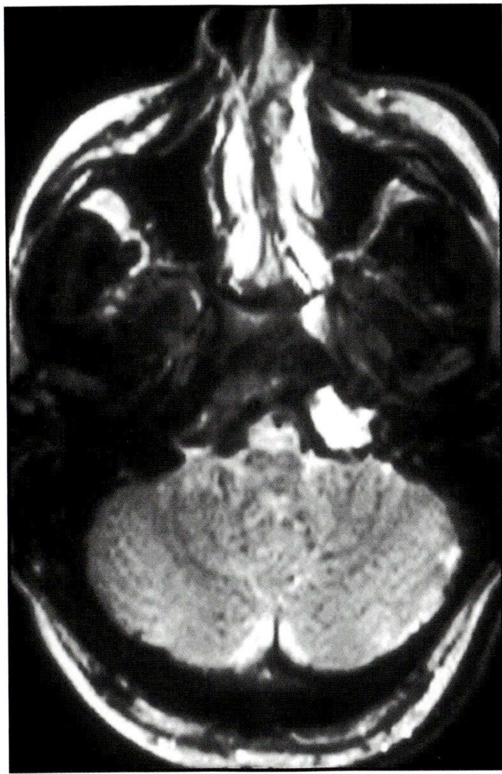

Fig. 14.48: Axial T2W MRI scan demonstrating that the lesion is also hyperintense on the T2W image

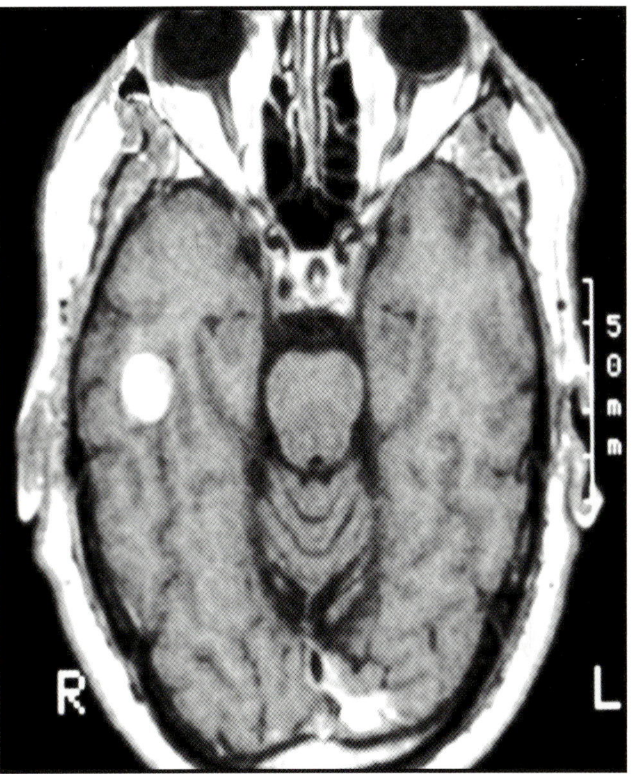

Fig. 14.50: Axial T1W MRI scan with an hyperintense lesion in the right middle cranial fossa

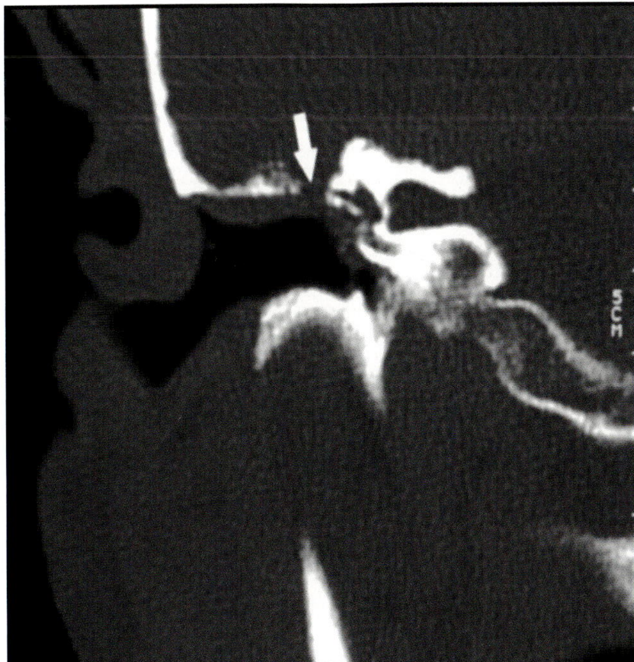

Fig. 14.49: Coronal CT scan of a patient with a cholesteatoma eroding through the middle fossa plate on the right side (white arrow)

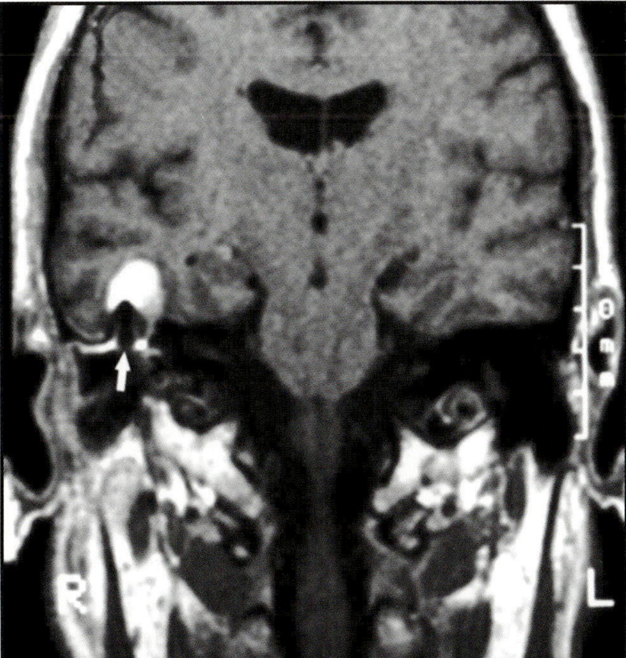

Fig. 14.51: Coronal view in the same patient with an hypointense area in the region of the defect and an hyperintense area superior to this (white arrow)

may extend and affect any of the structures in the temporal bone and CPA. A mass of soft tissue density with irregular erosion of bone are the features on CT. A lesion of high signal intensity is seen on MR imaging. Indium-labeled white cell scans will delineate the "hot spot" in the temporal bone and possibly the CPA. Loss of hearing, facial palsy and palsies of the last few cranial nerves may occur.

Wegener's Granulomatosis

The characteristic vasculitis in this condition tends to produce similar appearances on imaging to malignant otitis externa.

Benign Tumors of the Temporal Bone

Glomus Jugulare Tumors

Fisch types A, B and C involve the temporal bone but not the CPA (see lesions of CPA). The characteristic symptoms and signs and the features on imaging have already been described. A pulsatile mass in the middle ear may be caused by:
- Glomus tumors
- Lateral aberrant carotid artery
- High jugular bulb
- Middle ear adenoma.

These comprise the differential diagnosis (Moffat et al. 1989) and it is particularly important to exclude a lateral aberrant carotid artery (Fig. 14.52) and high jugular bulb (Fig. 14.53) in the management of these patients.

The "rising sun sign" may be seen in all of these conditions but typically in glomus tympanicum and glomus jugulare tumors (Fig. 14.54).

Glomus tympanicum tumors are confined to the middle ear (Fig. 14.54), arise out of the hypotympanum and do not erode the bone of the dome of the jugular bulb (Fig. 14.55) (Moffat et al. 1993).

Glomus jugulare tumors types B, C and D erode the jugular foramen (Figs 14.56 and 14.57).

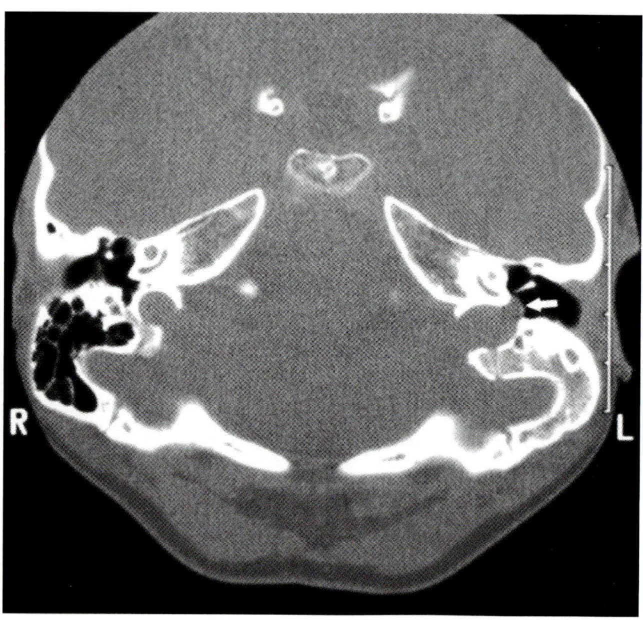

Fig. 14.53: Axial CT of high jugular bulb on the left side (white arrow)

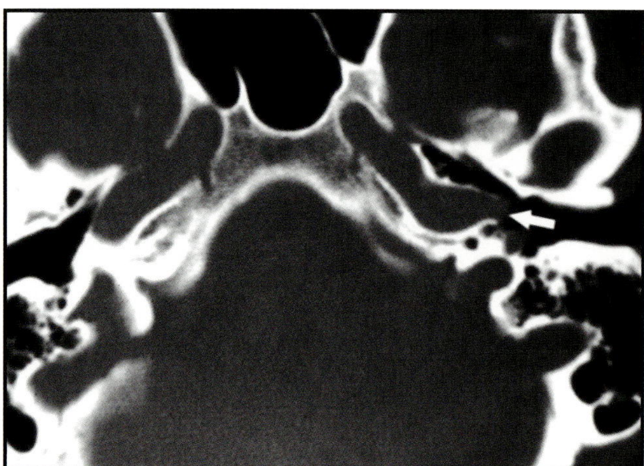

Fig. 14.52: Axial CT of temporal bones demonstrating an aberrant carotid artery on the left side (white arrow)

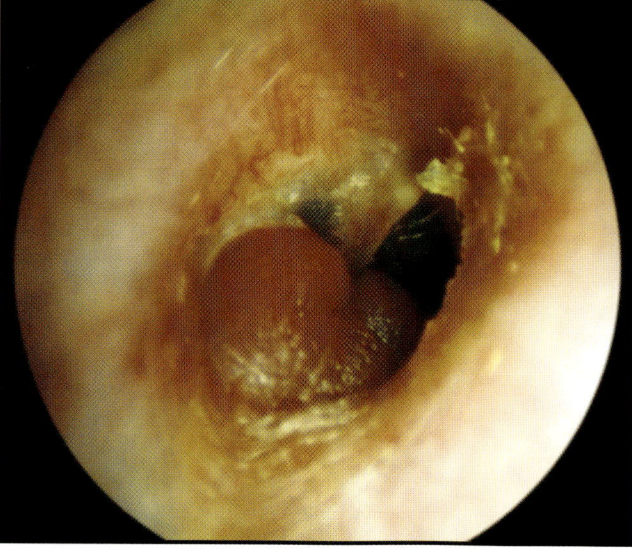

Fig. 14.54: Otoscopic view of "rising sun sign" seen in a glomus jugulare tumor

In non-chromaffin paragangliomas high resolution CT scanning delineates the exact extent of the bony erosion and MRI has the advantage of defining the soft tissue tumor mass in multiplanar images and allows assessment of the state of the carotid artery and defines intracranial extension (Fig. 14.58).

Extension into the neck (Figs 14.59 and 14.60) may erode the cervical vertebrae particularly in more aggressive tumors which tend to occur in the younger patient.

Carotid arteriography is still important for screening for concurrent, multicentric lesions, for defining the principle feeding vessels, the size and patency of the contralateral lateral sinus and purposes of preoperative or preradiotherapeutic embolization.

Figure 14.61 is a carotid arteriogram of a carotid body tumor showing the "Iyrebird sign" because the appearance is similar to the tail of a Iyrebird.

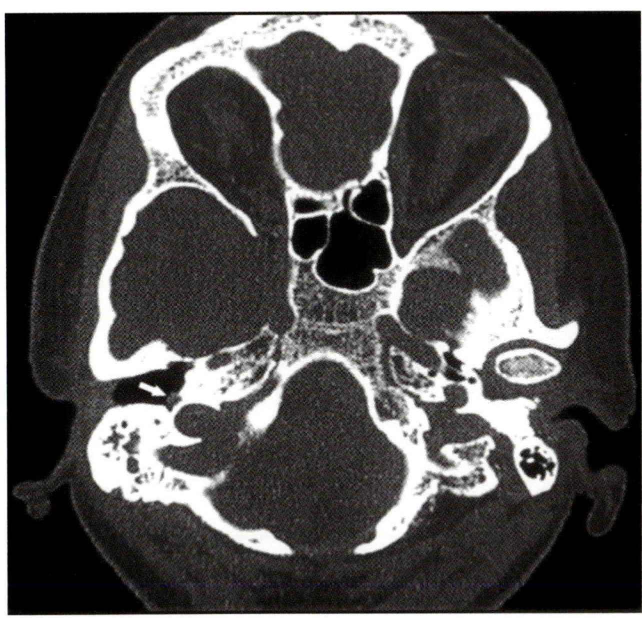

Fig. 14.55: Axial CT scan of right glomus tympanicum tumor (Fisch type A). There is no erosion of the jugular bulb (white arrow)

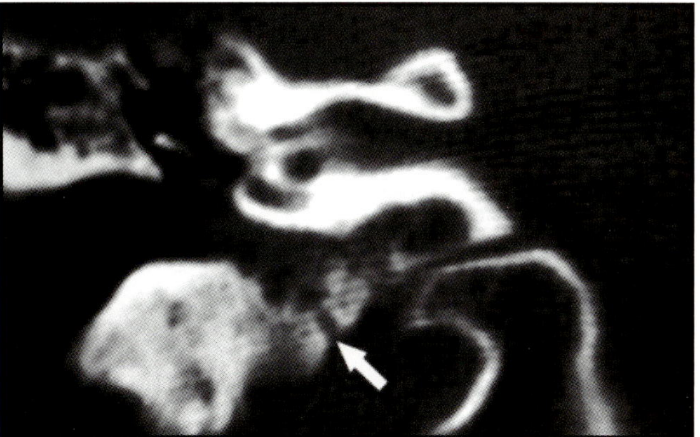

Fig. 14.57: Coronal CT with middle ear opacification due to a mass of soft tissue density eroding the dome of the jugular bulb (white arrow). This is an another example of a glomus jugulare tumor

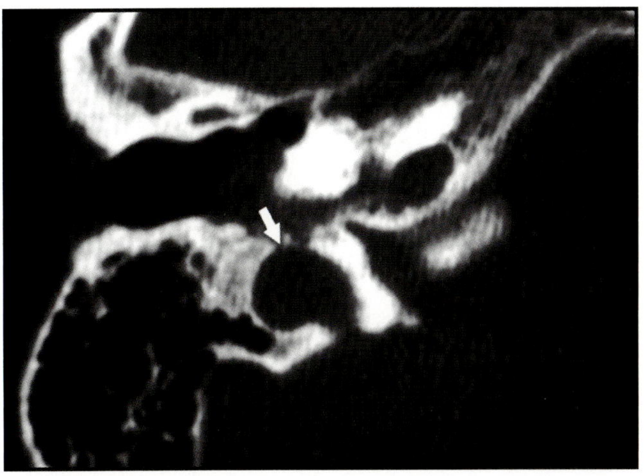

Fig. 14.56: Axial CT of glomus jugulare tumor on right side with erosion of the bone of the jugular bulb (white arrow)

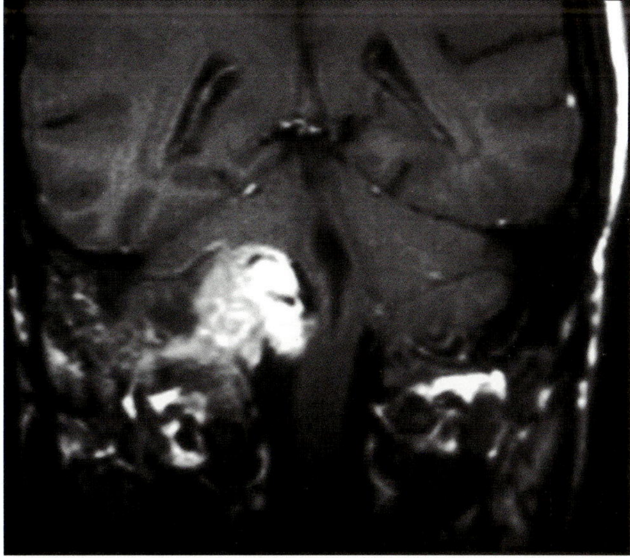

Fig. 14.58: Coronal T1W MRI scan of enormous Fisch type Di2 glomus jugulare tumor with marked brainstem compression and shift of the fourth ventricle

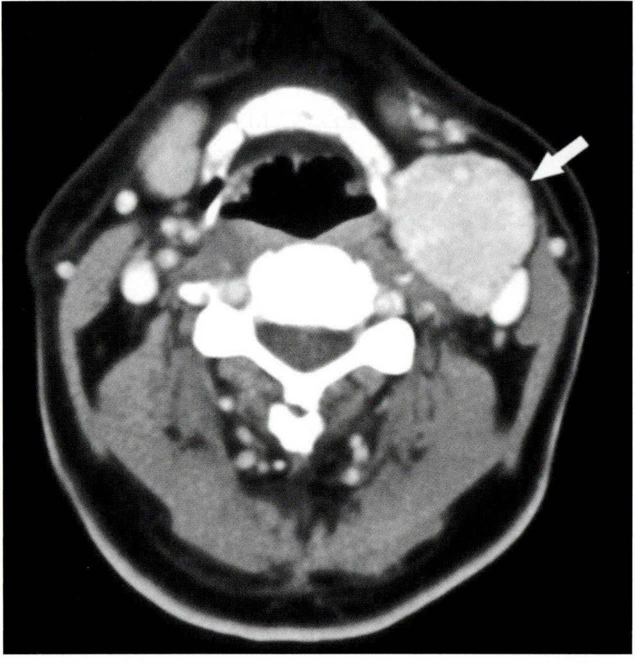

Fig. 14.59: Axial CT scan of the neck revealing the presence of a large soft tissue mass which is a glomus tumor (white arrow)

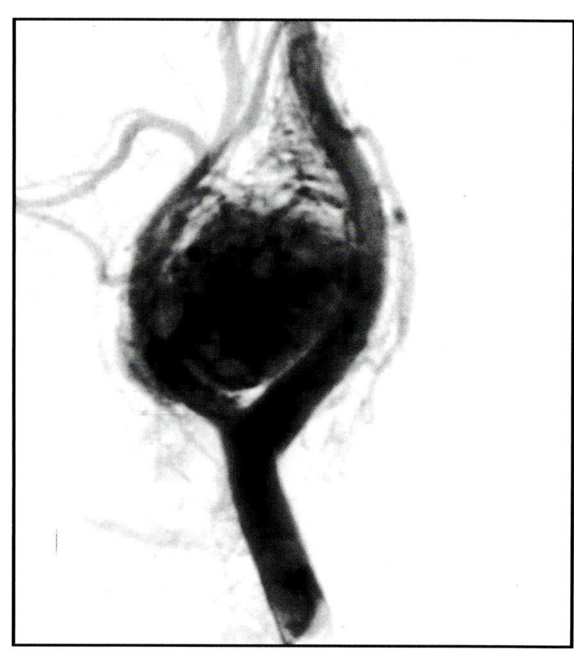

Fig. 14.61: Carotid body tumor producing the "lyre bird sign" on carotid arteriography

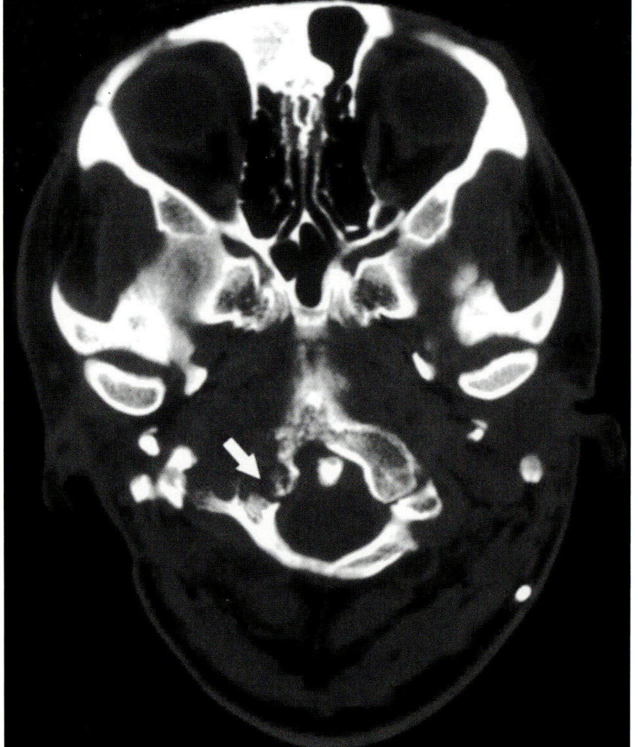

Fig. 14.60: Axial CT scan of the neck showing erosion of a cervical vertebra by a large glomus tumor in a young patient (white arrow)

Carcinoid Tumors

Carcinoid tumors (argentaffinoma) of the temporal bone are incredibly rare (Tabuchi, 2009). The small round, darkly staining cells are arranged in solid clumps or cylinders and acinar differentiation is unusual. If the cells are fixed freshly in formalin, special granules can be demonstrated with silver stains. Some carcinoid tumors are secreting and are associated with an endocrine syndrome characterized by episodic flushing, diarrhea, breathlessness and occasionally organic pulmonary stenosis. They are associated with the secretion of serotonin. They are benign tumors that pursue a very indolent course. CT scanning here in the axial plane reveals opacification with a mass of soft tissue density (Fig. 14.62). There is no bone destruction.

Glomus jugulare and carcinoid tumors look identical on imaging but have different immuno-histochemical characteristics which differentiate them.

Other Rare Benign Tumors

Solid

- Granular cell tumors
- Giant cell tumors (Yin et al. 2003)

- Adenoma of the middle ear (Mori et al. 2009)
- Myxoma of the middle ear (Zehlicke et al. 2008)
- Lipoma of the middle ear (Kasbekar et al. 2008)
- Chondroblastoma of the temporal bone (Tsutsumi et al. 2010)
- Cavernous lymphangioma (Hirai et al. 2010)
- Chondromyxoid fibroma (Thompson et al. 2009)
- Langerhans cell histiocytosis
- Extradural meningioma
- Endolymphatic sac tumor (Bell et al. 2010)

All these tumors are benign and patients present with a mass of soft tissue density in the temporal bone. They are distinguished histopathologically.

Cystic

- Cholesterol cyst of petrous apex (Ozturk et al. 2005)
- Aneurysmal bone cyst (Sabatini, 2005).

Primary Malignant Tumors of the Temporal Bone

Squamous Carcinoma

These difficult very aggressive malignant tumors of the temporal bone have a very poor prognosis and a low 5-year survival (Moffat et al. 1997). They have an incidence of 0.8 per million per year in males and are slightly more common in females with an incidence of 1 per million.

An exophytic, bleeding, painful mass in the external auditory canal (Fig. 14.63) or middle ear/mastoid are the characteristic features and facial nerve palsy may be a relatively early sign.

They have a propensity to spread superiorly through the tegmen or middle fossa plate (Fig. 14.64) and may invade dura (Fig. 14.65) and subsequently the temporal lobe of the brain.

In order to improve the 5-year survival, these tumors need radical excision by an extended temporal bone resection (Figs 14.66 to 14.68) with flap repair of the defect and postoperative radiotherapy (Moffat and Wagstaff 2003).

In the elderly, a very long procedure should be avoided and a scalp rotation flap may be necessary. Free-flap repair is very successful in the younger patient

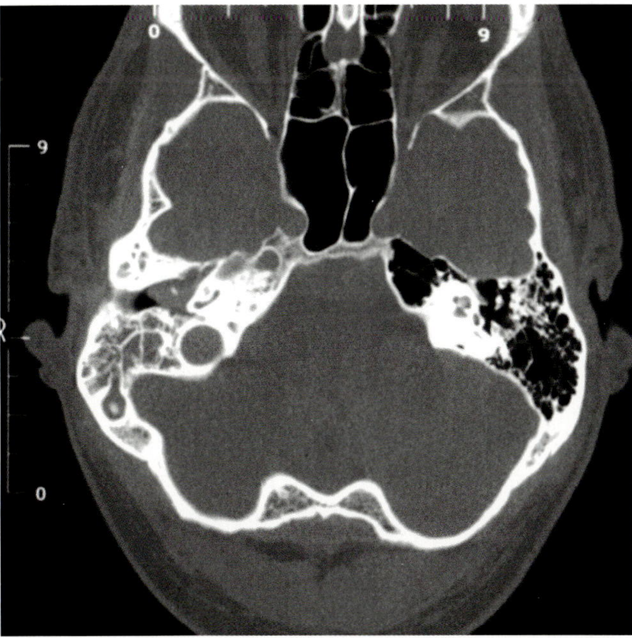

Fig. 14.62: Axial CT scan of a patient with a carcinoid tumor of the temporal bone. This presents as a mass of soft tissue density with no erosion of the bony trabeculae

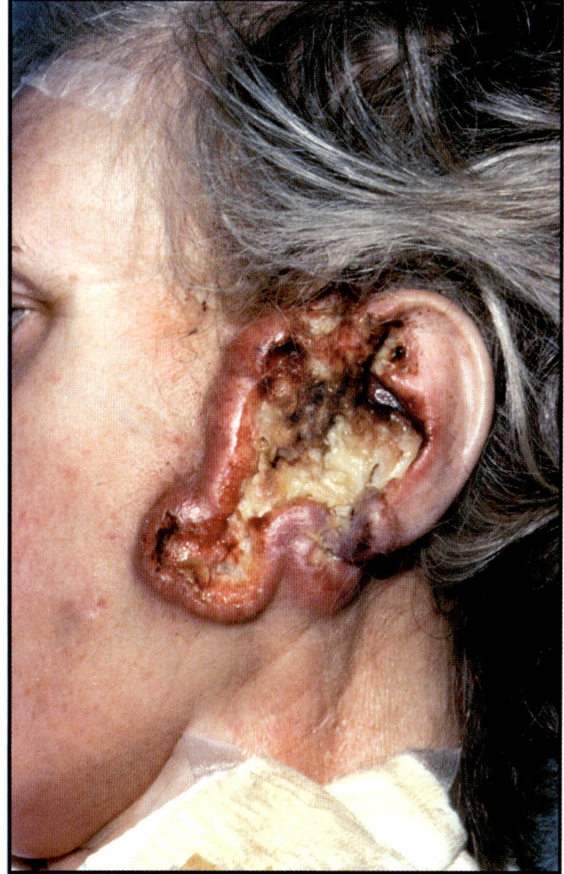

Fig. 14.63: Appearance of an advanced squamous carcinoma (SCC) of the temporal bone. Note the ulcerated fungating tumor with rolled edges

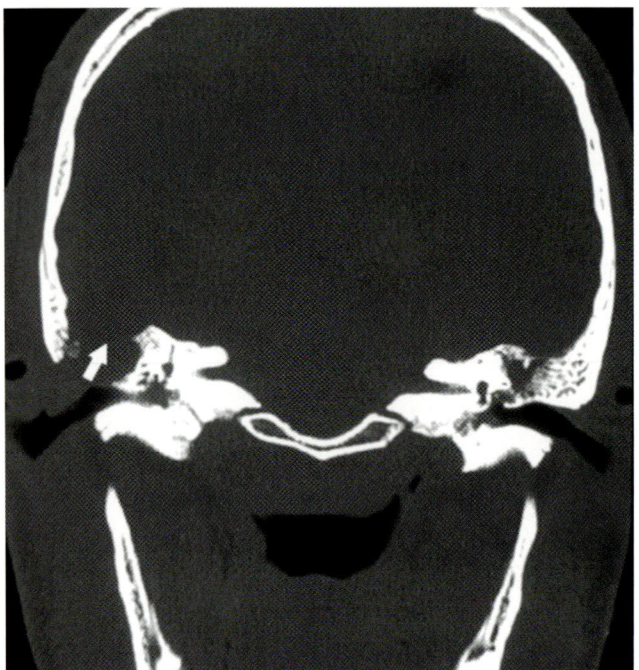

Fig. 14.64: Coronal CT of SCC of temporal bone. There is marked erosion of the middle fossa plate and extension into the middle cranial fossa (white arrow)

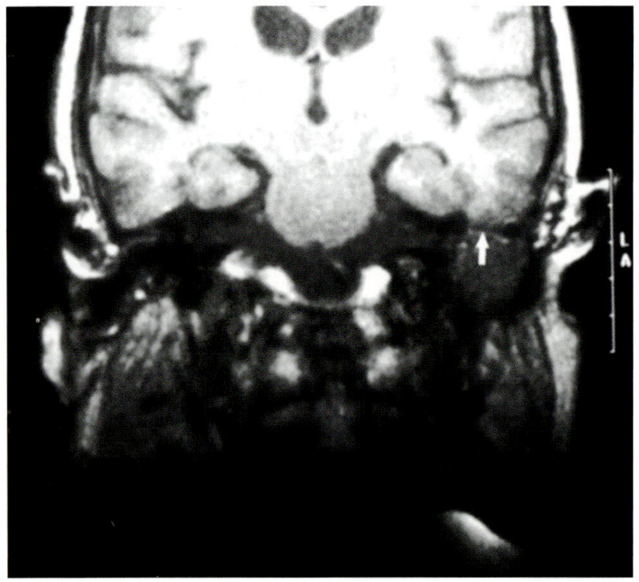

Fig. 14.65: Coronal T1W MRI scan of SCC of left temporal bone eroding into the middle cranial fossa and involving the dura and temporal lobe (white arrow)

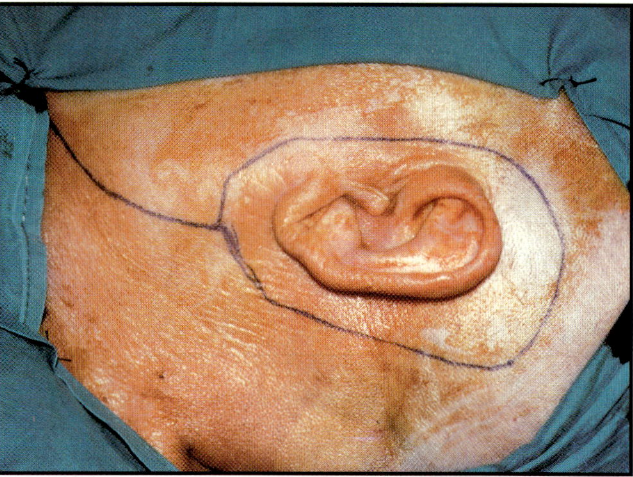

Fig. 14.66: Incision for extended temporal bone resection for SCC of temporal bone. An oval 10 × 8 cm is marked out on the skin with a tail into the neck in a skin crease

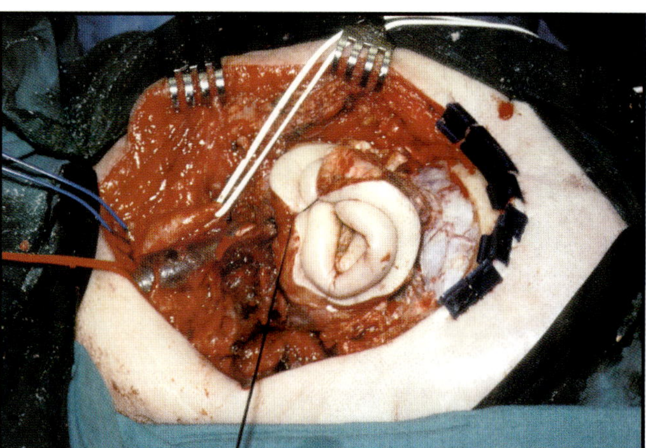

Fig. 14.67: Slings are placed around the great vessels to obtain vascular control and the whole temporal bone is excised along with the head of the mandible, glenoid fossa, ascending ramus of mandible and a total parotidectomy is also performed. It may be necessary to excise involved dura widely and also a part of the temporal lobe of the brain if this is involved by tumor. The venous sinus and the ninth, tenth and eleventh cranial nerves may also have to be sacrificed to obtain a clear margin

and the "modified Chinese flap" based on the anterior cubital artery (Figs 14.69 to 14.71) rather than the classical distal radial flap has been applied very successfully.

Free trapezius, anterolateral forearm and anterolateral thigh free flaps have been used more recently in the series and have an advantage that the donor site can be closed primarily and does not require split skin grafting (Moffat and Wagstaff, 2002).

Prosthetic ears can produce remarkable cosmesis but in some climates require a summer and a winter ear (Figs 14.72 and 14.73).

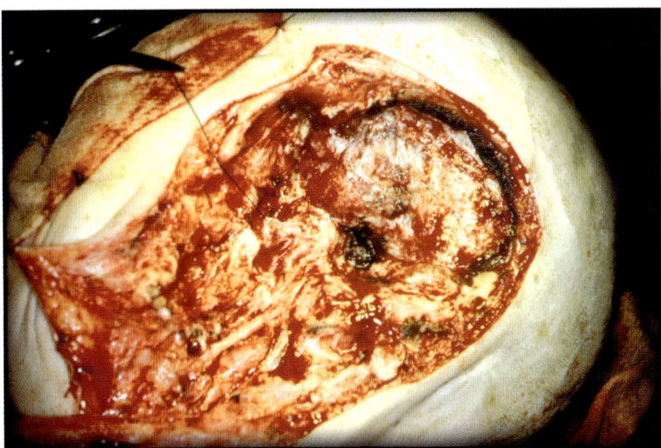

Fig. 14.68: This is the surgical defect after the resection. The dural defects are grafted with fascia lata and the wedge-shaped defect is obliterated with fat and fascia lata prior to flap repair

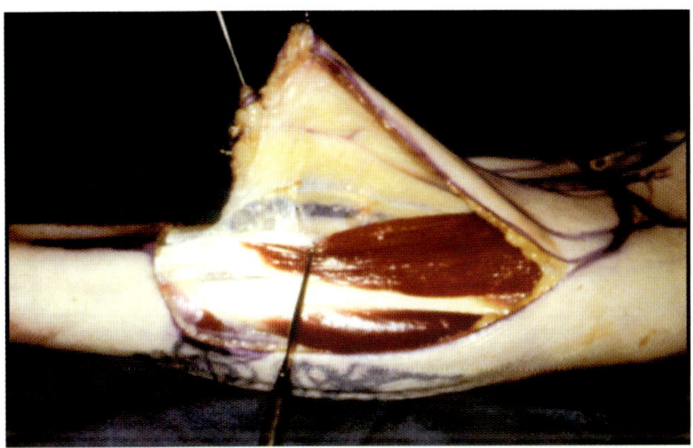

Fig. 14.69: Modified Chinese flap-based on the anterior cubital artery being raised

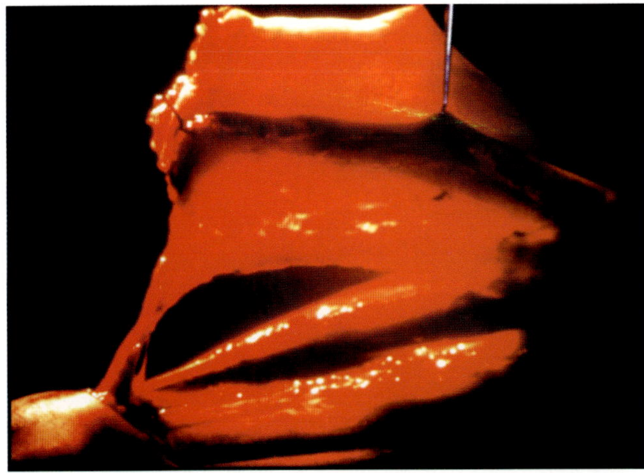

Fig. 14.70: Transillumination of the vascular pedicle

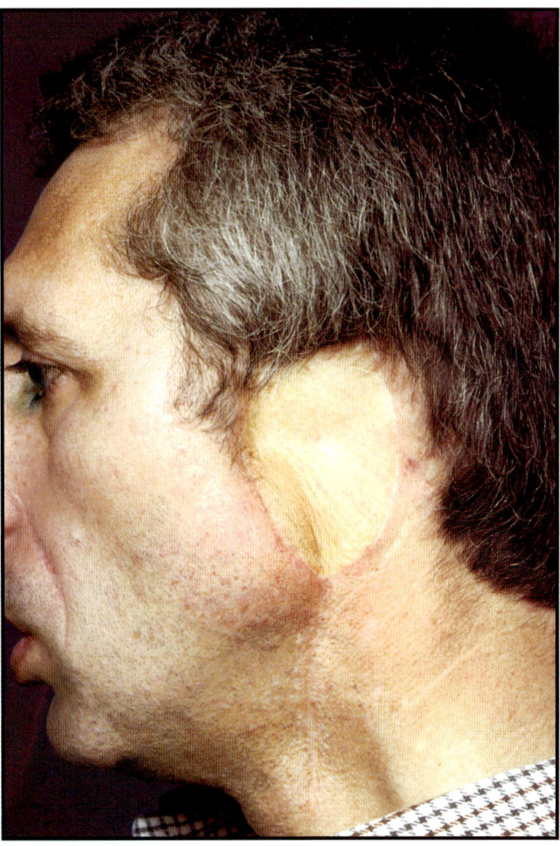

Fig. 14.71: The excellent cosmetic result of the free-flap repair

Chondrosarcoma

Chondrosarcoma of the skull base is a rare, aggressive, malignant tumor. Embryologically, the skull base ossifies predominantly endochondrally, whereas, the vault ossifies intramembranously. Cartilage rests around the foramen lacerum may be the progenitors of chondrosarcoma. There is an equal gender distribution and the tumors most commonly arise in the 4th and 5th decades and present with headache, hearing loss, dysphonia or diplopia. Cranial nerve deficits are common.

CT and MRI are used in a complimentary fashion in differential diagnosis and for the evaluation of the size and extent of the lesion. CT scanning delineates the bony destruction which occurs in 50% and in 60% and the isodense lesion shows areas of calcium stippling. There is only mild contrast enhancement.

MRI demonstrates the soft tissue component best and provides information on the surrounding neurovascular structures. Chondrosarcomas are usually of low to intermediate signal intensity on the

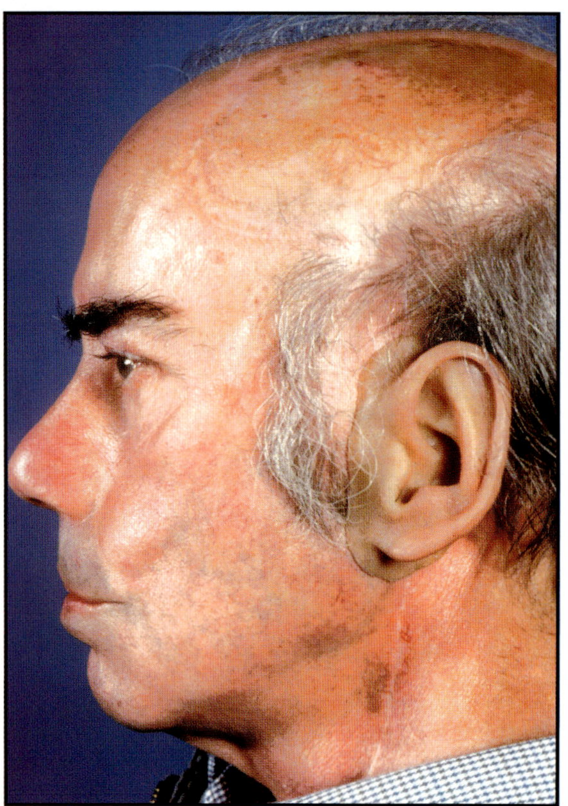

Fig. 14.72: Prosthetic ear has to be glued in place since there is no bone to osseo-integrate a titanium post. This is the summer ear

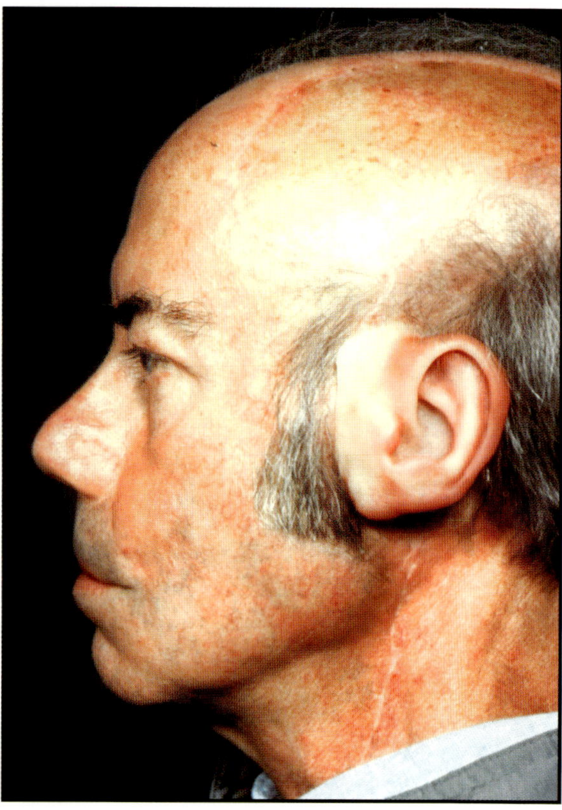

Fig. 14.73: In many climates, a winter ear is required since there is no bone to osseo-integrate a titanium post. This is the winter ear

T1 weighted sequence but are hyperintense on the T2W images. These MR imaging characteristics of a chondrosarcoma of the petrous apex and clivus are illustrated (Fig. 14.74). There is marked contrast enhancement with gadolinium DTPA.

Surgical excision is the treatment of choice for chondrosarcoma.

Chordoma

These are also rare and aggressive neoplasms which arise from the notochord. There are three types:
1. Conventional
2. Chondroid
3. De-differentiated (atypical).

The majority arise from the spheno-occipital synchondrosis. They occur twice as commonly in males as females and most often in the 4th and 5th decades of life. Headache and diplopia are the most common presenting symptoms and any of the cranial nerves can be affected.

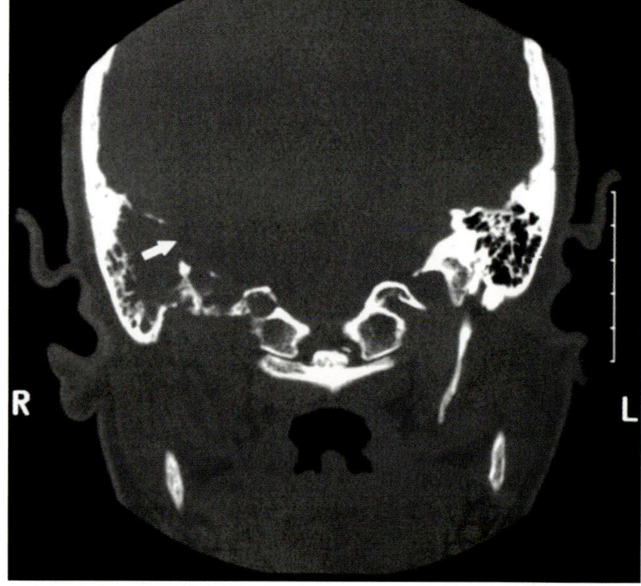

Fig. 14.74: The soft tissue mass eroding the right temporal bone is due to a metastasis and can be seen on this axial CT scan (white arrow)

CT and MR imaging assess the extent of bone erosion and the soft tissue mass, respectively. CT may show foci of calcification, bony sequestra and destruction without reactive sclerosis. Significant areas of low attenuation are common secondary to the high mucinous content.

MR imaging demonstrates a heterogeneous, predominantly low signal intensity mass on the T1-weighted image although it can be of high signal intensity if the mucin content is high. The signal is high on the T2-weighted image and the areas of low signal are due to degraded blood, bony sequestra and fibrous tissue. These radiological features of a chordoma can be clearly seen illustrated in Figure 14.75.

Radical surgical removal offers the best chance of disease free survival but adjunctive radiation therapy may be used postoperatively to improve outcome or for palliation. Chemotherapy is not effective in treatment of chordomas.

Rhabdomyosarcoma

Eighty percent of rhabdomyosarcomas present in children under the age of 12 with an average age at presentation of 4 years. Patients present with recalcitrant otitis media and mastoiditis with a mass in the region of the ear, aural polyp, otalgia, bleeding from the ear and deafness. Facial paralysis occurs in 14% of cases (Tsokos,1992) (Reid et al. 2006). CT scanning shows an infiltrative bony destruction and a soft tissue enhancing mass. MR imaging reveals homogeneous intermediate signal intensity that is hypointense relative to fat and isointense relative to muscle on the T1-weighted image and hyperintense on T2W sequences.

Five-year survival rates, which used to be very low (14% for head and neck tumors), have improved dramatically with multimodal therapy and now stand at 65%. Surgical intervention for deep tissue biopsy, radiation therapy and chemotherapy has increased disease-free survival.

Ewing's Sarcoma of the Temporal Bone

This is less common than rhabdomyosarcoma and exceptionally rare in the temporal bone. On CT imaging, the isodense mass surrounded by hypodense areas of hyperostosis enhances homogeneously. On MRI, it is hypointense on the T1-weighted image and of mixed intensity on the T2-wighted image. It enhances with gadolinium DTPA.

Secondary Malignant Tumors of the Temporal Bone

Secondary tumors in the temporal bone are present in 27% of patients with advanced malignancy (Figs 14.76 and 14.77) (Moffat et al. 1993). They are usually overshadowed by the primary growth and other metastatic lesions. The endochondral layer of the bone is resistant to invasion. The most common sites of origin are:
- Breast
- Kidney
- Lung
- Stomach
- Larynx
- Prostate
- Thyroid.

The most common sites for metastatic involvement of the temporal bone are:
- IAC
- Mastoid portion
- Tympanic portion
- Labyrinthine portion.

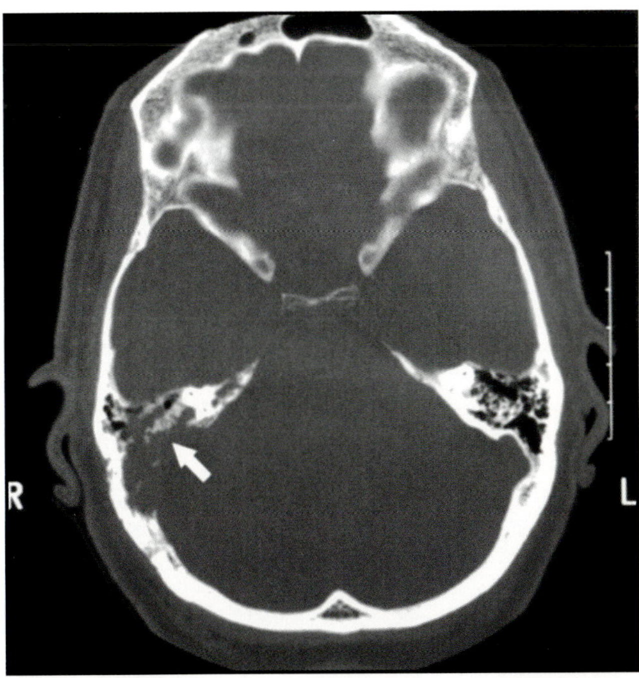

Fig. 14.75: The coronal CT image clearly demonstrates the extent of the bone erosion (white arrow)

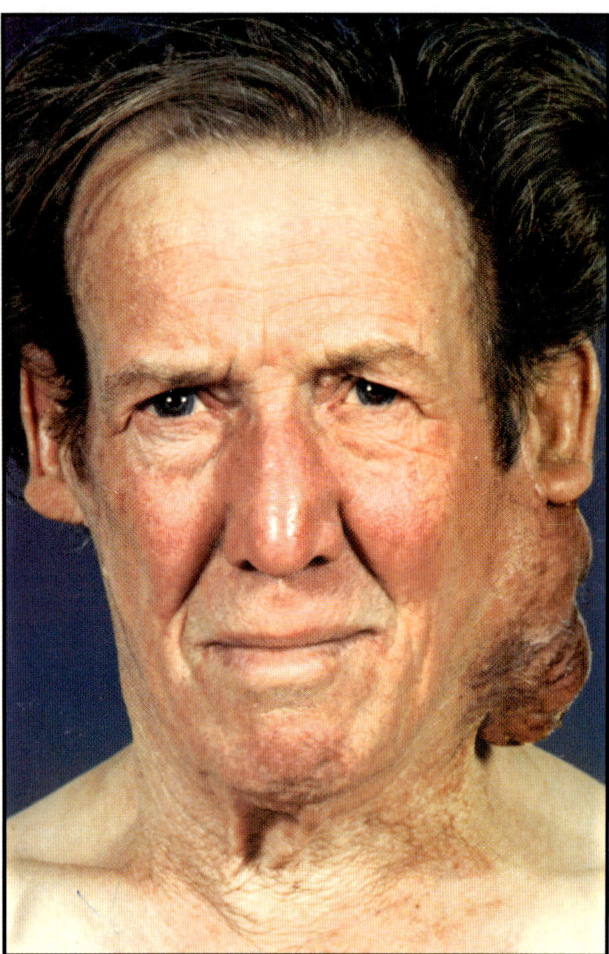

Fig. 14.76: Large malignant adenoid cystic carcinoma of the parotid salivary gland

Lesions of the Parotid

These may affect the pes anserinus or the distal intraparotid portion of the facial nerve.

Tumors of the Parotid

Primary Malignant

About 80% of occult primary lesions of the parotid are malignant (Figs 14.78A and B). Non-malignant lesions can produce a facial palsy due to pressure, kinking, inflammation and local toxic effects.

SURGICAL APPROACHES FOR FACIAL NERVE PALSY

The surgical approach depends upon the pathology, its site and extent and the results of high resolution imaging. The following surgical approaches may be utilized:

- Translabyrinthine
- Transcochlear
- Retrosigmoid
- Middle fossa
- Transmastoid
- Transmastoid-middle cranial fossa
- Infratemporal
- Lateral/subtotal/total petrosectomy
- Parotidectomy.

It is useful to adopt a combination of approaches in some instances.

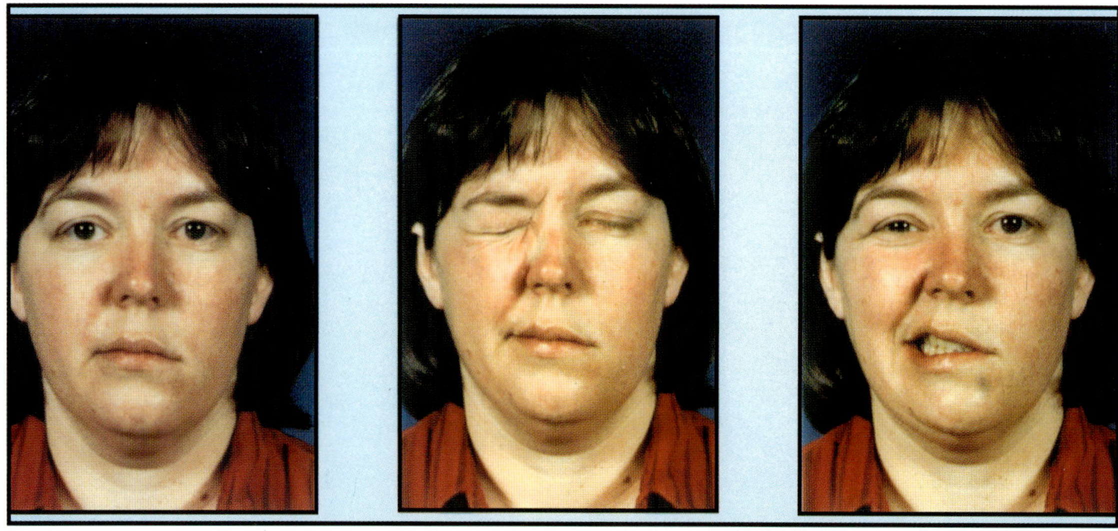

Fig. 14.77: House-Brackmann grade III facial palsy

FACIAL NERVE REHABILITATION

If more than 75% of the nerve can be preserved intact then recovery is likely to be satisfactory and at least a House-Brackmann grade III (Figs 14.79A and B) can be achieved with good eye closure. If more than 25% of the nerve is damaged it may be better to consider excision of the damaged segment with primary anastomosis if enough length can be obtained by taking the nerve out of the fallopian canal. If not or if a large segment of the nerve has to be excised then it may be necessary to consider grafting with greater auricular or sural nerve.

CONCLUSION

A total facial palsy is a very significant neurological deficit which leads to a considerable reduction in the patient's quality of life. This chapter has described in detail the presenting symptoms and signs and findings on imaging of all the interesting tumors which may result in a facial palsy throughout the length of the facial nerve. The surgical approaches which may be considered to excise the various pathologies have been mentioned but not described in detail since this was not the remit of this chapter. The clinical aspects of these tumors have been presented and are based on

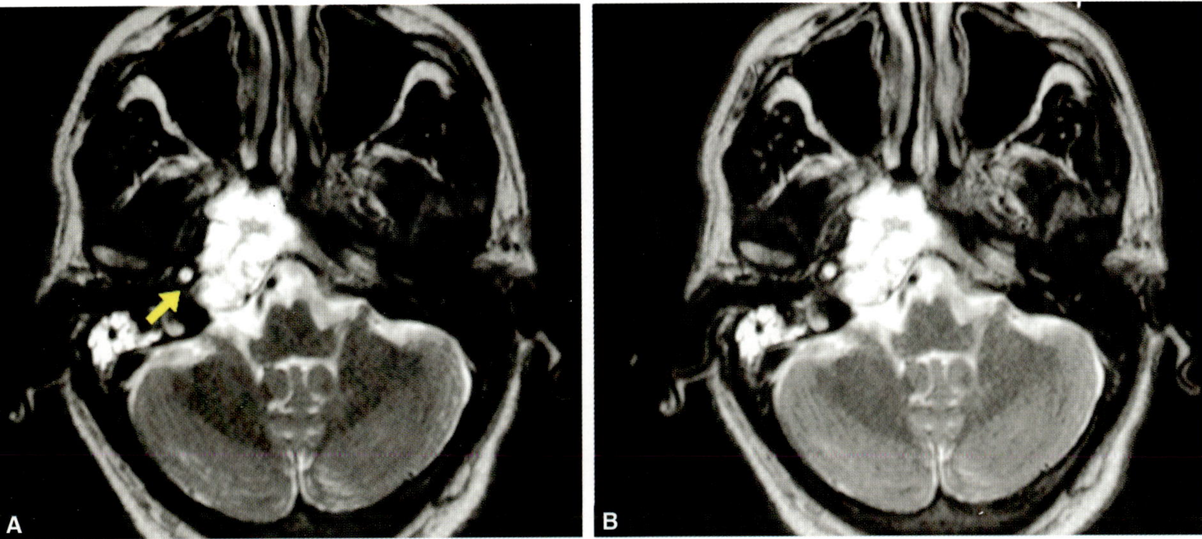

Figs 14.78A and B: Axial T2-weighted MRI scan of a chondrosarcoma in the anterior CPA and clival region. This heterogeneous lesion is mostly hyperintense. The high signal in the mastoid is due to fluid secondary to tumoral obstruction of the Eustachian tube

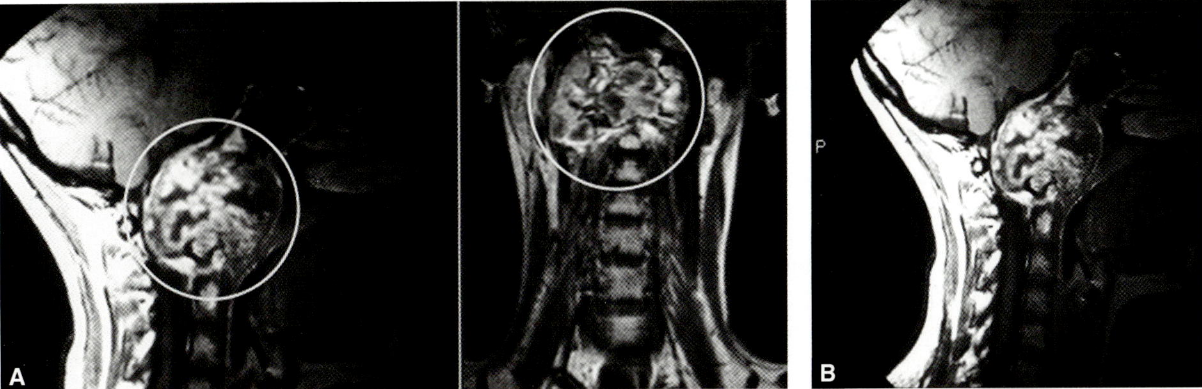

Figs 14.79A and B: Sagittal T2-weighted MRI scan illustrating the imaging characteristics of a large chordoma. Note the heterogeneity of the tumor which is largely hyperintense with some areas of hypointensity

the author's own experience in the Department of Otoneurological and Skull Base Surgery at Cambridge University Hospital over the last 23 years.

BIBLIOGRAPHY

1. Amirjamshidi A, Hashemi SM, Abbassioun K. Schwannoma of the greater superficial petrosal nerve. J Neurosurg. 2010;113(5):1093-8.

2. Atlas MD, Moffat DA, Hardy DG. Petrous apex cholesteatoma: diagnostic and treatment dilemmas. Laryngoscope. 1992;102(12 Pt 1):1363-8.

3. Baguley DM, Moffat D, Tsui YN. Audiological findings in medial and lateral acoustic neuromas. Br J Audio. 1989;23(2):158-9.

4. Baguley DM, Beynon GJ, Grey PL, et al. Audio-vestibular findings in CPA Meningioma. Proceedings of the 2nd International Conference on Acoustic Neuroma and 2nd European Skull Base Society Congress, Paris, April 22-6, 1995. Edited by JM Sterkers, R Charachon and O Sterklers Kugler Publications, Amsterdam/New York/Paris 1995;95-7.

5. Bakar B. The jugular foramen schwannomas: review of the large surgical series. J Korean Neurosurg Soc. 2008;44(5):285-94.

6. Bell D, Gidley P, Levine N, et al. Endolymphatic sac tumor (aggressive papillary tumor of middle ear and temporal bone): sine qua non-radiology-pathology and the university of Texas MD Anderson Cancer Center experience. Annals of Diagnostic Pathology. 2010(12). (Epub ahead of print).

7. Beynon GJ, Baguley DM, Moffat DA, et al. Positional vertigo as a first symptom of a cerebellopontine angle cholesteatoma: A case report. Ear Nose Throat J. 2000;79(7):508-10.

8. Borba LA, Araujo JC, de Oliveira JG, et al. Surgical management of glomus tumors: a proposal for approach selection based on tumor relationships with the facial nerve. J Neurosurg. 2010;112(1):88-98.

9. Brackmann DE, Doherty JK. CPA melanoma: diagnosis and management. Otology and Neurotology. 2007;28(4):529-37.

10. Brewis C, Bottrill ID, Wharton SB, et al. Glomus jugulare tumor with metastases to cervical lymph nodes. J Laryngol Otol. 2000;114(1):67-9.

11. Chang P, Moffat DA. Neurofibromatosis Type 2: A 15-year experience and current review. Australian J Otolaryngol. 2000;3(5):528-42.

12. Diwan AG, Agarwal SI, Lakade SM, et al. Facial paralysis due to arachnoid cyst. J Assoc Physicians India. 2005;53:544.

13. Evans DGR, Baser M O'Reilly, B Rowe, et al. Management of the patient and family with neurofibromatosis type 2: a consensus conference statement. Lancet, in press, 2003.

14. Grey PL, Moffat DA, Hardy DG, et al. Audio-vestibular results after surgery for cerebellopontine meningiomas. Am J Otol. 1996;17(4):634-8.

15. Guilemany JM, Alobid I, Gaston F, et al. Cerebellopontine angle and internal auditory canal metastasis from ductal carcinoma of the breast. Acta otolaryngol. 2005;125(9):1004-7.

16. Gunther M, Dankwardt-Lilliestrom N, Gudjonsson O, et al. Surgical treatment of patients with facial neuromas-a report of 26 consecutive operations. Otol Neurotol. 2010;31(9):1493-7.

17. Harada T, Irving RM, Moffat DA, et al. Molecular Genetic Investigation of meningioma. Human Molecular Genetics. 1995;3(2):347-50.

18. Hardy DG, Macfarlane R, Baguley DM, et al. Surgery for acoustic neuroma. An analysis of 100 translabyrinthine operations. J Neurosurg. 1989;71(6):799-804.

19. Hardy DG, Macfarlane R, Baguley DM, et al. Facial nerve recovery following acoustic neuroma surgery. Br J Neurosurg. 1989;3(6):675-80.

20. Hirai R, ileda M, Kishi H, et al. A case of middle-ear cavernous lymphangioma with facial palsy. J Laryngol Otol. 2011;125(4):405-9. Epub 2010 Dec 16.

21. Huoh KC, Cheung SW. Chorda tympani neuroma. Otol Neurotol. 2010:31(7):1172-3.

22. Huy PT, Kania R, Duet M, et al. Evolving concepts in the management of jugular paraganglioma: a comparison of radiotherapy and surgery in 88 cases. 2009;19(1):83-91.

23. Irving RM, Moffat DA, Hardy DG, et al. Somatic NF2 gene mutations in familial and non-familial vestibular schwannoma. Human Molecular Genetics. 1994;3(2):347-50.

24. Irving RM, Harada T, Moffat DA, et al. Somatic neurofibromatosis Type 2 gene mutations and growth characteristics in vestibular schwannoma. Am J Otol. 1997;18(6):754-60.

25. Kasbekar AV, Donnelly N, Axon P. Facial nerve palsy secondary to middle-ear lipoma. J Laryngol Otol. 2008;122(6):e14.

26. Knapp FB, Rieh E, Spreer J, et al. Primary B-cell non-Hodgkin lymphoma of the internal auditory canal: case report and literature review. HNO. 2008;56(6):633-7.

27. Marzo SJ, Zender CA, Leonetti JP. Facial nerve schwannoma. Curr Opin Otolaryngol Head Neck Surg. 2009;17(5):346-50.

28. Moffat DA, Saunders JE, McElveen JT, et al. Unusual cerebellopontine angle tumors. J Laryngol Otology. 1993;107:1087-98.

29. Moffat DA, Croxson GR, Baguley DM, et al. Brun's bidirectional nystagmus in cerebellopontine tumors. Clin Otolaryngol Allied Sci. 1988;13(2):153-7.

30. Moffat DA, Hardy DG, Baguley DM. The strategy and benefits of acoustic neuroma searching. J Laryngol Otol. 1989;103(1):51-9.

31. Moffat DA, Hardy DG. Surgical management of large glomus jugulare tumors: The infra and transtemporal approach. J Laryngol Otol. 1989;103(12):1167-80.

32. Moffat DA, Irving RM, Hardy DG. Sudden deafness in acoustic neuroma. J Laryngol Otol. 1994;108(2): 116-9.

33. Moffat DA, Ballagh RH. Rare tumors of the cerebellopontine angle. Clinical Oncology of the Royal College of Radiologists. 1995;7(1):28-41.

34. Moffat DA, Hardy DG, Grey PL, et al. The operative learning curve and its effect on facial nerve outcome in vestibular schwannoma surgery. Am J Otol. 1996;17(4):643-7.

35. Moffat DA, Baguley DM, Beynon GJ, et al. Clinical acumen and vestibular schwannoma. Am J Otol. 1998;19(1):82-7.

36. Moffat DA. Moffat Classification of Facial Nerve Function. A Supplemental Issue for The 11th Keio University international Symposium for Life Sciences and Medicine. Consensus Meeting on Systems for Reporting Results in Acoustic Neuroma. Keio Journal of Medicine. 2001;50 (Suppl 4):38-9.

37. Moffat DA, Quaranta N, Baguley DM, et al. Management strategies in neurofibromatosis type 2. Eur Arch Otorhinolaryngol. 2002;260(1):12-8.

38. Moffat DA, Quaranta N, Baguley DM, et al. Staging and management of primary cerebellopontine cholesteatoma. J Laryngol Otol. 2002;116(5):340-5.

39. Moffat DA, Wagstaff SA. Squamous cell carcinoma of the temporal bone. Current Opinion in Otolaryngology and Head and Neck Surgery. 2003;11(2):107-11.

40. Moffat D, De R, Hardy DG, et al. Surgical management of trigeminal neuromas: a report of eight cases. J Laryngol Otol. 2006;120(8):631-7.

41. Monem SA, Chiossone-Kerdel JA, Moffat DA. Lipoma of the cerebellopontine angle; a case report. In: Sanna M, Taibah A, Russo A, et al (Eds). Proceedings of the Third International conference on Acoustic Neuroma and other CXPA Tumors Monduzzi Editore, SpA. Bologna. 1999;823-30.

42. Monksfield P, Martinez Devesa P, Molyneux A, et al. Vertebral artery aneurysm causing cerebellopontine angle mass effect. Otol Neurotol. 2005;26(3):525-7.

43. Mori E, Kojima H, Wada K, et al. Middle ear adenoma diagnosed by recurrent facial paralysis. Auris Nasus Larynx. 2009;36(1):75-8.

44. Ozturk O, Inanli S, Sehitoglu MA. Facial paralysis in a patient with cholesterol cyst of the petrous temporal bone. Otolaryngol-Head Neck Surg. 2005;133(4):643.

45. Quaranta N, Chang P, Moffat DA. Unusual MRI appearance of an intracranial cholesteatoma extension: the 'billiard pocket sign'. Ear Nose Throat J. 2002;81(9):645-7.

46. Quaranta N, Baguley DM, Axon PR, et al. Conservative Management of Vestibular Schwannomas. In: Baguley DM, Ramsden RT, Moffat DA (Eds). Fourth International Conference on Vestibular Schwannoma and other CPA Lesions. Conference Proceedings. Immediate Proceedings Ltd. 2003. pp: 256-7.

47. Quaranta N, Chang P, Baguley DM, et al. Audiological Presentation of Cerebellopontine Angle Cholesteatoma. J Otolaryngol. 2003;32(4):217-21.

48. Ray A, Lammie GA, Shone G, et al. Venous angioma of the facial nerve: a case report. Surg Neurology. 2004;61(2):198-200.

49. Reid SR, Hetzel T, Losek J. Temporal bone rhabdomyosarcoma presenting as acute peripheral facial nerve paralysis. Pediatr Emerg Care. 2006;22(10):743-5.

50. Sabatini PR, Horenstein MG, Oliveri CV, et al. Aneurysmal bone cyst of the temporal bone associated with reversible hemifacial paralysis. Am J Otolaryngol. 2005;26(4):261-4.

51. Samii M, Nakamura M, Mirzai S, et al. Cavernous angiomas within the internal auditory canal. J Neurosurg. 2006;105(4):581-7.

52. Semaan MT, Slattery WH, Brackmann DE. Geniculate ganglion hemangiomas: clinical results and long-term follow-up. Otol Neurotol. 2010;31(4):665-70.

53. Ramina R, Neto MC, Fernandes YB, et al. Surgical removal of small petroclival meningiomas. Acta Neurochirurgica (Wien). 2008;150(5):431-8.

54. Shaida AM, McFerran DJ, da Cruz M, et al. Cavernous haemangioma of the internal auditory canal. J Laryngol Otol. 2000;114(6):453-5.

55. Schrock A, Laffers W, Bootz F. Solitary metastasis of lung carcinoma to the internal auditory canal. Am J Otolaryngol. 2006;27(3):214-6.

56. Tabuchi K, Aoyagi Y, Umaetomari I, et al. Carcinoid tumors of the middle ear. J Otolaryngol Head Neck Surg. 2009;38(3):e91-4.

57. Thompson AL, Bharatha A, Aviv RI, et al. Laryngoscope 2009;119(7):1380-3.

58. Towfighi J, Sheehan J, Isaacson J. Facial nerve neuroma associated with hemangioma of the geniculate ganglion: case report and review of the literature. Journal of Otolaryngology. Head and Neck Surgery 2008;37(5):E148-50.

59. Tsokos M, Webber BL, Parham DL, et al. Rhabdomyosarcoma: a new classification scheme related to prognosis. Arch Pathol Lab Med. 116: 847-55.

60. Tsutsumi S, mishima Y, Nonaka Y, et al. A case of chondroblastoma arising from the temporal bone. No Shinkei Geka. 2010;38(11);1019-24.

61. Yin S, Gong S. Giant cell tumor of temporal bone: a report of 7 cases. Lin Chuang Er Bi Yan Hou Ke Za Zhi. 2007;17(10):596-7,599.

62. Zehlicke T, Punke C, Bolze C, et al. Transient facial palsy in two cases of benign, very rare middle ear tumors (carcinoid tumor and myxoma). Neurologist. 2008;14(1):52-5.

15

Facial Nerve Schwannoma

Ricardo F Bento, Anna Carolina O Fonseca

INTRODUCTION

Facial nerve schwannomas (FNSs) are very uncommon tumors with an estimated prevalence of 0.15-0.8% (Saito et al. 1972) and their early diagnosis is still considered a challenge. FNSs are extremely slow-growing tumors that tend to occur during middle age and show a slight male dominance (Chao et al. 2009). The fact that the facial nerve is resistant to compressions and has the capacity to maintain normal function after episodes of paralysis causes delays in the diagnosis of this tumor or may even result in misdiagnosis as inflammatory palsy or Bell's palsy. Moreover, as there are few complementary exams which are helpful in diagnosis, early diagnosis requires a high degree of clinical suspicion therefore, it is safer to assume that each case of facial nerve dysfunction is an expression of tumoral compression, until proven otherwise. Bell's palsy is an exclusion diagnosis.

The facial nerve has a long and tortuous course. It originates in the pons and has a short intracranial portion. Subsequently, it follows an extratemporal pathway, where it leaves the stylomastoid foramen and innervates the facial muscles. FNS can arise at any point along the facial nerve, from the oligodendrocyte-Schwann cell junction to the most distal aspect of the extra-temporal facial nerve and may also involve the peripheral nerve branches within the parotid gland. Intraparotid FNSs are rare and unsuspected neoplasms, comprising only 0.2-1.5% of all facial neoplasms (Marchioni et al. 2007). Cerebellopontine angle (CPA) facial schwannomas are infrequent tumors, accounting for less than 20% of facial schwannomas and about 3% of CPA tumors (Lassaletta et al. 2002).

Tumors that affect the facial nerve can be intrinsic (schwannoma, hemangioma), which originate in the facial nerve itself or extrinsic (cholesteatoma, vestibular schwannoma and meningeoma), which arise from structures adjacent to the nerve.

FNS is the most common intrinsic tumor and is responsible for around 70% of the tumors that arise from within the facial nerve. About 5% of the cases of peripheral facial paralysis are caused by tumors and as many as 50% of the patients with facial nerve tumors do not present with facial paralysis when they consult a physician (O'Donoghue et al. 2005).

The peri-geniculate area and the horizontal and vertical portions of the facial nerve are most often affected (O'Donoghue et al. 2005). In a study at the University of São Paulo (Formigoni et al. 1980, Bento, et al. 1998, Bento, et al. 1999), the geniculate ganglion was the most affected site, (Figs 15.1A to C) followed by the tympanic (Fig. 15.2) and mastoid segments (Figs 15.3A and B). Usually, FNS would have already affected more than one segment at the time of diagnosis and rarely originates in one of the facial nerve branches. This tumor arises from the Schwann cells in the nerve sheath. Although Schwann cells can undergo cytological changes with nuclear pleomorphism and simulate aggressivity, they do not undergo mitosis and, therefore, they are benign (Fig. 15.4). Malignant schwannomas of the facial nerve have occasionally been reported (O'Donoghue et al. 2005). They are only considered when there are areas of markedly increased hypercellularity with many mitosis (Schaitkin, 2000).

Facial nerve hemangioma is the most important condition in the differential diagnosis of facial nerve schwannoma. Facial nerve hemangiomas are very rare and arise from the vascular plexus along the facial nerve and the geniculate ganglion is the most affected site. Unlike schwannomas, even small osseous hemangiomas can produce facial paralysis; therefore, they are usually diagnosed with a small size, which is a very important feature. Because of their vascular origin, even small tumors may cause facial nerve

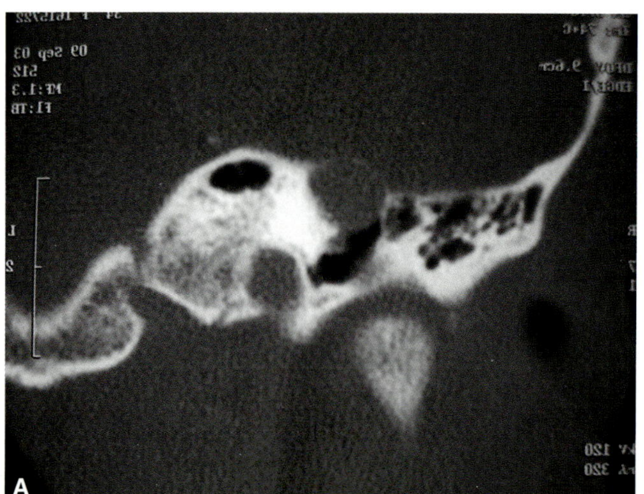

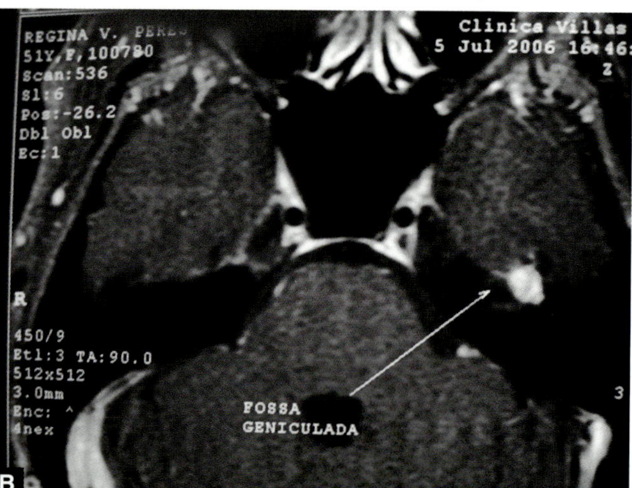

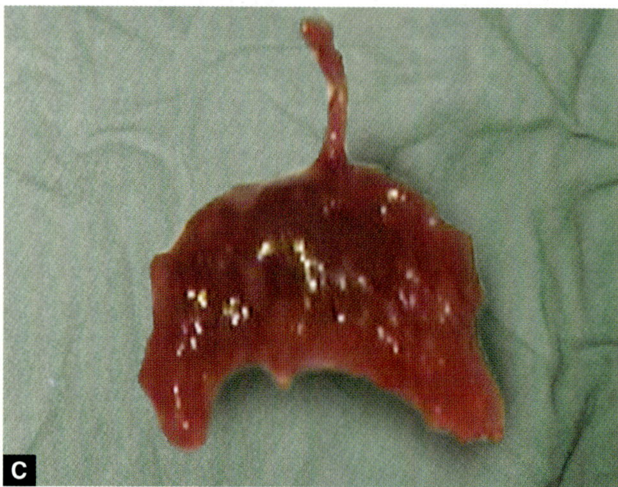

Figs 15.1A to C: Facial nerve schwannoma in the genicular ganglion area, (A) CT scan; (B and C) MRI and after removal showing the greater superior petrosal nerve

paralysis without compressing the nerve. Classically, the hemangioma is surrounded by newly formed bone, giving rise to its classic salt-and-pepper radiologic feature (Schaitkin, 2000). A FNS can be misdiagnosed as a vestibular schwannoma, especially when the tumor is confined to the internal auditory canal. There are no useful preoperative evaluation tools for precisely predicting the nerve origin of intracanalicular tumors (Park et al. 2007).

CLINICAL PRESENTATION

The two most common symptoms of FNS, facial weakness and hearing loss, are found in only half of the patients and tend to be found separately (McMonagle et al. 2008). Facial paralysis is the most

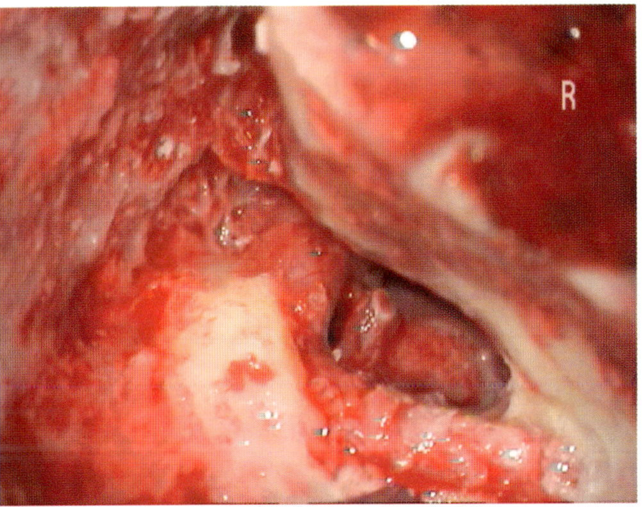

Fig. 15.2: Facial nerve schwannoma of the second portion, intratympanic cavity

important symptom of these tumors; therefore, utmost attention to the assessment of facial movement is essential in medical management. The unusual incidence of FNS, in addition to the high frequency of episodes of idiopathic peripheral facial paralysis, may result in misdiagnosis of FNS as a simple inflammatory episode.

The duration of the preoperative paralysis is the most important determinant of the outcome of any alternative approach for rehabilitation of facial function. It is of paramount importance to consider the possibility of a tumor in a patient with episodes of facial paralysis. Facial paralysis is usually presented as a slow progression of palsy over days or weeks, either before or followed by paresthesis or facial spasm. However, this cannot be considered as a rule for diagnosis. The practitioner will especially consider the diagnosis of FNS for a patient who presents with facial twitching (hyperkinesis) followed by a slowly progressive facial paralysis. However, FNS can present as sudden complete facial paralysis (Schaitkin, 2000). The recuperation of facial function after steroid treatment is also possible, thereby mimicking the characteristics observed in Bell's palsy.

Hearing loss can be caused by a tumor mass in the middle ear; conductive hearing loss occurs when the tumor affects the ossicular chain and the tympanic membrane and a sensorial hearing loss occurs when the labyrinth is eroded by the tumor. Although the incidence of otic capsule erosion has been reported to be 29%, the actual incidence of sensorineural hearing loss is not well-documented. The onset of facial nerve palsy is usually followed by sensorineural hearing loss

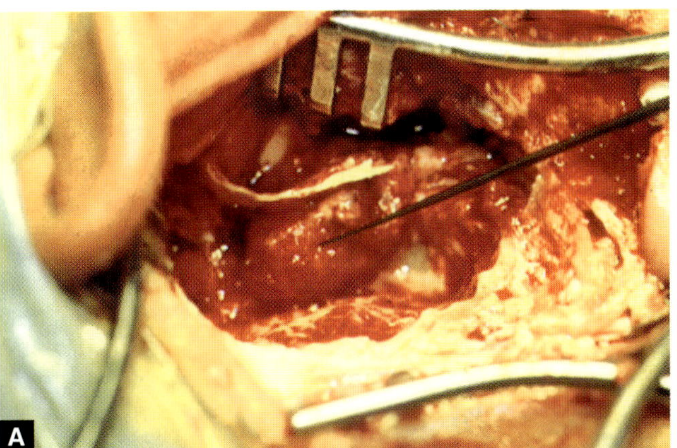

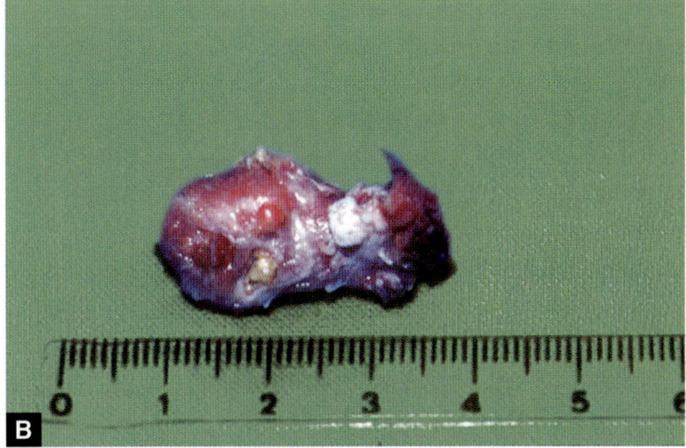

Figs 15.3A and B: FNS in the third portion of the facial nerve and after removal

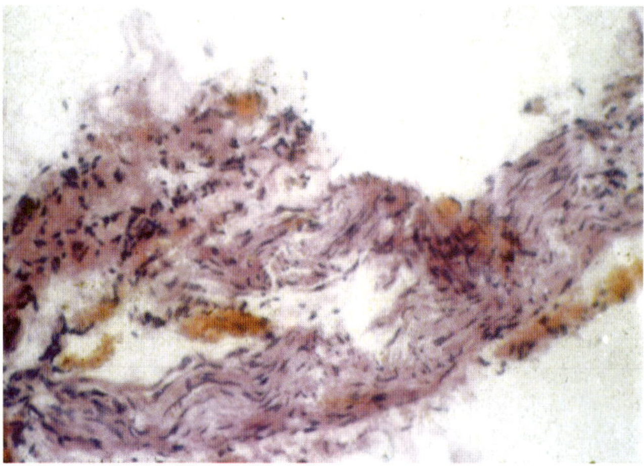

Fig. 15.4: Histologial section of a facial nerve schwannoma

secondary to a FNS in the internal auditory canal. This is in contradiction to the findings for acoustic tumors, which rarely affect the facial nerve preoperatively and certainly affect hearing first (Schaitkin, 2000). A good cochlear reserve is an important factor when planning surgery.

Other symptoms are uncommon and depend on the nerve segment involved. Imbalance can occur when the posterior labyrinth is affected; however, dizziness is rare. The involvement of other cranial nerves, especially V, VI, IX, X, XI and XII, depends on the tumor size and is presented more often in extrinsic tumors of the facial nerve. Headache and other neurological symptoms are usually absent. Physical examination of a patient with facial paralysis should entail facial nerve evaluation, otologic assessment, head and parotid exam. Neurologic and general physical examinations are also mandatory. The examiner must conclusively establish whether it is a peripheral or central paralysis. FNSs can produce peripheral paralysis even when they involve the intracranial segment of the nerve. The evaluation of facial paralysis is subjective and differences of opinion between examiners may occur. Therefore, the intensity (complete or incomplete), segment affected and presence of fasciculations or spasms should be taken into consideration. Although there are no pathognomonic aspects of facial paralysis to differentiate between a tumor and an inflammatory process, the above mentioned parameters can help the physician to identify if an event is different from that caused by Bell's palsy.

The otological exam involves an external ear inspection to search for masses, scars and ulcers. Otoscopy should rule out external auditory canal processes and tympanic membrane alteration. Middle ear mass may be identified in the first examination and this finding can be disregarded in some cases. Tuning fork tests, especially the Weber test, are important and easy to perform; these tests can categorize the hearing loss into the conductive or sensorial type. General examination of the neck and parotid gland are essential with the aim of detecting the presence of a mass or lymph node. Systemic and metastatic diseases should be ruled out as they may also affect the facial nerve.

DIAGNOSTIC STUDIES

Audiologic testing and radiologic investigation are not only important for the diagnosis but also for the management of FNS. Pure-tone audiogram and impedanciometry testing are sufficient for hearing evaluation and should be performed with an aim of diagnosing hearing loss and evaluating the best method to approach a tumor while preserving hearing ability. Other tests, such as eletrophysiological hearing evaluation, otoacoustic emission test or vestibular test are unnecessary and contribute neither to the diagnosis nor to the surgical planning, unless under clinical indication.

Advances in diagnostic imaging have contributed greatly to the diagnosis of FNS. Magnetic resonance imaging (MRI) and high-resolution thin-section computed tomography offer the possibility of reconstruction of images, which allows great accuracy in the differential diagnosis of small tumor lesions.

MRI is the first choice for ruling out or confirming a facial nerve mass and should be made very soon. High-resolution, gadolinium-enhanced MRI of all facial nerve segments is required for accurate diagnosis of these tumors (Kertesz et al. 2001). High-resolution computed tomography imaging is important for surgical planning after the tumor diagnosis. It can also aid in the localization of tumor margins and assessment of the involvement of adjacent structures (Kertesz et al. 2001). FNSs show specific findings in these image studies; therefore, these studies facilitate differential diagnosis. On MRI scans, FNSs present as heterogeneous lesions that are hypointense on T1-weighted images, isointense on proton-density images and hyperintense on T2-weighted images. These tumors show rapid enhancement with gadolinium. A pathognomonic finding is an enhanced enlargement of varying thickness along a significant length of the nerve (O'Donoghue et al. 2005).

More extensive FNSs that extend from the cerebellopontine angle-internal auditory canal (CPA-IAC) to the geniculate fossa show a "dumb-bell" shape. Geniculate ganglion and greater superficial petrosal nerve FNSs can present as a middle cranial fossa mass. Tympanic segment FNSs are often multilobular, dehiscence into the middle ear to present as avascular retrotympanic masses. Finally, mastoid segment FNSs can appear on MR imaging as locally aggressive masses that break into the surrounding mastoid air cells (Wiggins et al. 2006).

Currently, the diagnosis of FNS can be ascertained before surgery if the index of suspicion remains high; preoperative diagnosis can help avoid unexpected surgical discovery (Kertesz et al. 2001). This fact becomes very important because the prognosis is modified according to the histological type of the tumor; therefore, the medical decision is more precise, when the radiological study is performed properly.

Topodiagnostic tests and eletrophysiological examinations have a small role in FNS.

They are performed more for documentation purposes and do not have much clinical importance.

TREATMENT

Management of this clinical entity poses a true dilemma related to the timing of surgery, especially in patients presenting with good facial nerve function (Perez et al. 2005).

The treatment decision should be tailored according to the hearing function, tumor growth rate, surgical experience and most importantly, the degree of deterioration of facial function (Shirazi et al. 2007).

There are some principles that should be followed in the treatment of an intrinsic tumor of the facial nerve. Regardless of the type of facial nerve reconstruction performed after tumor resection, the patient will not show recovery better than a House-Brackmann (HB) (House and Brackmann, 1985) grade III palsy (Saleh et al. 1995). If the treatment is deferred till the nerve has shown clinical degeneration, the likelihood of achieving this outcome reduces (Schaitkin, 2000). For this reason, only tumors that cause facial paralysis greater than HB grade III should be resected, unless there is a suspicion of malignancy or the intracranial component is too big. Preoperative hearing level evaluation is very important for surgical planning, not only on the tumor side but also on the contralateral side.

FNS presenting with normal facial function or facial paralysis better than HB grade III can be monitored through annual MRI studies. Surgery is only performed if there is an important intracranial component or if there is no certainty over the benign nature of the lesion. In a study that demonstrated the frequency and location of nerve fibers within FNS, Hajjaj and Linthicum emphasized the importance of imaging to determine the type and extent of middle ear masses before performing any surgical intervention (Hajjaj, 1996).

If the facial nerve paralysis has developed to more than HB grade III, surgery is recommended to obtain a good postoperative facial functional recovery (Kim et al. 2003).

Surgery can be performed using many surgical approaches. This choice is made according to the size and position of the tumor and also the hearing status in both ears. FNS in the mastoid or tympanic portion can be approached by a canal wall up (CWU) mastoidectomy. However, the approaches for the geniculate ganglion and the labyrinthine portion of the facial nerve are chosen according to the hearing status. If the patient has good hearing, middle fossa approach is indicated; if not, the segments can be reached through mastoidectomies associated with labyrinthectomies. In this procedure, the intracranial segment of the facial nerve or the intracranial component of the tumor is removed by a translabyrinthine approach that results in complete hearing loss.

FNSs of the extralabyrinthine portion are operated on by traditional approaches to the parotid gland and in some cases, mastoidectomies, to extend the removal of the intratemporal component.

Angeli and Brackmann presented evidence to support a conservative approach as an alternative to surgical removal in cases of unsuspected facial neuroma in patients with normal facial function. A wide decompression is employed to allow the tumor to grow outside the natural bony canal minimizing compression of the nerve fibers and neighboring structures. This is accomplished by removing bone around the tumor and around the nerve just distal and proximal to the tumor (Angeli and Brackmann, 1997).

Facial nerve reconstruction after tumor removal can be performed according to the size of the neural defect. In some cases, it is possible to resect the tumor with some neural integrity. In such cases, no reconstruction is necessary. However, in the majority of the cases, a neural suture or an end-to-end anastomosis should be performed. Other options are nerve transposition or the use of grafts (sural or auricular nerve) (Fig. 15.5). When the use of grafts is impossible because of the nonexistence of a proximal stump, functional restoration should be performed through hypoglossal-facial anastomosis. If there is no distal stump (extratemporal), like in parotid tumors, a facial aesthetical procedure should be performed.

The most important determinant of the outcome, in terms of facial nerve dysfunction, is the duration of the preoperative paralysis (O'Donoghue et al. 2005). Recovery of facial movement after grafting the facial nerve is not influenced by graft length or graft type. Prolonged preoperative facial dysfunction has a negative influence on recovery after grafting (Dort and Fish, 1991).

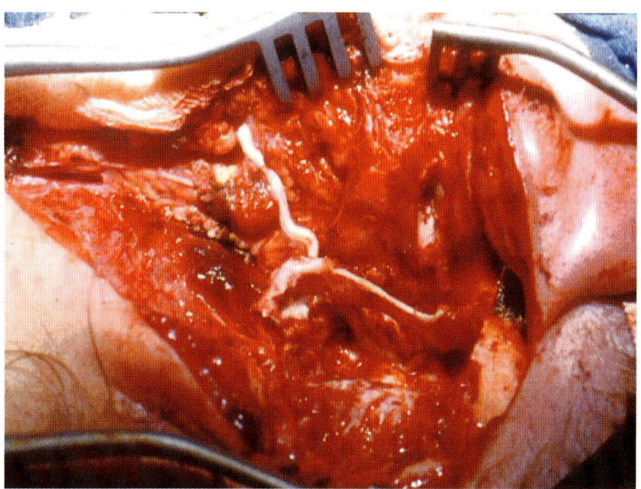

Fig. 15.5: Facial nerve graft after tumor removal, from the second portion until the facial nerve trunk after stylomastoid foramen

BIBLIOGRAPHY

1. Angeli SI, Brackmann DE. Is surgical excision of facial nerve schwannomas always indicated? Otolaryngol Head Neck Surg. 1997;117(6):S144-7.
2. Bento RF, D'Antonio WA, De la Cortina RAC, et al. Neurinoma do nervo facial: relato de quatro casos. In: Congresso de Otorrinolaringologia da FMUSP, 1., São Paulo. 1999.
3. Bento RF, Miniti A, Bogar P. Facial nerve schwannoma-five case reports and their management. In: Yanagihara N; Murakami S. New horizons in facial nerve research and facial expression. Haia, Holanda: Kugler Publications. 1998. pp. 473-6.
4. Chao WC, Liu TC, Ng SH, et al. Facial nerve schwannoma. Otolaryngol Head Neck Surg. 2009;141(1):146-7.
5. Dort JC, Fisch U. Facial nerve schwannomas. Skull Base Surgery. 1991;1:51-6.
6. Formigoni LG, Mendonça Cruz, OL Médicis da Silveira, et al. Neurilenome du nerv facial en trajet intraparotidien: présentation d'un cas. Revue de laryngologie, otologie, rhinologie. 1980;101(1-2).
7. Hajjaj M, Linthicum FH Jr. Facial nerve schwannoma: nerve fibre dissemination. J Laryngol Otol. 1996;110(7): 632-3.
8. House JW, Brackmann DE. Facial nerve grading system. Otolaryngol Head Neck Surg. 1985;93:146-7.
9. Kertesz TR, Shelton C, Wiggins RH, et al. Intratemporal facial nerve neuroma: anatomical location and radiological features. Laryngoscope. 2001;111(7):1250-6.
10. Kim CS, Chang SO, Oh SH, et al. Management of intratemporal facial nerve schwannoma. Otol Neurotol. 2003;24(2):312-6.
11. Lassaletta L, Roda JM, Frutos R, et al. Facial nerve schwannoma of the cerebellopontine angle: a diagnostic challenge. Skull Base. 2002;12(4):203-7.
12. Marchioni D, Alicandri Ciufelli M, Presutti L. Intraparotid facial nerve schwannoma: literature review and classification proposal. J Laryngol Otol. 2007;121(8):707-12. Epub 2007 Mar 23.
13. McMonagle B, Al-Sanosi A, Croxson G, et al. Facial Schwannoma: results of a large case series and review. J Laryngol Otol. 2008;122(11):1139-50.
14. O'Donoghue GM, Nikolopoulos T. Tumors of the Facial Nerve. In: Brackman DE, Jackler R (Eds). Neurotology. (2nd edn). Elsevier:Mosby. 2005. pp. 1258-69.
15. Park HY, Kim SH, Son EJ, et al. Intracanalicular facial nerve schwannoma. Otol Neurotol. 2007;28(3):376-80.
16. Perez R, Chen JM, Nedzelski JM. Intratemporal facial nerve schwannoma: a management dilemma. Otol Neurotol. 2005;26(1):121-6.
17. Saito H, Baxter A. Undiagnosed intratemporal facial nerve neurilemmomas. Arch Otolaryngol. 1972;95(5):415-9.

18. Saleh E, Achilli V, Naguib M, et al. Facial nerve neuromas: diagnosis and management. Am J Otol. 1995;16:521-6.

19. Schaitkin BM. Facial nerve schwannoma. In: Jackler R, Driscoll CLW (Eds). Tumors of the ear and temporal bone. Philadelphia: Lippincott Williams & Wilkins. 2000. pp. 276-89.

20. Shirazi MA, Leonetti JP, Marzo SJ, et al. Surgical management of facial neuromas: lessons learned. Otol Neurotol. 2007;28(7):958-63.

21. Wiggins RH 3rd, Harnsberger HR, Salzman KL, et al. The many faces of facial nerve schwannoma. AJNR Am J Neuroradiol. 2006;27(3):694-9.

16

Plastic-Surgical Repair of the Paralyzed Face

Narendra Pandya, Ashok Shah

INTRODUCTION

The face plays a very important role in communication. In facial nerve paralysis, the face is paralyzed and all expressions are lost. The patient loses the power of communication, develops an inferiority complex and is depressed. Facial paralysis results in severe psychological, cosmetic and functional disabilities.

The goals in the treatment of facial paralysis are:
- To achieve normal appearance at rest
- Symmetry with voluntary motion as well as with involuntary emotional control of the ocular, oral and nasal sphincters
- No significant functional deficit secondary to the reconstructive surgery (Grabb and Smith, 1997).

Functional recovery takes priority in the reconstruction. It is of utmost importance, in view of the possibility of corneal ulceration and blindness, to prevent eye complications in the patient with facial paralysis. The treatment of facial paralysis requires the skill of many specialists like neurosurgeon, neurologist, ophthalmologist, otolaryngologist and plastic surgeon. A multiple or combined surgical approach depending on the cause, time interval and wound characteristics often gives best results.

A wide range of procedures is available but a totally paralyzed face can never be made normal by any of the modern and recent surgical methods of reconstruction. The surgeon must employ a number of concepts depending on the etiology, the time interval, the wound characteristics and the availability as well as the necessity of neuromuscular substitution. No single surgical method can correct a complex deformity and results of surgery are not always gratifying (Mahaluxmivala, 1998). Unfortunately, despite decades of efforts and advances, there is a need and scope for the development of additional procedures for the multiple and complex problems associated with a paralyzed face.

ANATOMY

A fundamental knowledge of the surgical anatomy of the parotid gland and facial nerve is essential for the surgeon reconstructing patients with facial paralysis. In infants, the facial nerve lies more superficially.

Intratemporal Facial Nerve

The facial nerve is formed by supranuclear and infranuclear fibers from the facial nucleus. It leaves the pons and enters the facial canal of the temporal bone. The facial nerve gives greater superficial petrosal nerve, (supplies secretomotor fibers to the lacrimal gland, taste sensations from the soft palate), nerve to the stapedius muscle (sound vibrations) and chorda tympani nerve (provides secretomotor fibers to the sub-maxillary and sublingual glands and taste fibers from the anterior two-thirds of the tongue).

Extratemporal Facial Nerve

The larger superficial segment of the parotid gland lies lateral to the facial nerve branches and the smaller deep portion lies medial to these branches. The facial nerve emerges from the skull through the stylomastoid foramen, gives muscular rami to various muscles and enters the parotid gland. In the parotid gland, the nerve splits into two main divisions, the temporofacial and the cervicofacial portions. The two divisions sub-branch to form five main branches:

1. Temporal
2. Zygomatic
3. Buccal
4. Mandibular
5. Cervical.

These branches supply the muscles of facial expression. There is an extensive arborization and interconnections in distal area.

Facial Muscles

Orbicularis oculi muscle acts as a sphincter to close the eyelids and play a vital role in protection of the eye. Orbicularis oris, levators and depressors of lips acts as a sphincter of the mouth and play a vital role in speech, eating and drinking. Other facial muscles also play a vital role in facial and emotional expressions.

ETIOLOGY AND CLASSIFICATION

The various etiologic factors involved may be broadly classified into three major groups:

1. Intracranial
2. Intratemporal
3. Extracranial.

Intracranial

- Vascular abnormalities
- CNS degenerative diseases
- Intracranial tumors
- Trauma to the brain
- Congenital abnormalities and agenesis.

Intratemporal

- Bacterial and viral infections
- Trauma
- Tumors invading the middle ear, mastoid and facial nerve.

Extracranial

- Parotid tumors
- Trauma
- Malignant tumors of the mandible, pterygoid region and skin.

The Clinical Problem

Functions of the facial muscles are vital for portion of the eyes, oral continence, clear speech and emotional expressions.

Paralysis of orbicularis oculi causes corneal exposure, desiccation and lower eyelid ectropion. Paralysis of orbicularis oris affects patient's ability to speak, eat and drink properly. Because of paralysis of all facial muscles, patient cannot express his emotions and because of lack of emotions the patient is frequently treated as mentally disabled rather than physically disabled.

EVALUATION

A careful history is obtained, including the onset and duration of the condition and the degree of recovery. Various topognostic tests like hearing test, balance tests, Schimer test, stapes reflex, submandibular flow test and taste tests are done. Additionally, the physician examines the face at rest and in motion, noting muscular tone and symmetry and analyzing the various mimetic muscles. Motor function is tested by asking the patient to wrinkle the forehead, close the eyelids tightly, show the teeth, pucker the lips and grimace. The platysma muscle and depressors can be tested by having the patient draw the lower lip and angle of the mouth downward. Paralysis of the buccinator and orbicularis oris muscles results in speech impairment, drooling and inability to whistle or puff out the cheeks. An assessment of other cranial nerves, particularly the fifth is also performed. Paralysis of other cranial nerves may increase the morbidity of facial nerve paralysis. Cranial nerves should also be assessed of possible donor motor nerves.

Various electro-diagnostic tests of facial nerve and muscles are performed to establish a physiologic baseline of neuromuscular status (Mahaluxmivala, 1998). Tomographic, angiographic and neurological investigations add valuable information about intra-temporal lesions.

LOCATION OF THE LESION

Supranuclear paralysis involves only paralysis of the lower facial muscles contralateral to the side of the lesion. Lesions in the pons, intratemporal or extra-temporal portion result in weakness of the entire ipsilateral half of the face, including the forehead. Intratemporal lesions can be identified by Schimer's test (lacrimal gland function), intolerance to loud sound (stapedius branch) and applying galvanic current and noting metallic taste on normal side and electric shock on affected side of the tongue. In extratemporal lesion, patient loses movements of facial muscles and facial expressions.

CHOICE OF PROCEDURE

Dynamic reconstruction and neural reconstruction are almost always preferred to static methods, except under special circumstances (McCarthy, 1990). Two essential elements are required for facial movement:
1. An intact facial nerve
2. Functional facial muscles.

If the facial muscles are healthy, the requirements for reinnervation are:
- A viable ipsilateral facial nerve nucleus
- A proximal nerve segment capable of supporting axonal regeneration
- A distal nerve segment through which axons may regenerate to the facial muscles.

However, significant muscular degeneration may preclude reanimation without the transfer of new muscular tissue to the face. Lacerations and iatrogenic injuries of the facial nerve are best repaired immediately. It is within the first three weeks after injury that the neural and muscular elements have the best chance of complete recovery. Muscles degenerate after 1-2 years of paralysis but they are capable of functioning again if the regenerating nerve reaches them, i.e. via nerve grafting or nerve crossover procedure, which are the procedures of choice. If the muscle is not reinnervated, it undergoes atrophy with disappearance of contractile elements. There is often a combination of neural and muscular deficit requiring transfer of both elements for reanimation. After two years, muscles degenerate hence muscle transfer or static reconstruction are more suitable techniques (McCarthy, 1990).

TREATMENT

Aims of the treatment are to:
1. Protect the eye
2. Full function of the face at rest and during expression, but this is rarely achieved.
3. Symmetry of oral fissure.
4. Control of oral and ocular sphincter function, and
5. Spontaneous and natural expression of emotions.

Reconstruction can be either dynamic or static.

MANAGEMENT

Non-Surgical Management

While surgery is being planned, it is very important to protect the eye and maintain the lubrication of the eye.

Dynamic Reconstruction

Neural Repair

1. *Direct nerve repair and grafting*: The most effective means of rehabilitating the paralyzed face is to re-establish the neural pathway by direct approximation or autogenous nerve grafting. Each of these approaches requires adequate mimetic muscle function. Usually good results are obtained up to one year following facial paralysis. Direct nerve approximation is indicated in any instance in which the main trunk can be re-approximated with no tension (Grabb and Smith, 1997). However, immediate facial nerve grafting is used to overcome loss of the main trunk, peripheral branches or a nerve

segment. Obviously, if the distal part of the facial nerve including the mimetic muscles is ablated, nerve grafting is unrealistic; muscle transposition is the preferred treatment in such cases.

Branches from the cervical plexus from the ipsilateral or contralateral side are most frequently used for facial nerve autografting and they are sutured to the terminal branches of the temporal, zygomatic, buccal and mandibular divisions. The sural nerve is an alternative donor site. The nerve graft should be sutured without any tension and it should lie in a healthy, well-vascularized area free of scar tissue. The fascicular repair with atraumatic technique by using operating microscope gives the best results and the timing of repair is of utmost importance, the ideal situation being at the time of the primary ablative procedure. The time interval for return of facial movement varies from 6-24 months, depending on the length of the graft. The quality of return is always mass movement. There is always a deficit in emotional expression.

2. *Cross-face nerve grafting (Facio-facial anastomoses)*: The procedure is based on cross-innervations from the non-paralyzed side by means of sural nerve grafts that connect the reservoir of peripheral healthy facial nerve fascicles to the corresponding branches of specific muscle groups on the paralyzed side (Cohen, 1994).

Fascicular repair is used and the length of the grafts varies from 6-8 cm. Most authors prefer a two-stage procedure, allowing the nerve axons to grow to the opposite side and then resecting the neuroma to demonstrate the success of the axon regrowth before suturing the graft to the paralyzed side. This procedure has limited applications (except when combined with micro-neuromuscular muscle transfers) and the overall results were disappointing when compared to those obtained with classic procedures.

Operative technique: In this the buccal branches of the facial nerve on the nonparalyzed side is sutured microsurgically to the corresponding branches of the facial nerve on the paralyzed side (or to the nerve of a vascularized muscle) by using the sural nerve graft. This procedure is done in two stages.

Sacrifice of facial nerve branches, on the normal side does not produce long-term weakness and may even be beneficial in equalizing the two sides.

The primary disadvantage is long operating time and the time required for return of function. The facial muscles undergo further atrophy during the time required for axonal growth through the long nerve grafts. The greatest disadvantage of this technique is that only 50% of all nerve fibers of the facial nerve can be used from the normal side and they are joined to about 50% of the paralyzed side, thereby limiting the amount of axonal input.

In general, the distinct disadvantages include the following:
- There are two suture lines for each nerve graft, increasing the probability of a greater loss of sprouting axons
- A longer time is required for reinnervation from these long grafts, during which there may be further muscle atrophy
- The greatest disadvantage is the reduced axonal input to accomplish powerful reinnervation if one is not to sacrifice too much function on the normal side
- Technical difficulty in identifying distal branches of the facial nerve
- Postoperatively mass movements are seen.

The cross-face nerve graft is only another alternative to the classic procedures of hypoglossal facial nerve crossover and muscle transposition.

3. *Nerve crossover*: The surgical technique is straightforward and has the advantage of requiring only one anastomosis of nerves that are a satisfactory physical match (McCarthy, 1990).

Nerve crossovers are used when direct anastomoses or grafting is not feasible when facial paralysis is resulting from intracranial lesions or disorders of the temporal bone. Commonly used nerves are glossopharyngeal, accessory, phrenic and hypoglossal nerves. The hypoglossal-facial nerve crossover is the most popular crossover operation in use today.

Nerve crossover techniques are advantageous because they are simple, require only a single suture line and serve as a powerful source of innervations. The main disadvantage is that they result in associated, uncoordinated movements, loss of emotion on face and in loss of function of the donor nerve.

Muscle Repair

1. *Muscle transfers*: Transfer of muscle to the paralyzed face is usually done under following circumstances:
- After long-standing muscle atrophy
- As an adjunct to the mimetic muscles to provide new muscle and myoneurotization
- In combination with a nerve graft or crossover nerve implanted in the transposed muscle. Masseter and temporalis muscle transposition are most commonly used.

Masseter muscle transposition (Fig. 16.1): This muscle is ideally suited to give motion to the lower half of the face (De Castro and Zani, 1993). Commonly, three muscle slips are sutured to the dermis of the lower lip, oral commissure and upper lip. Over-correction must be accomplished. The patient maintains voluntary control over the muscle and can activate it by clenching the teeth.

Temporalis muscle transposition (Figs 16.2A and B): For facial rehabilitation, the temporalis muscle has enjoyed more popularity than the masseter because of its position, its facility for greater excursion of movement and its adaptability to the orbit (Breidahl et al, 1996). The technique that is now most widely employed involves two temporal musculofascial strips, which are woven around the zygoma (Figs 16.3A to C). These musculofascial strips are used to reconstruct upper lip, lower lip and both eyelids. Additional fascial strips can also be anchored to ala of the nose. The technique has several advantages, one of which is that the muscle provides good muscle bulk to compensate lack of fullness on the paralyzed side, in the severely atrophic face. Furthermore, there is direct muscular insertion on the structures to be moved giving greater range of mobilization and direct muscular insertion enhances chances of myoneurotization.

This procedure is better suited for ocular paralysis but facial movements are not physiological.

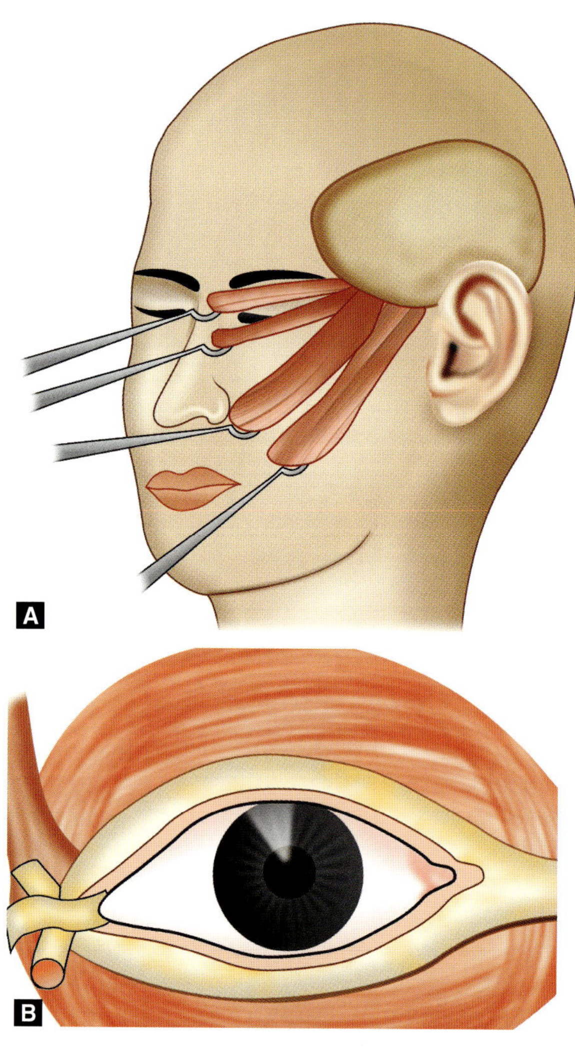

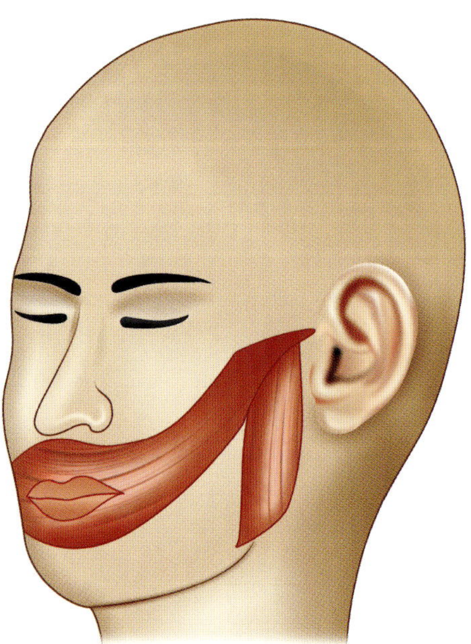

Fig. 16.1: Masseter muscle transposition

Figs 16.2A and B: (A) Temporalis muscle transposition. Four or five muscle slips are transposed to the upper and lower eyelids, upper lip and nasolabial fold, lower lip and commissure. Over correction is essential; (B) Technique of transplantation of temporalis: muscle and facia to upper and lower eyelids

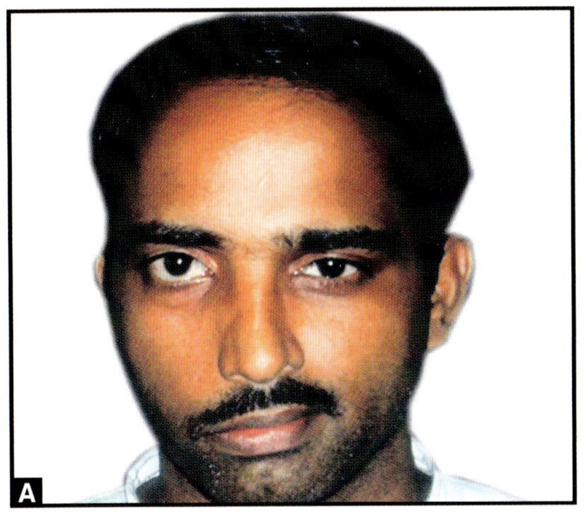

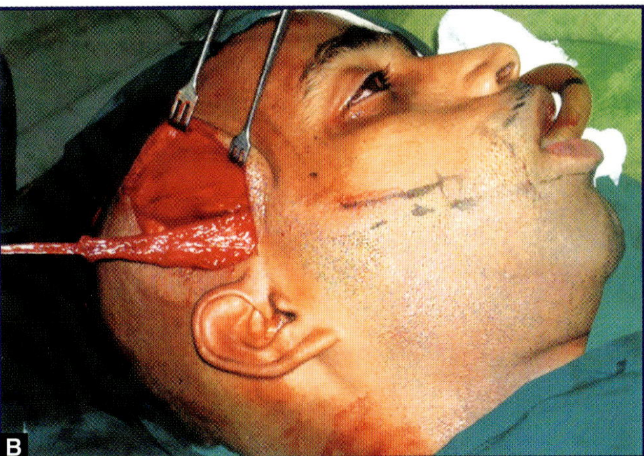

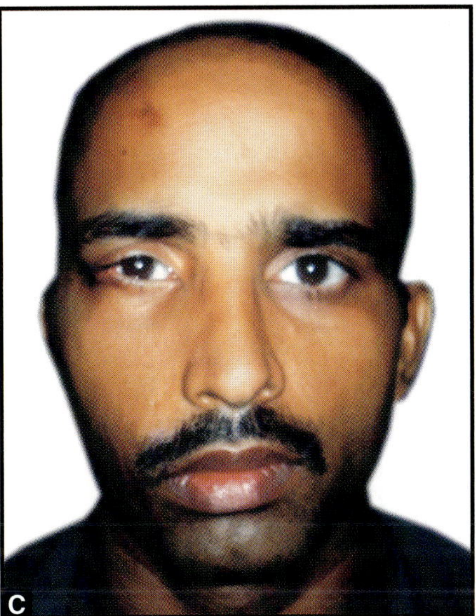

Figs 16.3A to C: Temporalis muscle transposition. (A) Preoperative; (B) Temporalis muscle with epicranium attached; (C) Postoperative

Because the impulse for muscle movement in temporalis and masseter transfers originates from the trigeminal nerve, facial movements are produced upon chewing, clenching the teeth and moving the mandible. The basic advantage of masseter and temporalis transfer is the introduction of a large volume of living and dynamic muscle into the face, simplicity of the technique, possibility of myoneurotization and no loss of other significant functions.

2. *Free muscle graft*: In the past, free autogenous muscle graft was also used. The muscle is denervated 14 days before transplantation, full length of the muscle is preserved and denervated muscle is placed in direct contact with normal, vascularized muscle at the recipient site. The main disadvantages of this procedure are that it is a multistage procedure and it is necessary to intervene on the non-paralyzed side.

With the present high success rates of micro-neurovascular muscle transfer, the technique of free muscle grafting has little or no place in the reconstruction of the paralyzed face (McCarthy, 1990).

3. *Free microneurovascular muscle transfer*: The most recent contribution to reanimation of the paralyzed face is the micro-neurovascular muscle transfer, combined with cross face nerve graft, ipsilateral nerve graft or split hypoglossal anastomosis. This technique provides new, vascularized muscle to the

face that can produce pull in various directions and accomplish more normal facial animation. The advantage over the muscle transfer technique is that the transferred muscle can be reinnervated by a cross face nerve graft, thereby enhancing control of voluntary facial movement. There are certain limitations and at present, it is another alternative in the surgeon's armamentarium of facial reanimation.

Choice of donor muscle: The ideal donor muscle has following criteria:

- Excursion should be equal to the normal side of the face
- Reliable vascular and nerve pattern of a size similar to that of the recipient
- Removal of the muscle should not leave any functional deficit
- Location should be such that two surgical teams should be able to operate simultaneously.

Gracilis muscle (O'Brien et al. 1980): It has a predictable, adequate neurovascular pedicle with adequate bulk. The muscle can be split longitudinally and anterior third of the muscle can be used.

Pectoralis minor muscle (Georgiade, 1992): Its flat shape facilitates insertion in the face. The proximity of the upper chest makes simultaneous two-team dissection difficult.

Latissimus dorsi muscle and serratus muscle: They have a predictable neurovascular pedicle and longitudinal intramuscular pattern.

Rectus abdominis and platysma muscles: These muscles can also be used.

All of the aforementioned muscles leave minimal or no functional deficit when sacrificed.

Operative technique: The operative procedure is usually divided into two stages. The first stage consists in one or more cross-face nerve graft and about 9-12 months later the vascularized muscle is transferred and its neural element is sutured to the distal end of the cross-face nerve graft (Terzis, 1987).

It is important to emphasize that movement of the face after microneurovascular muscle transfer is never normal. Microneurovascular muscle transfer is an alternative surgery for facial paralysis.

The main advantage of the technique is that facial movement is provided and controlled by the contralateral facial nerve, providing for better symmetry and perhaps a more definitive smile. Many disadvantages, however, still exist:

- There are at least two operative stages with a long surgical time
- There are two donor site scars
- Usually two years elapse before return of facial movement
- Complete eyelid closure, forehead movement, oral sphincter and depressor lip function are almost never restored
- The technique is not free of synkinesis and deficit of involuntary emotional expression, common to most other rehabilitative techniques.

4. *Muscle transplantation in the absence of seventh nerve:* When seventh nerve is not available from normal side in case of bilateral paralysis and mobius syndrome, this method is very useful. Here, innervations of the segmental gracilis muscle transplant is done by using motor nerve to masseter.

Static Methods of Reconstruction

The static methods of reconstruction of the paralyzed face are the well-known techniques of suspension with fascia lata, tendon or alloplastic materials. Materials varying from wire, silk, stainless steel and tantalum are also used. Static slings are used to achieve symmetry at rest without providing animation.

Face lifting and stabilization with dermal flaps have also been used. Reactivation of the facial muscles by neural reconstitution or muscle transposition supersedes any type of rehabilitation by suspension or skin stretching, except perhaps in the elderly or debilitated patient. Static techniques can, however, be complementary to dynamic reconstruction.

Suspension (Figs 16.4 and 16.5A to C): Fascia lata is used as a sling for support of orbicularis oris and lower eyelid. Tendon provides longer lasting support with less stretching than fascia lata for correction of severe ectropion.

Mechanical devices: Various mechanical devices like gold weights (Fig. 16.6), springs (Fig. 16.7) and magnets are used for eyelid closure.

Selective neurectomy: Selective sectioning of the intact facial nerve in order to accomplish a more balanced face.

Selective myectomy: Various techniques for selective myectomy of the facial muscles to accomplish better balance in repose and during facial expression.

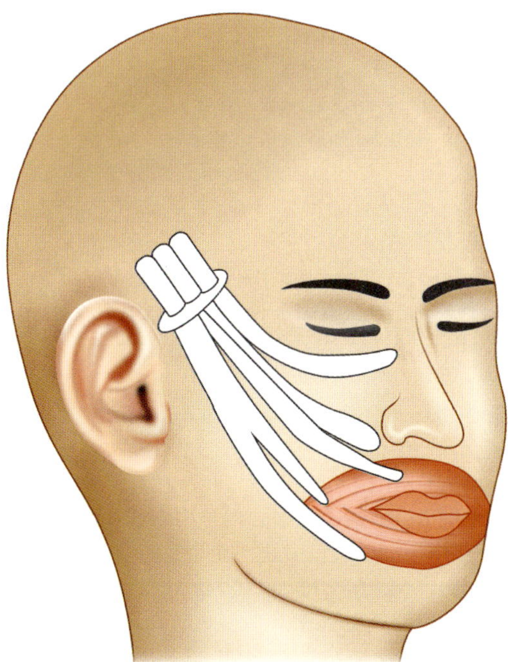

Fig. 16.4: Fascia lata suspension. The circumoral fascial strip and fascial sling to the lower eyelid is anchored to the temporal fascia by using fascia lata

Surgery for correction to camouflage the deformity: Various surgical procedures are used to camouflage the deformity. These procedures include excision of nasolabial skin, nasolabial dermofat sling, face-lift, brow-lift and excision of redundant skin and mucosa.

Endoscopic surgery: With the development of endoscopic surgery, endoscopically assisted brow lifts can also be done.

Botulinum toxin: Clostridium botulinum toxin (Botox) is a neurotoxin that temporarily interferes with acetylcholine release from motor nerve endplates, causing skeletal muscle paralysis. The effect lasts for 4-6 months. Botulinum toxin has been useful in the treatment of facial paralysis by weakening the contralateral side to allow centering of the mouth, more symmetry on smiling and treatment of hypertrophied platysmal bands.

SUMMARY

There are many options of treatment, which are available for the patient with facial nerve paralysis. The treatment goals are directed to the functional and cosmetic deficits that are present and are individualized to suit the patient's needs.

The first goal is to prevent eye complications secondary to corneal exposure. The second goal is to provide functional and cosmetic restoration of the eye, nose and mouth. These procedures should ideally provide static and dynamic symmetry to the face and allow the patient spontaneous facial animation.

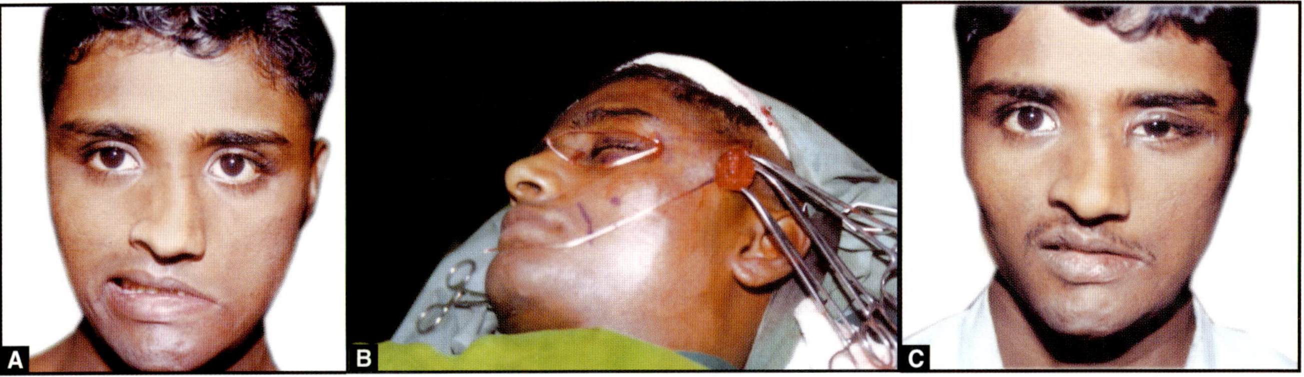

Figs 16.5A to C: Fascia lata suspension. (A) Preoperative; (B) Fascia lata to be anchored to orbicularis oris and lower eyelid. (C) Postoperative

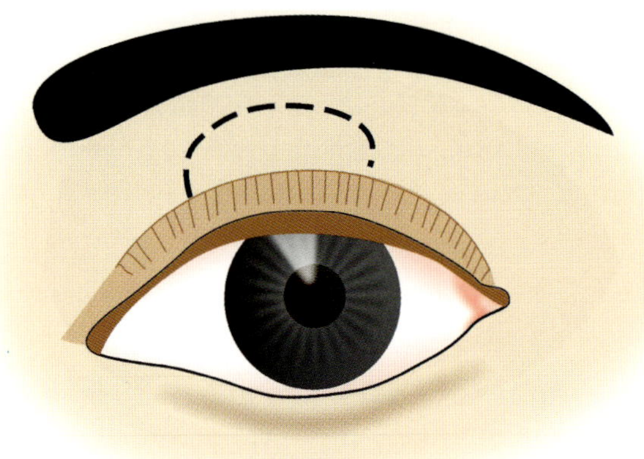

Fig. 16.6: Weights to aid lid closure. Weight inserted superficial to tarsal plate and deep to orbicularis oculi

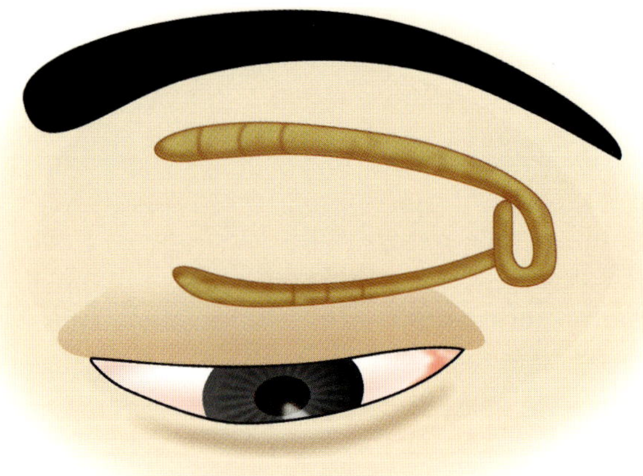

Fig. 16.7: Spring to help eyelid closure. Upper limb sutured to periosteum of supraorbital rim. Lower limb sutured to tarsal plate at eyelid margain

BIBLIOGRAPHY

1. Breidahl AF, Morrison WA, Donato RR. A modified surgical technique for temporalis transfer. Br J Plast Surg. 1996;49(1):46-51.
2. Cohen Mimis. Facial reanimation. Mast Plast Reconstr Surg. 1994;1045-59.
3. De Castro Correia P, Zani R. Masseter muscle rotation in the treatment of inferior facial paralysis. Plast Reconstr Surg. 1993;52(4):370-3.
4. Georgiade Gregory S. Facial paralysis: Principles of treatment. Textbook of Plastic, Maxillofacial and Reconstructive Surgery. 1992;581-96.
5. Grabb, Smith. Reconstruction of the paralyzed face. Plast Surg Lippincott - Raven. 1997;545-57.
6. McCarthy Joseph G. Facial Paralysis. Plast Surg. 1990;2237-319.
7. O'Brien BM, Franklin JD, Morrison WA. Cross-facial nerve grafts and microneurovascular free muscle transfer for long established facial palsy. Brit J Plast Surg. 1980;33(2):202-15.
8. Rayment R, Poole MD, Rushworth G. Cross-facial nerve transplants: why are spontaneous smiles not restored? Br J Plast Surg. 1987;40(6):592-7.
9. Sam M Mahaluxmivala. Facial reconstruction. Plastic Surgery-a compendium. 1998;59-64.
10. Stephen J.Mathes. Facial Paralysis. Plastic Surgery, 2nd edition. Saunders Publisher. 2006. pp. 883-916.
11. Terzis JK. Reconstructive Micro reconstruction of nerve injuries. 1987. pp. 170-4.
12. Tolhurst DE, Bos KE. Free revascularized muscle grafts and facial palsy. Plast Reconst Surg. 1982;69(5):760-1.

17

Threadlift Facelift in Paralyzed Face

Mohan Jagade, Ganeshan

INTRODUCTION

Threadlift technique has been described as another method to achieve static suspension. Through a multivector approach, sutures are placed, resulting in functional and aesthetic improvements. The suture technique is less invasive than other static techniques. It can be accomplished percutaneously and several types of sutures have been employed for this method.

THREADLIFT

Facial contouring is an achievable objective without surgery utilizing Non-Surgical Skin Tightening (NSST) and/or the threadlift facelift procedure.

The threadlift facelift procedure is a minimally invasive procedure that utilizes sutures to mechanically lift the skin. The threadlift facelift sutures have cogs or knots and cones on one side of the suture. The cogs or cones are able to engage the soft tissue and create a lifting effect to the face and neck.

HISTORY AND EVOLUTION OF THREADLIFT FACELIFT

Since the early 1990's, surgeons have been evaluating new surgical techniques for lifting the cheeks and jowls.

In 1992, Ruff started working on an idea of a barbed suture for cosmetic applications. Ruff took the idea of a barbed suture and applied it to an absorbable suture material made of polydioxanone. The advantage of using an absorbable polymer suture is that it does not need to be removed and it does not need knots to make it secure. The barbed configuration anchors the suture into the tissue and provides adequate tissue adhesion while the wound heals under minimum residual tension and pressure (Ruff GL, 1994)

Aptos is derived from the Greek "Anti" plus "Ptosis" (Lycka B et al. 2004; Jan, Lee S, Isse N. 2005, Khawaja HA, Hernandez-Perez E. 2005; Vazquez GD. 2005). It is a barbed thread that adheres to the dermis and acts as a gathering stitch. The aptos thread is based on the concept that the skin can be lifted and held in a suspended position with barbs alone without affecting the underlying muscle or bone. The barbed adherence is performed without suturing or anchoring to fascia muscle or bone. The thread itself is a polypropylene suture with barb sutures in two directions. The bidirectional configuration of sutures hold tissue in both inferior and superior direction, giving greater adherence (McKenzie AR. 1967). Ruff has independently developed a different concept of barbed suture for facial suspension. Having used the model of the porcupine quill (erethizon dursaton) as a multi-barbed suture that maintains a hold or grasp on soft tissue through an even and spiral diffusion of barbs on each quill, Ruff began work on the "quill suture" in the early 90's as a closure technique for surgical wounds. It was found to be self-anchoring with no knots, giving a faster and more efficient closure with broadly distributed tension. The "contour suture" (Contour Threads™ monograph-Surgical Specialties Corporation) was thus developed as a unidirectional barbed monofilament suture with a different pattern of insertion and anchored superiorly to a fixed structure.

The success of this novel suture requires the suture geometry to be well characterized and monitored during manufacture for two reasons: quality control (measuring the uniformity of the barb geometry) and the need to determine the effect of tissue holding capacity and the barb geometry. The monofilament sutures contain up to 78 barbs manufactured in a spiral pattern around the circumference of the suture. The barbs are divided into two groups facing each other in opposite directions around the mid-point. The two sets of barbs divide the suture into sections, right and left.

Using image analysis techniques, the geometry of the barbs has been characterized by defining the (depth of cut (Dc), length of cut (Lc), the distance between the cuts and the number of cuts per unit length (McKenzie AR. 1967). θ → Cut angle.

The length of the cut is a calculated value using the following formula:

$$Lc = \frac{Dc}{\sin(180 - \theta)}$$

These values are measured, recorded and analyzed statistically on a routine basis. The barbs are deployed using a controlled, uniform and mirrored geometry.

Summers, in 1998, performed a series of facelift procedures using the Mid-Face Sling technique.

In Russia, Sulamandize developed the Aptos (antiptosis) technique for facial rejuvenation using modified sutures. The original Aptos facelift technique did not require any incisions but was not as secure as the Mid-Face Sling described by summers. To achieve increased stability, Summers places a small 1.5 inch incision in the hair-bearing scalp to secure the Aptos facelift threads (Sulamandize M et al. 2001). Additionally, Summers uses a multiplanar approach, placing the sutures in the soft tissue layers around the skin, muscle and fat (adipose). This enables variable elevation of each tissue layer, optimizing the results for each individual patient. Subsequently Bhangoo, Woffles Wu (cited Wu WT, 2004) and Shumrick, Rocardo (2004) have contributed immensely to thread lift procedure.

A barbed surgical suture is configured to grip the tissue through which it is inserted (Monheit G. 2005; Fukaya M. 2006; Horne DF, Kaminer MS. 2006; Paul MD. 2008). The suture has a generally flat and elongated suture body with a multiplicity of barbs located along one or both of the lateral edges. The barbs are of sufficient size and appropriate geometry for fastening the tissue and achieving closure of an incision or wound without the need for tying knots in the suture. The barbed surgical suture may be configured as a single-ended suture with all of the barbs aligned to allow the suture to move through tissue in one direction only. Alternately, it may be configured as a double-ended suture with the barbs on a first end portion aligned to allow the suture to move through tissue in one direction and the barbs on a second end portion aligned to allow the suture to move through tissue in the opposite direction. The suture needles may be permanently or temporarily attached to the barbed surgical suture or alternatively, the suture needle may be integrally formed with the barbed surgical suture. Various methods are described for manufacturing the barbed surgical suture by stamping, cutting or progressive die cutting the suture out of flat material or by chemically etching the suture out of flat material and or by injection molding. Optionally, specialized coatings are recommended to enhance the performance of the barbed surgical suture.

Like a conventional suture, a barbed suture may be inserted into tissue using a surgical needle.

Sulamandize and Mikhailov used conical barbs arranged sequentially along the length of a thread and oriented in a direction opposite to that of the thread tension, with the distance between barbs being not less than 1.5 times the thread diameter.

Ruff recommended a device for positioning a barbed suture in order to close a wound. The insertion device has a tubular body for receiving a barbed suture and preferably also has a handle to facilitate manipulation of the device by the surgeon. This is useful where the suture portion being inserted includes barbs facing a direction opposed to the direction of insertion.

In my experience, I prefer that in a heavily set individual the thread should be relatively superficial as opposed to a thin statured individual where the thread can be placed deep to get the desired lift without folding the skin. Unlike typical facelift techniques, the threadlift facelift does not remove any skin, so it is not a good procedure for individuals with very loose skin. Between two and six threadlift threads are used on each side of the face to elevate the sagging cheeks and jowls. Once the Threadlift threads are placed under the skin, the Aptos cogs form a support structure for the tissues of the face. Over a period of about 6 weeks, the Threadlift threads will be stabilized as new collagen is formed around the cogs. The Threadlift facelift and necklift procedure is performed under local anesthesia in about one hour and the results are seen immediately. These threads can be removed and re-implanted which is the main advantage as this procedure can be revised without much morbidity to the patients. Re-implantation is done by cutting the anchoring needle and removing the suture by the other end and lastly putting a separate needle for anchoring.

Threadlift is not a substitute but a supplement to facelift procedure. In this context one patient who had first opted for facelift but later denied it as it takes 4-5 hours was then offered a Threadlift procedure which is a "Lunch Break Therapy". Having got convinced she underwent the Threadlift Surgery and opted for the facelift after 3 years, wherein during the facelift when we lifted the skin the Threads implanted previously were found to be thin and hardly perceptible. This indicates that initially it's the threads that provide the necessary anchorage and later on it's the fibrosis around the threads that provide the optimum sustained lift.

Tightening can be done in a previously placed facelift suspension suture. Therefore, in some patients, it is possible to return at a later time to further lift the cheeks and jowls even more. Because all patients age at different rates, it is impossible to predict how long the Threadlift facelift and neck lift results will last in any particular patient. However, I am in accordance with Summers' long-term experience with the Mid-Face Sling procedure, he believes that the Endo-Aptos Threadlift Facelift procedure may provide beneficial results lasting up to 5 years or more.

THREADLIFT FACELIFT RISKS

Some bruising is possible, but other side effects associated with facelift surgery (swelling, numbness, muscle weakness, scars) are very unusual or completely unexpected. Dimpling of the skin is possible, but when noticed at the time of the procedure, can be resolved quickly and painlessly. Dimples or surface irregularities noted later may require a minor procedure to release the dimple. These dimples can be avoided by deploying the threads well. Minor facial asymmetry is possible and a small degree of asymmetry may be acceptable. However, significant asymmetry may result from disengagement or breakage of the Threadlift threads. In this case, a new threadlift thread may be placed or an existing threadlift thread may be tightened to restore the desired contour. The most significant concern is that the threadlift thread may be felt or seen under the skin. This may occur if the threadlift thread is too close to the surface of the skin or if the skin thins with advancing age or weight loss. In this scenario, the offending Threadlift thread may be removed and a new Threadlift thread can be inserted (Silva-Siwady JG et al. 2005).

The following specific risks and complications of the one hour threadlift facelift procedure are listed below within particular risk categories:

After the Threadlift Facelift

Following the threadlift facelift procedure, patients can reduce their risk of bruising and swelling if they keep their head elevated, keep cool compresses over the cheeks and avoid straining or strenuous activities. To reduce the risk of disengagement or breaking of the threadlift threads, the face/cheeks should not be pulled down for 6 weeks. For example, facial massages are to be avoided and patients should take care when

COMMON (70%)	
Bruising	Most bruising typically resolves completely within 3–4 days
Swelling	Visible swelling typically resolves within one week.
	This can be minimized by preoperative administration for 3 days of Arneca Forte (Barakshar medicine) and Bromelein (An extract from pineapple)
RARE (<5%)	
Palpable thread	May be removed/replaced if problematic
Breakage of thread	Suspension typically not affected. May be replaced if necessary
Asymmetry	Correction of new asymmetry is possible with tightening of existing threads or placement of additional threads.
VERY RARE (1%)	
Hair loss	Loss of 5–10 hair follicles in the incision should be completely hidden
Scarring	Scarring from needle punctures is rare
Early loss of support	Additional threads can be placed for enhanced support.
UNEXPECTED (<1%)	
Contour irregularity	Typically resolves spontaneously or is correctable
Visible thread	Visible threads should be removed/replaced. Colorless threads can be used in such cases.
Bleeding	May require drainage
Nerve injury	Resolution may occur over time
Cheese wire cutting through	Seen as a complication in loop lift (Curl lift).

washing their face or shaving not to stretch their cheeks and jowls downward. Also he is cautioned not to yawn or open mouth fully and forcefully for 14 days.

About 3-4 weeks after the procedure, body will grow collagen fibers around the threadlift threads, effectively locking the threadlift sutures into place. This provides long-term support and gives an opportunity to re-tighten sutures in future.

All Threadlift facelift procedures fall under one general category—suture suspension lifts.

The best features to find in a suture suspension lift include:

1. Easy insertion
2. Lack of palpability
3. No visible suture
4. Adequate and symmetric suspension
5. Durability and longevity of suspension
6. Ability to adjust amount of lift post-operation

TYPES OF THREADLIFT

Bidirectional Threadlift Without Incision

Aptos threadlift: The Aptos threadlift facelift procedure was originally developed by Sulamandize, a Russian physician, in the 1990's. The Aptos threadlift facelift procedure involved insertion of a polypropylene suture with bi-directional barbs. The Aptos Threadlift suture was inserted using a needle and was not secured to deeper tissue. (Adamyan A et al. 2002)

Later, a needleless thread was created; it had converging prominences and could be introduced subcutaneously through a conducting needle; it also needed a more simplified manipulation, without needing a significant incision. Accordingly, the optimal skin marking was developed for each area of the face, with full consideration for different anatomical, functional and pathological features of the different areas and pathologies. This technique of thread lifting became popular very soon and came to be called the Aptos thread.

Unidirectional Threadlift Requiring Incision

Initially the thread were called contour threads, the new facelift thread is called a "Silhouette Suture". Silhouette sutures do not have sharp barbs, which can weaken the suture. A barbed suture is created when cuts are made in the shaft of conventional sutures, which then weakens the inherent strength of the thread itself. Silhouette sutures are made from 3-0 polypropylene substrate, which allows for smaller knot tying in the temporal area and also utilizes clear, flexible, absorbable cones. Over time the cones are completely absorbed and tissue grows around and through the small knots to allow for long-lasting tissue suspension.

STUDY DISCUSSION FOR THREADLIFT

Evaluation of Functional Outcome in Facial Reanimation

(*Courtesy by:* House J 1983, Chee GH, Nedzelski JM 2000. Brenner MJ et al. The Nottingham system 1994).

Several grading systems have been developed to quantify the extent of facial paralysis and the outcome of reanimation of the face. In our study, facial dysfunction was measured by House's well-established standard grading system (House, 1983). The degree of dysfunction is clearly defined on a scale from 1 to 6.

Because the Contour Thread™ barbs may be released with intense pressure, patients must initially avoid strenuous exercise or movements that could dislodge the tightened skin from the barbs along the sutures. Data from the manufacturer demonstrate that in laboratory rats these sutures develop a fibrous capsule that becomes well integrated into the dermis and subcutaneous tissue over several months. Theoretically, a similar process in human skin could lead to a secure and long-lasting cosmetic effect.

CONCLUSION OF THREADLIFT PROCEDURE

1. The postoperative satisfaction grade was much better and significant with threadlifts .
2. The time required for performing the surgery too was less in threadlifts
3. The postoperative recovery time too was less in thread lifts making it a day care surgery .
4. Postoperative complications and morbidities were comparatively less in threadlifts
5. All thread lifts were done under simple local anesthesia
6. No special training is required in the threadlift procedure except the finesse in surgery
7. Even the patients post-threadlift donot require any learning for animation

Based on the objectives of the comparative analysis it was found that the newer techniques of threadlift gave better results in respect of facial symmetry, good symmetrical smile, good oral competence, good cosmetic satisfaction and an excellent surgical time taking just half to one-hour and the patient can go home in an hour after the threadlift procedure.

- Patient is made upright and against gravity, cheek is pulled by fingers.
- The pull is judged to balance the otherside unparalyzed face. This gives us an idea as to how much pull on the thread is required.
- Along the lines of pull, it is marked by marking ink. This forms the 'Vectors'.
- The procedure is done under local anesthesia with 2% Lignocaine and 1:200,000 Adrenaline. It is infiltrated along the vector markings and some infiltrated in the temporal region where incisions will be taken.
- Two small parallel incisions perpendicular to the vectors , are taken in the temporal region (As this is the area of scalp that does not bald both in males as well as females).
- These small incisions are taken to accommodate the anchoring needle.

The thread is inserted through the dermal tissue and **'Snaked'** while palpating to come out just before the nasolabial fold.

- After the needle is taken out the thread is pulled out till the first Barb.
- The needle is cut and a similar needle is inserted through the same incision towards the angle of mouth.
- Both threads are held on the cheek side by one hand and the other hand pushes the cheek tissue up along the threads, this opens the cones or barbs and lifts the skin at the angle of mouth and nasolabial fold. Tension is applied to balance with the otherside of the unparalyzed face—deployment of thread.
- Anchoring needle is used to anchor the thread in the subcutaneous tissues and brought through the second incision.
- The two threads are tied together and while tying, again tension is applied onto the threads.
- This knot is buried, over which the skin is sutured with an absorbable material.

- After which skin is cleaned and Tincture Benzoin is applied, over which sterile micropore dressing is applied to overcorrect the pull, it acts as a dressing and also allows the underlying skin to breathe through the micropores.

- After half an hour of observation, patient can go home.
- Patient is post procedure warned not to yawn and open the mouth fully or forcefully for 14 days, after which the micropore dressing is removed (Figs 17.1 and 17.2).

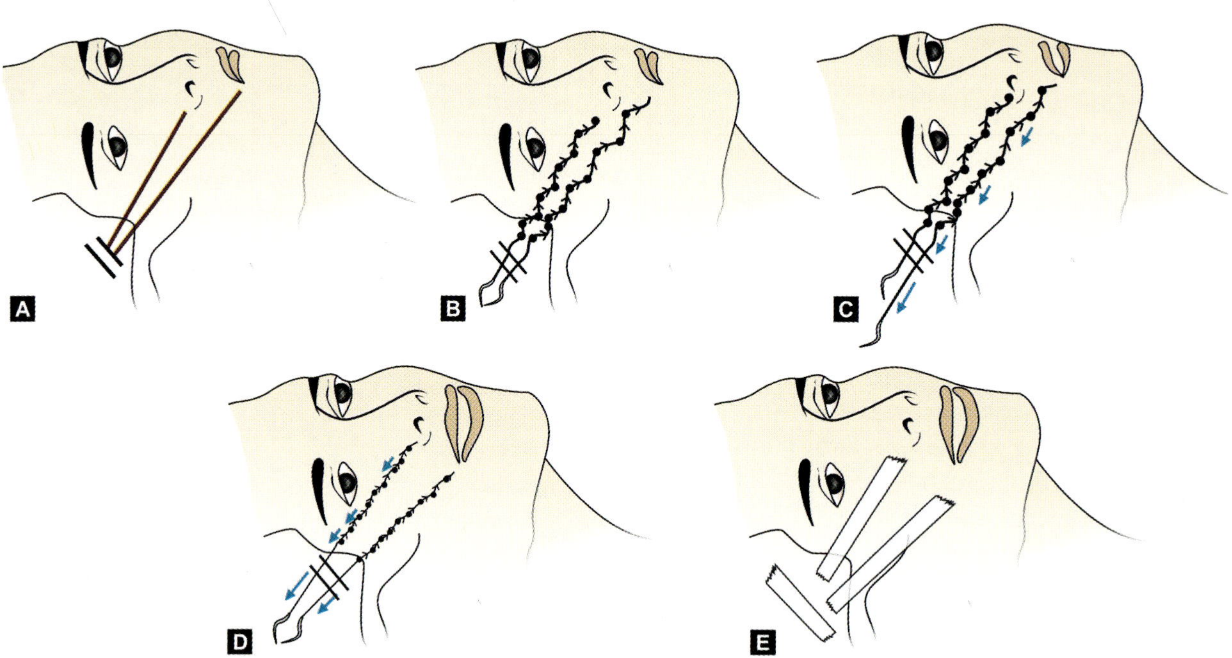

Figs 17. 1A to E: (A) Skin incision and vectors; (B) Threads snaked in; (C) Tension applied to one thread; (D) Deployment and anchoring of both threads; (E) Micropore dressing given

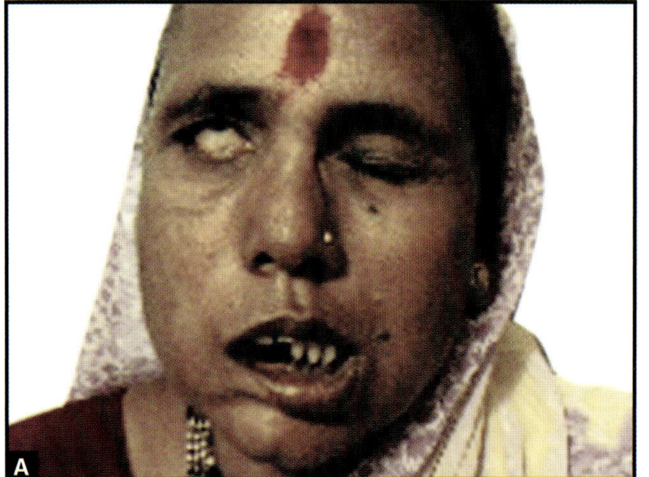

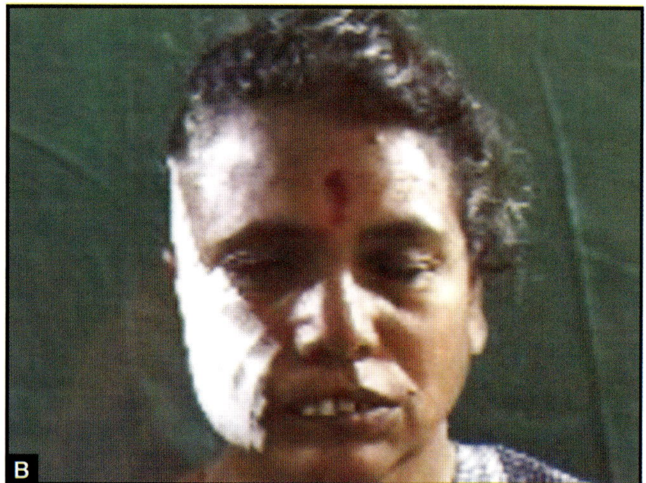

Figs 17.2A and B: (A) Preoperative photograph of patient operated for 8th nerve schwanoma four years back giving rise to right facial nerve paralysis; (B) Postoperative (after threadlift) photograph of the same patient as in 17.2A, patient is able to close the right eye easily with the check pulled upwards

BIBLIOGRAPHY

1. Adamyan A, Skuba N, Sulamandize M, Khusnutdinova Z. Morphological foundations of facelift using APTOS filaments. Annals of Plastic Reconstructive and Aesthetic Surgery. 2002;3:19-27.
2. Bhangoo - Personal Communication.
3. Brenner MJ, Neely JG. Approaches to grading facial nerve function. Semin Plast Surg 18(1):
4. Chee GH, Nedzelski JM. Facial nerve grading systems. Facial Plast Surg. 2000;16(4):315-24.
5. Contour Threads™ monograph - Surgical Specialties Corporation.
6. Fukaya M. A new method of face lift using barbed threads: X-tosis. J Jpn Soc Aesthet Surg. 2006;43:173.
7. Horne DF, Kaminer MS. Reduction of face and neck laxity with anchored, barbed polypropylene sutures (Contour Threads). Skin Therapy Lett. 2006;11(1):5-7.
8. House J. Facial nerve grading systems. Laryngoscope. 1983;93:1056-69.
9. Khawaja HA, Hernandez-Perez E. Transcutaneous face-lift. Dermatol Surg. 2005;31(4):453-7.
10. Lee S, Isse N. Barbed polypropylene sutures for midface elevation: early results. Arch Facial Plast Surg. 2005;7(1):55-61.
11. Lycka B, Bazan C, Poletti E, et al. The emerging technique of antiptosis subdermal suspension thread. Dermatol Surg. 2004;30(1):41-4.
12. McKenzie AR. An experimental multiple barbed suture. Prelimenary report. J Bone Joint Surg Br. 1967;49(3):440-7.
13. Monheit G. Suspension for the aging face. Dermatol Clin. 2005;23(3):561-73, viii.
14. Murty GE, Diver JP, Kelly PJ, et al. The Nottingham system: objective assessment of facial nerve function in the clinic. Otolaryngol Head Neck Surg. 1994;110:156-61.
15. Paul MD. Barbed sutures for aesthetic facial plastic surgery: indications and techniques. Clin Plast Surg. 2008;35(3):451-61.
16. Ruff GL. Barbed tissue connector, US Patent 6. 241, 747, 2001 June 5.
17. Ruff GL. Insertor for Barbed tissue connector, US Patent 5, 342, 376, 1994, August 30.
18. Silva-Siwady JG, Diaz-Garza C, Ocampo-Candiani J. A case of Aptos thread migration and partial expulsion. Dermatol Surg. 2005;31(3):356-8.
19. Sulamandize MA, Fournier PF, Paikidze TG, et al. Removal of facial soft tissue ptosis with special threads. Dermatol Surg 28(5):367-71.
20. Sulamandize MA, Paikidze TG, Sulamandize GM, et al. Facial lifting with "APTOS" threads: Featherlift. Otolaryngol Clin North Am. 2005;38(5):1109-17.
21. Vazquez GD. Facial percutaneous suspension. Plast Reconstr Surg. 2005;116(2):656-60.
22. Wu WT. Barbed sutures in facial rejuvenation. Aesthet Surg J. 2004;24(6):582-7.

18

Facial-Hypoglossal Nerve Jump Anastomosis for Reanimation of the Paralyzed Face

JJ Manni

"The human face is the most exciting area in the world."

— *Johan Kaspar Lavator (1741-1801)*

INTRODUCTION

Preservation of the facial nerve function is a major challenge to the surgeon involved in temporal bone and cerebello-pontine angle surgery. Despite advances in intraoperative facial nerve monitoring, damage to the facial nerve still occurs. A large variety of surgical techniques are available for facial reanimation, with specific indications. Primary end-to-end anastomosis of the facial nerve stumps results in the most optimal functional recovery. To ensure a tensionless facial nerve anastomosis, a nerve graft or facial nerve rerouting, is often needed. End-to-end anastomosis of the intracranial segment is difficult because the facial nerve lacks epineurium at this area. Moreover, the constant pulsation of the brainstem and the flow of CSF in a deep and narrow wound hamper the technique of anastomosis.

When the proximal stump of the facial nerve is not available for anastomosis, transposition of other cranial nerves to the distal facial nerve stump is a preferred technique. This technique is also indicated when, despite anatomical preservation of the facial nerve, functional recovery does not occur and the muscles of facial expression are still functional.

Transposition of the hypoglossal nerve and end-to-end anastomosis directly to the facial nerve is a popular, effective and reliable technique with constant and satisfying results. However, the complete transection of the hypoglossal nerve inevitably results in homolateral paralysis of the tongue with atrophy, which interferes with mastication, speech and swallowing in particular when the function of muscles of facial expression is less than normal. Moreover, it is emotional for the patient to decide to sacrifice another cranial nerve after having lost the vestibular, acoustic and occasionally the lower cranial nerves or trigeminal nerve as a result of cerebello-pontine angle surgery. Postoperative difficulty in swallowing that was attributed to tongue dysfunction was a complaint of 10-12% of patients (Conley and Baker, 1979). Pensak et al. (1986) reported that 74% of patients in their series had some functional difficulty while eating, of which 21% were debilitating. Hammerschlag (1989) observed both speech and swallowing problems in 45%. In an effort to reduce the adverse effects, Rubin et al. (1984) inter-digitated the midline tongue musculature using a Z-plasty technique. Other techniques used to reduce the postoperative tongue atrophy were anastomosing of the ansa hypoglossi to the distal stump of the hypoglossal nerve or longitudinal splitting of the hypoglossal nerve and performing a split XII-VII anastomosis. The results of all these methods were not always encouraging. [Conley and Baker (1979), Kessler et al. (1959), Ueda et al. (1994), Arai et al. (1995)].

In 1991, May et al. described a technique wherein the hypoglossal nerve and the facial nerve are anastomosed with the interposition of a free nerve graft, end-to-end to the distal facial nerve stump and end-to-side to the hypoglossal nerve. The latter is cut in transverse direction for approximately 50% of its diameter. The procedure is indicated in patients with an intact homolateral hypoglossal nerve, an inaccessible central facial nerve stump and a preserved distal facial nerve stump. The activity of the muscles of facial expression should have the potency to be reversible. With this technique, the authors observed good facial reanimation and rarely atrophy or impaired movement of the homolateral side of the tongue.

SURGICAL TECHNIQUE

The skin incision starts from the insertion of the lobule of the ear slightly curved backward and downward over a distance of approximately 4 cm. The greater auricular nerve is identified and dissected to obtain a graft of about 6 cm length. The facial nerve stump is identified and transected near the styloid foramen together with mobilization of the lateral posterior border of the parotid gland. The hypoglossal nerve is identified just beneath the digastric muscle where it crosses the carotid artery bifurcation and internal jugular vein and it is followed anteriorly to the ansa hypoglossi. The distal end of the graft of the greater auricular nerve is interpositioned end-to-end to the distal stump of the transected facial nerve and the other end sutured end-to-side to the obliquely transected (up to half its diameter) hypoglossal nerve proximal to the ansa hypoglossi (Figs 18.1A to K). Monofilament 10-0 nylon suture material is used for interrupted epineural tension-free approximation under the operating microscope. Occasionally, a penrose drain is left in the wound. Usually the patient is discharged the second day following the operation. In most of the patients a gold weight is placed on the upper eyelid, after release of an existing tarsorrhaphy.

PHYSIOTHERAPY

The patients are advised to follow a physiotherapy program as soon as initial movements in the face appear during tongue movement. The goal of these exercises is to promote facial expression and movements in relation with emotions and expression.

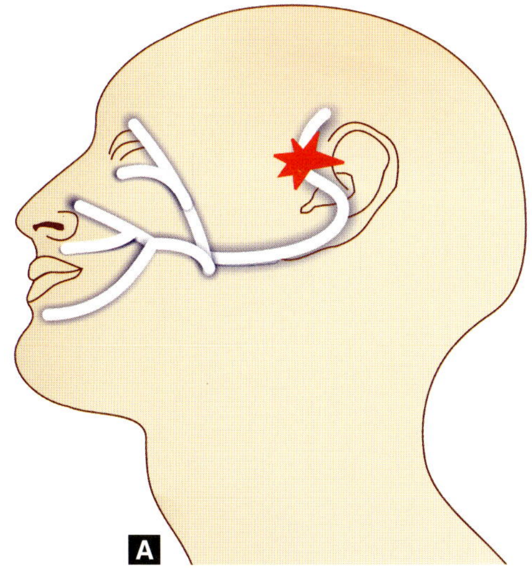
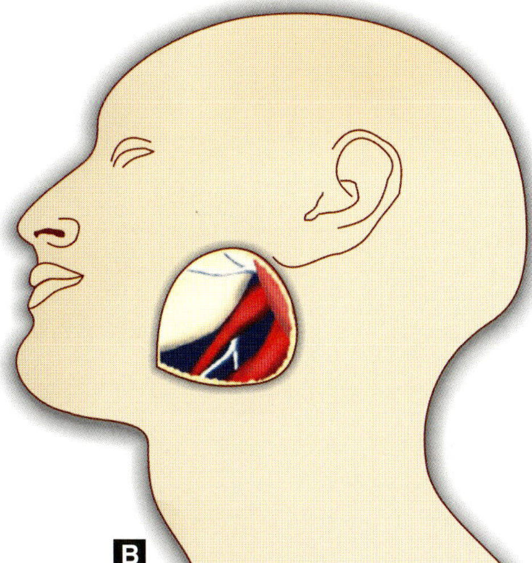

Figs 18.1A and B

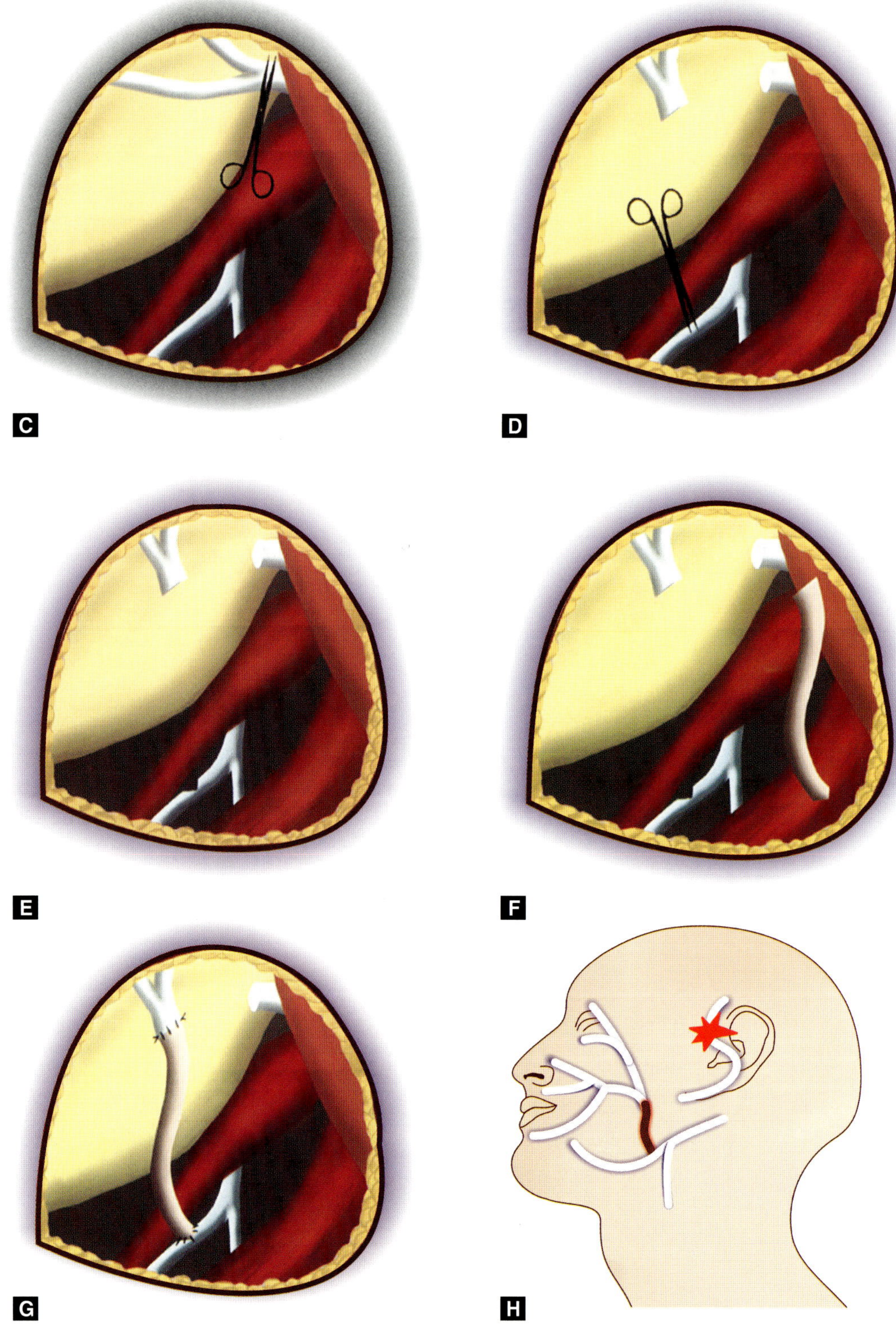

Figs 18.1C to H

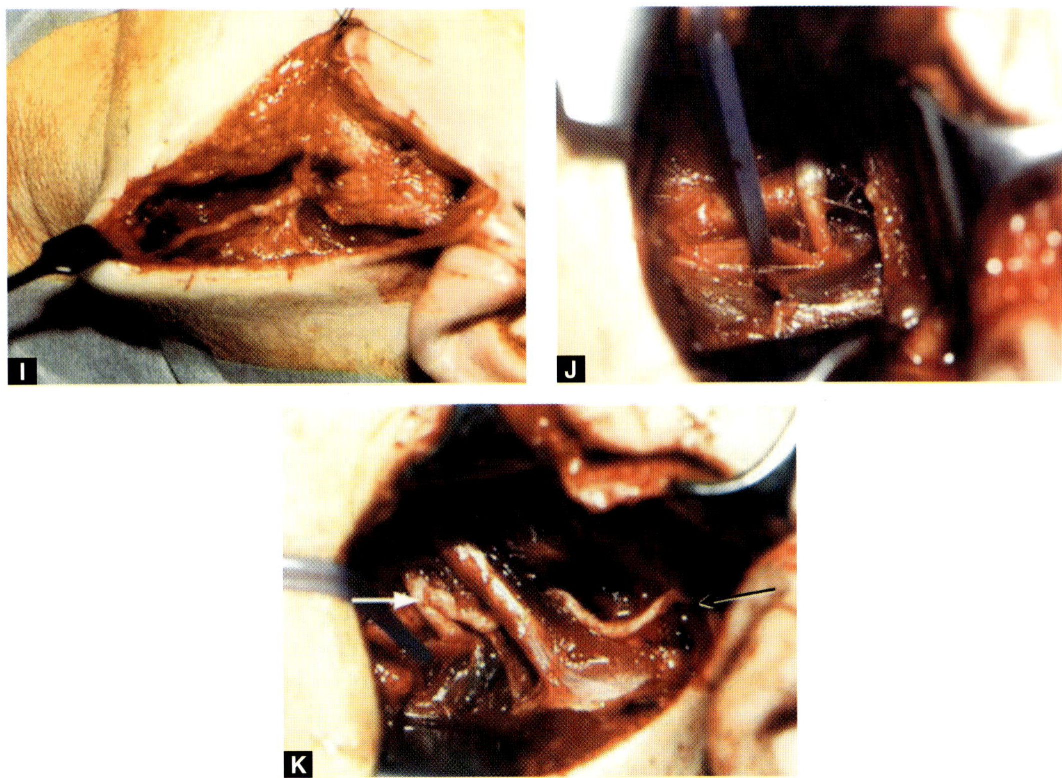

Figs 18.1I to K

Figs 18.1A to K: (A) Facial paralysis not recovered after acoustic neuroma surgery; (B) Overview of regional anatomy; (C) Cutting facial nerve main stem; (D) Transverse cutting of hypoglossal nerve distal from ansa hypoglossi; (E) Result of D; (F) Prepared free graft of greater auricular nerve; (G) End-to-end anastomosis to peripheral facial nerve main stem and side-to-end to hypoglossal nerve; (H) An overview of NVII-NXII jump anastomosis with free nerve graft, (I) *Intraoperative view.* After skin incision preparation of the free graft of the greater auricular nerve; (J) *Intraoperative view.* Preparation of hypoglossal nerve and ansa hypoglossi crossing the carotid artery; (K) *Intraoperative view.* Free nerve graft anastomosed end-to-side of hypoglossal nerve (white arrow) and end-to-end to peripheral facial nerve stem (black arrow) guided underneath digastric muscle (see text)

PERSONAL EXPERIENCE

The medical records of all patients who underwent hypoglossal facial nerve anastomosis with interposition of a free nerve graft were reviewed. Facial reanimation was assessed in 29 patients who completed 24 months of follow-up. The causes of facial nerve paralysis are summarized in (Table 18.1). These 29 patients were placed into three groups related to the interval between the onset of facial paralysis and the hypoglossal facial nerve graft anastomosis: Group 1 with an interval from 4 to 12 months, Group 2 with an interval from 12 to 24 months and Group 3 with an interval of more than 24 months. Group 1 comprised 19 patients (13 females and 6 males) their ages ranged from 11 to 71 years with a mean age of 42.9 years.

Group 2 included 6 patients (5 females and 1 male) their ages ranged from 28 to 62 years with a mean age of 41.9 years. Group 3 consisted of 4 patients (1 female and 3 males) their ages ranged from 30 to 62 years with a mean age of 46.7 years. For the evaluation of tongue mobility and appearance, all 29 patients were

Table 18.1: Etiology of facial paralysis	
Acoustic neuroma	25
Cerebral infarction	1
Middle ear malignancy	1
Supralabyrinthine intracranial cholesteatoma	1
Plexus chorioideus papilloma	1
Total number of patients	**29**

assessed 6 to 24 months after the operation. Facial nerve function was established using the House-Brackmann (HB) facial nerve grading system (House and Brackman, 1985) (Table 18.2).

RESULTS

Improved facial tone and symmetry preceded initial facial movements. In all patients, facial movements appeared at 4-18 months and were usually first observed in the mid-face. We observed that the longer the duration before the operation, the poorer the result. When the duration of paralysis exceeded 2 years, recovery of the muscles of facial expression was poor. Synkinesis was observed in most patients, but no mass movements or gross hypertonia was present. Initial anesthesia due to ablation of the greater auricular nerve appeared insignificant to all patients. Problems with speech, mastication or swallowing were not seen. In a small percentage of patients, slight asymmetry due to reduction in the size of the homolateral tongue was observed. Another small percentage of patients showed no improvement at all.

COMMENTS

- End-to-end anastomosis of the facial nerve stumps either by direct suturing or by interpositioning of a free nerve graft results in the best functional recovery. When the proximal stump is unavailable

or when the anatomically preserved facial nerve after cerebellopontine angle or temporal bone surgery has not regained function and the muscles of facial expression are still viable, transposition of other cranial nerves to rehabilitate these muscles can be considered. The concept of transposition of an alternative motor nerve dates back to 1879, when Drobnik anastomosed the spinal accessory nerve to the facial nerve. Other (cranial) nerves used for transposition are:

- Hypoglossal nerve
- Facial nerve (cross face anastomosis)
- Phrenic nerve
- Glossopharyngeal nerve.

The major disadvantage of donor nerve techniques is that a functional nerve has to be sacrificed, leaving the patient with functional loss. Results of facial nerve reinnervating surgery are related to the duration of the paralysis, i.e. the functional state of the muscles of facial expression. The functional recovery of denervated muscles is time dependent (Table 18.3) (Stennert, 1979). In addition, the duration of the neurotization also has to be considered. The different steps in neurotization and their duration are summarized in (Table 18.4) (Seckel, 1990; Reynolds

Table 18.2: House-Brackmann facial nerve system

Grade description	Characteristics
I Normal	Facial function in all areas
II Mild dysfunction	Slight weakness noticeable on close inspection; may have very slight synkinesis. At rest: normal symmetry and tone.
III Moderate dysfunction	Gross: obvious but not disfiguring difference between two sides: noticeable but not severe synkinesis, contracture, and/or hemifacial spasm. At rest: normal
IV Moderately severe dysfunction	Gross: obvious weakness and/or Disfiguring asymmetry and tone.
V Severe dysfunction	Gross: only barely perceptible motion. At rest: asymmetry
VI Total paralysis	No movement

Table 18.3: Relation of duration of denervation of muscles of facial expression and expectation of successful rehabilitation

Duration of denervation	Functional recovery
1 year	Absolutely certain
2-2 years	Seemingly certain: recommendable
2-3 years	Probable with delay and decrease in functions
3-5 years	Increasingly questionable; patient must be notified
5+ years	Improbable; not to be recommend

Table 18.4: Duration of the different stages in neurotization

Stages	Duration
Sprouting of cranial stump	± 1 month
Passage of nerve suture site	± 1 month
Passage of distal nerve (nerve graft)	± 1 mm/day
Motoric endplate electromyographic activity	± 1 month

and Woolf, 1992). Taking into account both the duration of facial paralysis and the duration of reneurotization, the decision to perform hypoglossal facial nerve interpositional graft anastomosis is to be taken at latest 1 year after the onset of paralysis in order to obtain the best results. In the presence of an anatomically intact facial nerve and postoperative facial paralysis, nerve function usually showed signs of recovery within 12 months after acoustic neuroma surgery (Kunihiro et al. 1994; Fenton et al. 1999). One may argue that facial nerve regeneration may take up to 18 months before any significant sign of recovery is noted. However, it is questionable if results of recovery will appear as good as with hypoglossal facial nerve graft anastomosis performed at around 12 months after injury, in the absence of clinical and electromyographic signs of recovery. When paralysis lasts more than 2 years, the atrophy of the muscles of facial expression has progressed so far that surgical techniques other than facial nerve re-innervating procedures have to be considered.

Our study confirms the favorable functional results of this technique. Three quarters of our patients achieved HB Grade II and III. The results appear at least as good as the classical, direct hypoglossal-facial nerve anastomosis (Conley and Baker, 1979; Hammerschlag, 1999; Brudney et al. 1998; Kunihiro et al. 1994) and preserves tongue function. The best results were ascertained in patients undergoing surgery within 12 months after facial nerve injury. This was also shown by others using the classical direct end-to-end anastomosis between both nerves (Conley and Baker, 1979; Stennert, 1979; Kunihiro et al. 1994).

In the present study, the recovery of the temporal branch of the facial nerve was very poor. This may be related to the observation of Chang and Shen (1984) that the temporal branch contains a relatively small number of fibers. However, ineffective function caused by cross-innervation of antagonistic muscles in this region and canceling out each other's activity, a process called "autoparalysis", may play a role (Stennert, 1985). We observed less synkinesis with the jump technique in comparison to the classical end-to-end anastomosis. This may be related to the reduced re-innervation. Another explanation could be that, the routinely included physiotherapy may result in more efficient use of the facial musculature.

BIBLIOGRAPHY

1. Arai H, Sato K, Yanai A. Hemihypoglossal-facial nerve anastomosis in treating unilateral facial palsy after acoustic neurinoma resection. J Neurosurg. 1995;82:51-4.
2. Brudney J, Hammerschlag PE, Cohen HL, et al. Electromyographic rehabilitation of facial function and introduction of a facial paralysis grading scale for hypoglossal-facial nerve anastomosis. Laryngoscope. 1988;98(4):405-10.
3. Chang CGS, Shen AL. Hypoglossalfacial anatomosis for facial palsy after resection of acoustic neuroma. Surg Neurol. 1984;21(3):282-6.
4. Conley J, Baker D. Hypoglossal-facial nerve anastomosis for reinnervation of the paralysed face. Plast Reconstr Surg. 1979;63(1):63-72.
5. Fenton JE, Chin RYK, Shirazi A, et al. Prediction of postoperative facial nerve function in acoustic neuroma surgery. Clin Otolaryngol Allied Sci. 1999;24(6):483-6.
6. Gidley PW, Gantz BJ, Rubinstein JT. Facial nerve grafts: from cerebellopontine angle and beyond. Am J Otol. 1999;20(6):781-8.
7. Hammerschlag PE. Facial reanimation with jump interpositional graft hypoglossal facial anastomosis and hypoglossal facial anastomosis: evolution in management of facial paralysis. Laryngoscope. 1999;109(2 Pt 2 Suppl 90):1-23.
8. House JW, Brackmann DE. Facial nerve grading system. Otolaryngol Head and Neck Surgery. 1985;93:146-7.
9. Kessler LA, Moldaver J, Pool JL. Hypoglossal-facial anastomosis for treatment of facial paralysis. Neurol. 1959;9:118-25.
10. Kunihiro T, Kanzaki J, Yoshihara S, et al. Analysis of the prognosis and the recovery process of profound facial nerve paralysis secondary to acoustic neuroma resection. ORL J Otorhinolaryngol Relat Spec. 1994;56(6):331-3.
11. Kunihiro T, Matsunga T, Kanzaki J. Clinical investigation of hypoglossal-facial nerve anastomosis. Eur Arch Otolaryngol. 1994;(suppl):3730-5.
12. Manni JJ, Beurskens CHG, Velde van de C, et al. Reanimation of the paralyzed face by indirect hypoglossal-facial nerve anastomosis. Am J Surg. 2001;182(3):268-73.
13. May M, Sobol SM, Mester SJ. Hypoglossal-facial nerve interpositional-jump graft for facial reanimation without tongue atrophy. Otolaryngol Head Neck Surg. 1991;104(6):818-25.
14. Pensak ML, Jackson CG, Glasscock ME, et al. Facial reanimation with the twelve-seven anastomosis. Otolaryngol Head Neck Surg. 1986;94:305-10

15. Reynolds ML, Woolf CJ. Terminal Schwann cells elaborate extensive processes following denervation of the motor endplate. J Neurocytol. 1992;21:50-66.

16. Rubin L, Mishrike YY, Speace G. Reanimation of the hemi-paralytic tongue. Plast Reconstruct Surg. 1984;84:192-6.

17. Seckel BR. Enhancement of peripheral nerve regeneration. Muscle Nerve. 1990;13:785-800.

18. Stennert E. Hypoglossal facial anastomosis: its significance for modern facial surgery II. Combined approach in extra-temporal facial nerve reconstruction. Clin Plast Surg. 1979;6(3):471-86.

19. Stennert E. The autoparalytic syndrome as cause of permanent loss of function of the frontalis muscle. In: Portmann M (Ed). Facial Nerve. New York:Masson; 1985. pp. 291-5.

20. Ueda K, Harri K, Yamada A. Free neuromuscle transplantation for the treatment of facial paralysis using hypoglossal nerve as a recipient motor source. Plast Reconstruct Surg. 1994;94(6):808-17.

19

Facial Reanimation and Facial-Hypoglossal Neurorrhaphy

Laura Hetzler, Rohan R Walvekar

INTRODUCTION

Facial paralysis is a devastating occurrence regardless of etiology. The social and emotional implications of no longer being able to express oneself naturally can be more distressing than the cause of paralysis. The human face is what we recognize as our personal identity and its expressions are a separate and distinct language. Loss of these expressions leaves our patients with only verbal communication lacking their individual thumbprint of personality.

Loss of facial motion is best approached systematically. Static or dynamic reconstruction of deficient facial function may be elected based on the remaining anatomy or based on the patient himself. In most cases, a combination of interventions that may include dynamic procedures for the lower face and static therapy for the upper face have the best results. Facial reanimation is dependent upon the anatomical and functional status of the proximal and distal facial nerve as well patient goals and desires. Consequently, an individualized approach is imperative to a successful outcome.

The use of facial-hypoglossal neurorrhaphy was first described by Korte in 1901 (Korte W, 1903). The technique has since been modified to avoid complete sacrifice of the ipsilateral hypoglossal nerve in an effort to reduce morbidity and to optimize surgical results. Anecdotally, some believe that in more robust patients, a complete transfer of the hypoglossal nerve can lead to excessive grimacing and movement that may lead to a less optimal functional result. Possible techniques for facial-hypoglossal neurorrhaphy include a direct end to end anastamosis, end to side anastamosis, jump graft or a split hypoglossal technique.

The hallmark of facial hypoglossal neurorrhaphy is the preservation of tone in the paralyzed face. This bears tremendous benefit in an aging population where the main goal may be simple maintenance of symmetry. Benefits may appear as early as 6 months, following the procedure with some patients reporting improved mobility for up to 2-3 years (Sobol SM et al. 1991; Conley J et al. 1979). Refining the results of facial hypoglossal transfer will often involve bio-feedback exercises and motor re-education to learn voluntary control of movement and limit facial grimacing that can occur with mastication.

Facial hypoglossal neurorrhaphy can be used in combination with other dynamic procedures including staged cross facial nerve grafting with subsequent free muscle transfer. The cross facial graft and the facial-hypoglossal portions of the procedure may be performed in the same surgical setting followed by the free tissue transfer at the appropriate later date. The objective of this combined technique is that the facial hypoglossal component will offer tone with the cross facial/free tissue portion granting more elegant facial motion.

The hypoglossal nerve can be used as a donor in other dynamic techniques of reanimation including hypoglossal transfer to free tissue. An in-depth discussion on this particular indication is beyond the scope of this chapter. However, it is mentioned simply to imply that we must weigh all options for risk and benefit with specific reference to the viable anatomy, individual patient desires, health status and expectations.

INDICATIONS AND PATIENT SELECTION

Facial-hypoglossal neurorrhaphy is most often employed when there is ample distal facial nerve available without proximal facial nerve viability. A common scenario for this procedure is with facial nerve sacrifice in acoustic neuroma surgery. In this situation, the pulsations of cerebral spinal fluid on a fresh neurorrhaphy and the technical difficulty of suturing in the cerebellopontine angle often make facial-hypoglossal transfer an attractive option for reanimation.

In patients with an intra-temporal extracranial defect, all attempts should be made to perform a primary repair or cable graft. If this cannot be done due to a poor proximal segment, the distal facial nerve may be mobilized for other dynamic reanimation procedures including facial-hypoglossal grafting.

The technique of facial hypoglossal neurorrhaphy mandates intact and functioning motor end-plates. Prolonged or chronic paralysis greater than 2 years is often considered a contraindication. Complete electrical silence on electromyography (EMG) implies inactive motor end plates and thus any dynamic procedure for reanimation that utilizes the native facial nerve and its musculature is futile. The author has seen benefit if facial-hypoglossal transfer is performed up to 2 years following facial paralysis.

Individuals with concomitant injury to cranial nerves IX and X are not considered candidates for facial-hypoglossal neurorrhaphy as any additional cranial nerve XII weakness could result in severe swallowing dysfunction and oral incompetence.

PREOPERATIVE PLANNING

In preparation for facial-hypoglossal grafting, preoperative counseling should be given to include possible poor result, excessive result with grimacing and synkinesis, tongue weakness or dysarthria.

Operative approach and incisions will be dictated by any prior scars or concomitant procedures to be performed at that time. If the neurorrhaphy is performed at the time of tumor extirpation, the most appropriate incision to allow complete removal of the tumor takes precedence. If the surgeon suspects that mobilizing any significant length of the facial nerve from the temporal bone will not be possible, consideration of donor nerve harvest to perform a jump graft must be discussed preoperatively. Donor nerves frequently used for jump grafting are the great auricular nerve, medial antebrachial cutaneous nerve and the sural nerve.

Adjunctive static procedures are often recommended to optimize surgical results, particularly when ocular protection is in question. A gold or platinum weight can be implanted for expected lagophthalmos without any significant addition to surgical time or added morbidity. If lower lid laxity is present preoperatively and sacrifice of the facial nerve is expected, support of the lower lid with a horizontal tightening procedure is suggested. The author's preference is a lateral tarsal strip procedure. Midface support such as with a static sling is also a viable option and should be discussed.

Standard preoperative photos are prudent in any facial reconstructive procedure.

SURGICAL TECHNIQUES

Fundamental understanding of neural repair is crucial. The epineurium is ideally preserved on the separate nerves. It is paramount that the neurorrhaphy be completed in a tension free fashion for optimal results. The facial nerve should be identified as far out as the division of the facial nerve into its upper and lower division or the "pes" to allow for appropriate mobility and reflection. Identification may be difficult as the nerve can suffer atrophy with prolonged paralysis. Clean sectioning of the distal facial nerve is best performed with a new scalpel on a supported surface. If possible, preserving an epineurial cuff will allow for improved suture technique and more optimal alignment of axons end to end rather than the bunching and divergence past one another once neurorrhaphy is complete.

The hypoglossal nerve is easily found high in the neck and deep to the posterior belly of the digastric muscle (Fig. 19.1). The nerve is often crossed by the occipital artery which may need to be divided to allow for better exposure and mobilization. The ranine plexus of veins is often visible overlying the hypoglossal nerve and the ansa hypoglossi may be seen descending into the neck as part of the cervical plexus. The descendens hypoglossi is accepted anatomically as a cervical root contribution to the hypoglossal nerve and not originating from the hypoglossal nucleus in the brainstem. Consequently, it is typically recommended that the surgical division of the hypoglossal nerve should be planned distal to the descendens hypoglossi to allow for the majority

of motor nerve fibers to be from the hypoglossal nerve and thus directed to tongue mobility (Fig. 19.2).

Ideally, the facial nerve is divided near the second genu and mobilized from the temporal bone. Care must be taken near the stylomastoid foramen where interdigitaton of the periosteum and the epineurium can occur. This provides ample length to the facial nerve to extend inferiorly without tension to the hypoglossal nerve (Fig. 19.3). As mentioned previously, in situations where the nerve cannot be found within the mastoid and must be reflected inferiorly from the stylomastoid foramen, a jump graft may be necessary. This is not always the case. In some instances the hypoglossal nerve may be split and reflected superiorly avoiding the need for an interposition jump graft.

Sectioning of hypoglossal nerve should not be performed through more than 1/3 of the total diameter as this allows for less morbidity associated with ipsilateral tongue weakness and less likelihood of

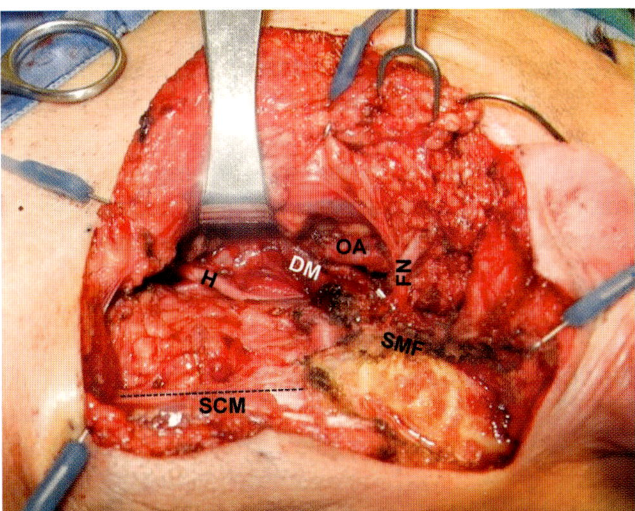

Fig. 19.1: Proximity of the hypoglossal nerve to the facial nerve trunk (FN) with the posterior belly of the digastric muscle (DM) retracted anteriorly, the hypoglossal nerve (H) can be seen lateral to the carotid artery. The proximity of the facial nerve trunk as it exits the stylomastoid foramen (SMF) is depicted here. The occipital artery (OA) is seen branching from the external carotid system between the neural trunks. (SCM - Sternocleidomastoid muscle; anterior border depicted by dashed line)

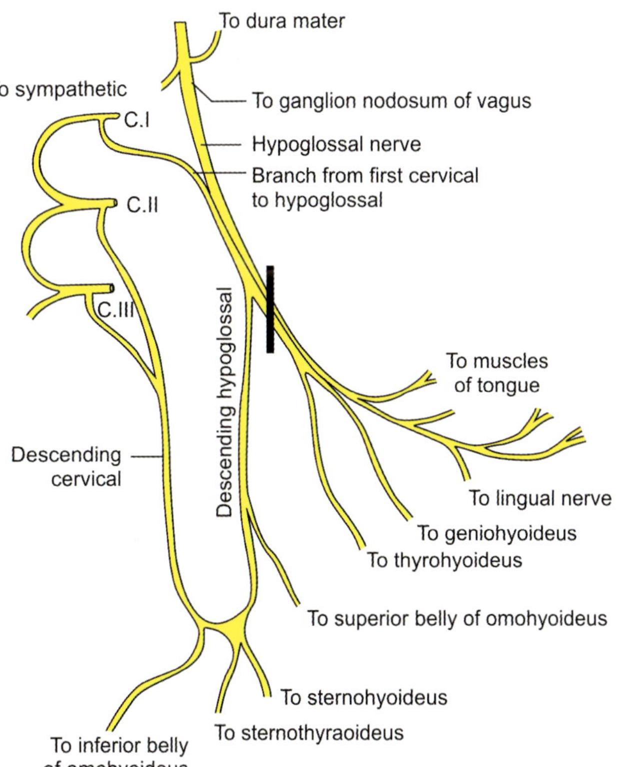

Fig. 19.2: Illustration showing the origin of the descendens hypoglossi and the components of the hypoglossal nerve. The black line depicts the recommended site for surgical division of the hypoglossal nerve for facial hypoglossal anastamosis

spasm and grimacing (May M et al. 1991). The stump of the facial nerve may then be sewn into the beveled division of the hypoglossal nerve in the retrograde direction (Fig. 19.4). If a jump graft is being used, the interposition nerve is sewn into the hypoglossal nerve in an identical fashion and the opposite end is sewn end-to-end to the facial nerve.

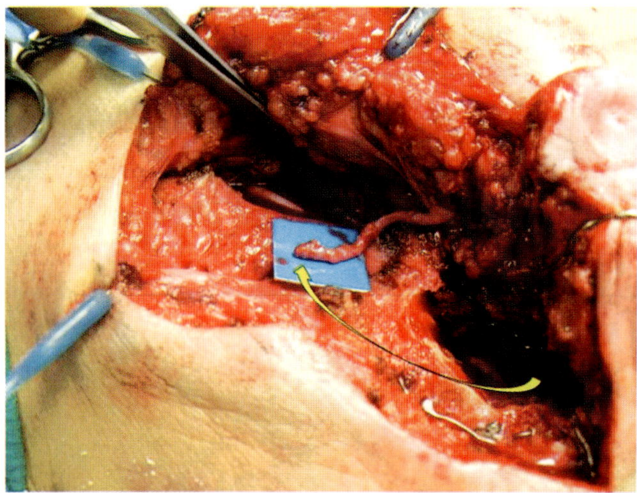

Fig. 19.3: Length of facial nerve following decompression. The facial nerve has been transected at the second genu and reflected inferiorly. Care is taken to release the nerve from the soft tissue at the stylomastoid foramen extending to the pes.

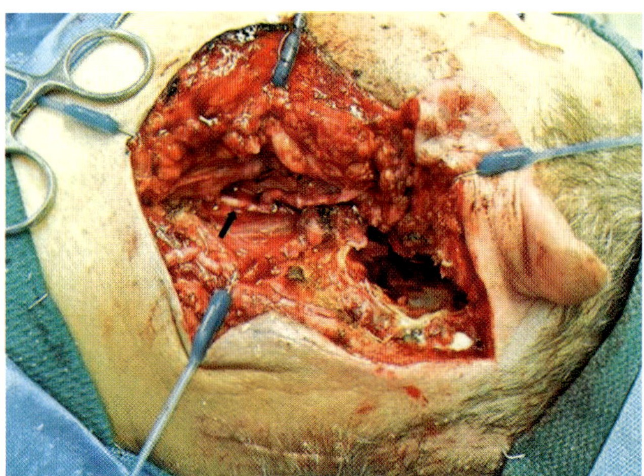

Fig. 19.4: Tension free neurorrhaphy. The transected proximal facial nerve is then coapted to the beveled incision into the recipient hypoglossal (black arrow points to anastamosis). The hypoglossal is only transected to approximately one-thirds to one-half of its diameter with the facial nerve sutured in a retrograde direction. The neurorrhaphy is performed with ample laxity to allow for mobility and contraction.

Division of the hypoglossal nerve may be performed in a split fashion with teasing of the transected nerve fibers into a separate neural trunk. This may then be reflected to the facial nerve trunk and decrease the need for a jump graft. Lin et al. recently reported no difference in whether or not a jump graft was used (Lin V, et al. 2009).

Postoperative Care

Drainage of the wound bed is to the surgeon's preference. Postoperative antibiotics are preferred if there is oral contamination during the procedure however not required in a clean case.

PITFALLS AND COMPLICATIONS

The most common complication following facial hypoglossal transfer is a disappointing result that fails patient expectations. Consequently, preoperative expectations must be managed to ensure an understanding that rarely can be coordinated for facial motion be obtained. Patients with the best result are highly motivated and undergo significant rehabilitation and bio-feedback to achieve their goals. Some may experience excessive function related to grimacing and synkinesis. This can be particularly problematic. Tongue mobility is often adequate with a split hypoglossal technique allowing greater than half of the hypoglossal nerve fibers to continue to enter the tongue.

BIBLIOGRAPHY

1. Conley J, Baker D. Hypoglossal-facial nerve anastomosis for reinnervation of the paralyzed face. Plast Reconstruct Surg. 1979;63(1):63-72.
2. Korte W. Ein Fal von Nerven Fropfung: des Nervus facialis auf den Nervus hypoglossus. Dtsch Med Wochenschr. 1903;29:293.
3. Lin V, Jacobson M, Dorion J, et al. Global Assessment of outcomes after varying reinnervation techniques for patients with facial paralysis subsequent to acoustic Neuroma Excision. Otol Neurotol. 2009;30(3):408-13.
4. May M, Sobol SM, Mester SJ. Hypoglossal-facial nerve interpositional-jump graft for facial reanimation without tongue atrophy. Otolaryngol Head Neck Surg. 1991; 104(6):818-25.
5. Sobol SM, May M. Hypoglossal-facial anastomosis: its role in contemporary facial reanimation. In: Rubin LR, Ed. The paralyzed face. 1st ed. St. Louis: Mosby-Year Book; 1991. pp. 137-43.

20

Facial Nerve and the Petrous Apex

James Lin, Rohan R Walvekar, Daniel W Nuss

PERTINENT ANATOMY

The petrous apex is the medial most portion of the temporal bone. Laterally, its broad base consists of the bony labyrinth, cochlea and petrous carotid artery. The roof of the petrous apex is comprised of the floor of the middle cranial fossa that is medial to the arcuate eminence and the greater superficial petrosal nerve (GSPN). Its posterior face is the anterior bony boundary of the cerebellopontine angle which lies medial to the operculum, lateral to the clivus and superior to the inferior petrosal sinus which runs into the jugular bulb. Within the petrous apex is the internal auditory canal which transmits the three branches of the 8th cranial nerve, the facial nerve and the intermediate nerve. The petrous apex is traversed along its superior-most area by the abducens nerve through Dorello's canal. The superior petrosal sinus runs along its posterosuperior surface while the inferior petrosal sinus runs along its inferomedial surface. Both sinuses connect the cavernous sinus (anteromedial and adjacent to the petrous apex) to transverse-sigmoid-jugular venous system. Most petrous apices contain only bone marrow

and lack pneumatization.

The intracanalicular facial nerve assumes an antero-superior location relative to the 8th nerve branches. At the fundus or lateral end of the internal auditory canal, the facial nerve is separated from the more posterior superior vestibular nerve by the vertical crest also known as "Bill's Bar." At this point, the nerve has entered its bony tunnel in the temporal bone known as the fallopian canal. The first portion of the facial nerve in the fallopian canal is known as the labyrinthine segment where the bony canal is most narrow at 0.5-2.5 mm and encased within a fibrous ligament and least forgiving in the case of a traumatized, edematous nerve (Kefalidis G et al. 2010).

The labyrinthine facial nerve ascends in its bony canal and then becomes intimately involved in the geniculate ganglion. From the geniculate, the GSPN exits anteriorly and medially while the fibers of the main trunk of facial nerve turn at an acute angle in a posterior direction to enter its tympanic segment. The geniculate ganglion radiologically is dehiscent without bony covering in about 15% of temporal bones (Isaacson B et al. 2007).

Because of the central location of the petrous apex, diseases of the petrous apex can be present for long periods of time prior to the onset of symptoms. Headache and upper as well as lower cranial neuropathies may be associated with petrous apex disease. Its central location within the skull base also makes it a difficult area to access surgically.

DISEASES OF THE PETROUS APEX

Several different disease entities may involve the petrous apex. This chapter attempts to include the most pertinent ones.

Infectious Disorders

Petrous Apicitis

Petrous apicitis typically results from acute or chronic otitis media with medial spread and can be life-threatening when it occurs. The classic Gradenigo's triad of abducens palsy, otorrhea, and retro-orbital pain occurs rarely with petrous apicitis. Also, given that the apex contains the carotid artery; petrous apicitis can also lead to constriction of the carotid artery and/or cavernous sinus thrombosis. In this era of modern antibiotics, the mainstay of treatment is pressure equalization tube and long-term culture-directed intravenous antibiotics. Petrosectomy may be required and is reserved for recalcitrant or progressive disease (Visosky AM et al. 2006). Simple ventilation of the petrous apex via apicotomy in such cases may be inadequate.

Figures 20.1 to 20.3 demonstrate radiological findings of an adult patient who had right otitis media complicated by petrous apicitis. The patient presented with fevers, headache and retro-orbital pain with ipsilateral abducens palsy. Intravenous antibiotics, placement of a pressure equalization tube and a short course of corticosteroids led to resolution of the abducens palsy within days.

Skull Base Osteomyelitis

Skull base osteomyelitis is a more widespread infection of the base of the skull that may or may not include the petrous apex. The etiology is more diverse and additionally includes otitis externa, particularly in the

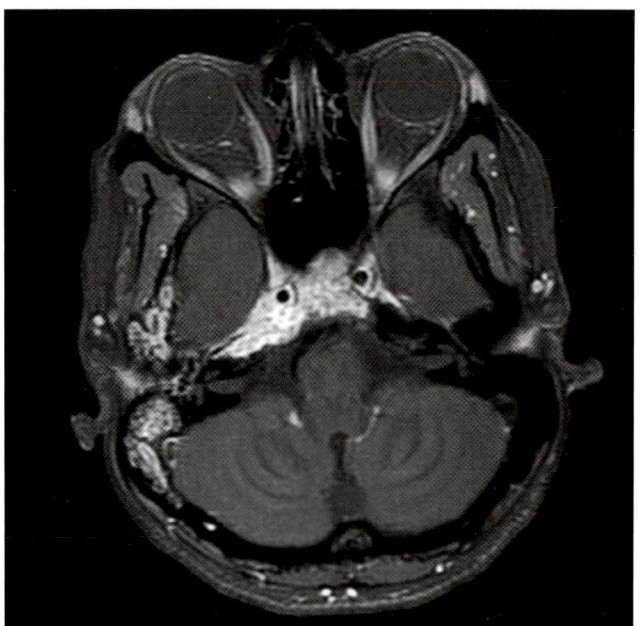

Fig. 20.1: Petrous apicitis. A contrasted T1-weighted fat suppressed axial MRI of a middle aged female with right petrous apicitis. Note the diffuse enhancement of the right petrous apex and clivus as well as the right mastoid air cells and bone along the zygomatic root

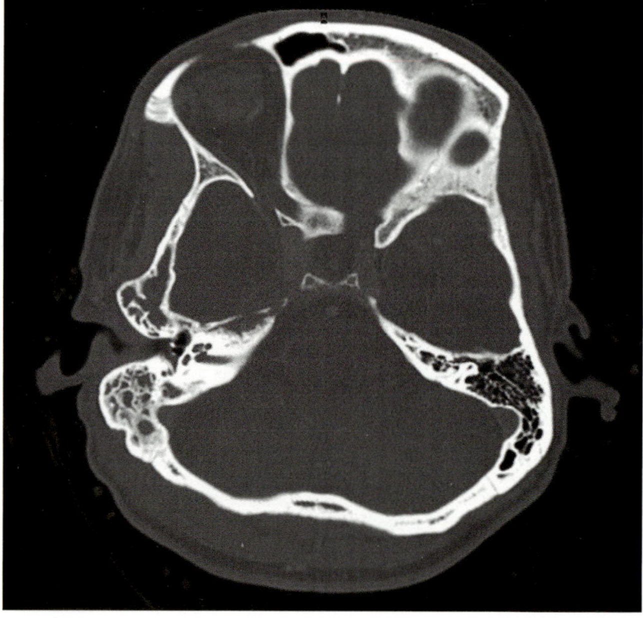

Fig. 20.2: Petrous apicitis. Demonstration of the high resolution contrasted axial CT scan of same patient from Figure 20.1. Note the opacification of the right mastoid, zygomatic root as well as petrous apex on the right

immuno-compromised or diabetic patient. The treatment protocol remains the same. Initial management includes culture-directed intravenous antibiotics for several weeks and surgical debridement is reserved for recalcitrant or progressive cases only. The course and success of treatment may be followed by patient symptomatology, imaging studies, radionuclide studies and lab indices (Erythrocyte Sedimentation Rate, C-reactive protein, White blood cell count). A multidisciplinary approach with early inclusion of an infectious disease specialist is recommended. In the author's experience, the work-up of an erosive skull base lesion requires biopsy-proven exclusion of a neoplastic process. The biopsy also provides specimens that can be sent for culture. Multiple surgical interventions may be required to acquire a representative biopsy and for debridement. Figures 20.4 to 20.7 depict a middle-aged female who experienced left excruciating facial pain and developed neuropathies involving cranial nerves V, VI, IX, X and XI due to widespread skull base osteomyelitis. She had multiple endoscopy directed biopsies in two separate states within the United States prior to being evaluated in our clinic. Further biopsies and culture at our institution

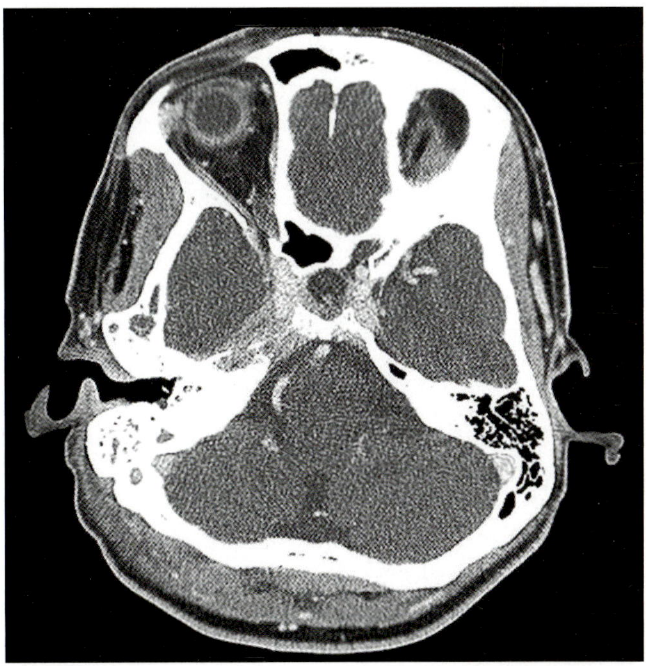

Fig. 20.3: Petrous apicitis. This figure shows the contrasted head CT in soft tissue windows of the same patient from the prior two figures. Note the continuous enhancement through bony dehiscence along the right petrous apex and the region of the cavernous sinus

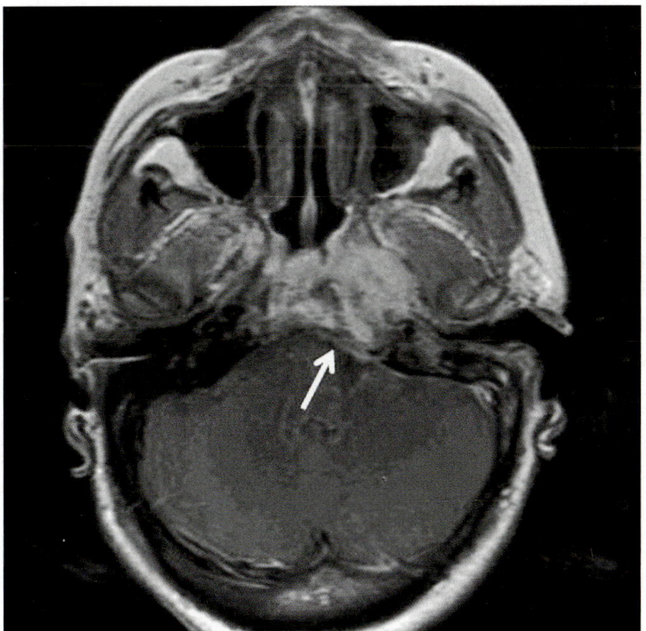

Fig. 20.4: Chronic skull base osteomyelitis. This is the axial T1-weighted MRI with gadolinium of a middle aged female with long standing left facial pain. Note the diffuse enhancement along the clivus and left petrous apex region and the subtle enhancement of the dura along the clivus and petrous apex (white arrow).

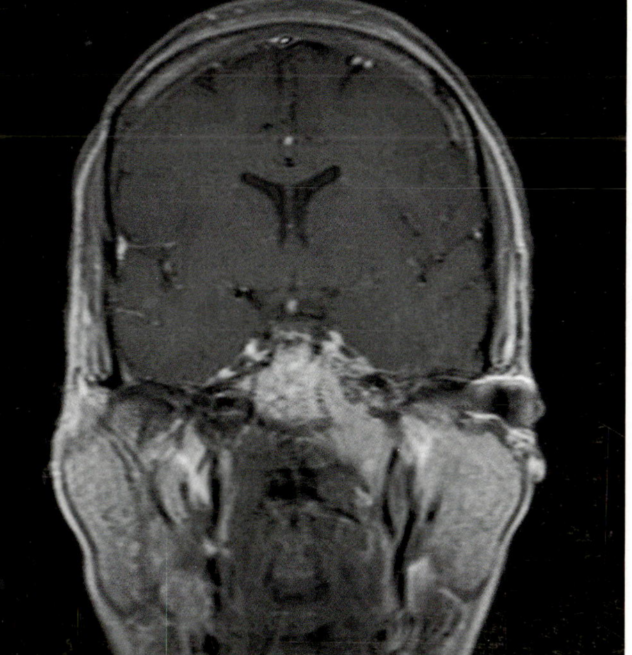

Fig. 20.5: Chronic skull base osteomyelitis. This figure demonstrates the T1-weighted coronal MRI with gadolinium of the patient from the Figure 20.4. Note the diffuse enhancement of the soft tissues deep to the left nasopharynx.

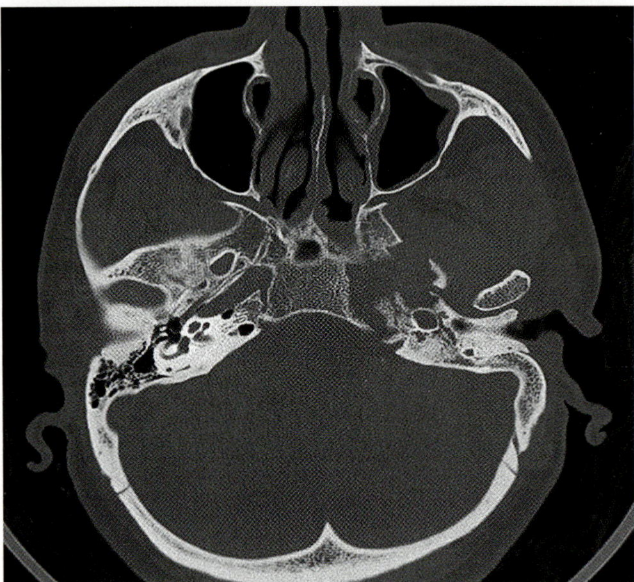

Fig. 20.6: Chronic skull base osteomyelitis. Axial temporal bone CT of the patient from Figures 20.4 and 20.5. Note the bony erosion of the left petrous apex compared the normal right side. Also note the asymmetry of mastoid pneumatization versus the right side; this finding suggests that the skull base osteomyelitis may have had an otogenic source.

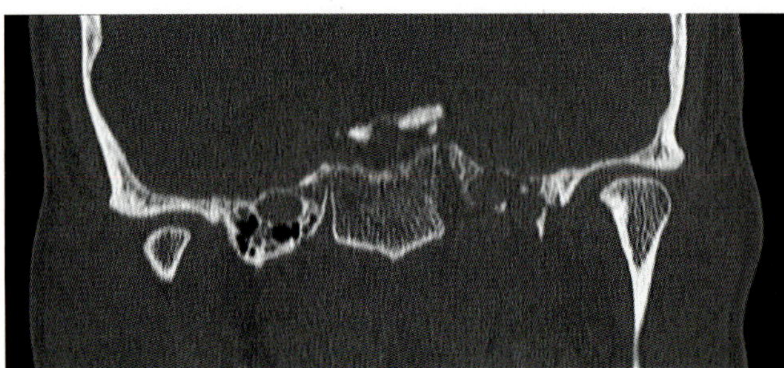

Fig. 20.7: Chronic skull base osteomyelitis. Coronal CT scan of the patient from Figures 20.4 to 20.6. Note the bony erosion of the left petrous apex surrounding the intratemporal internal carotid artery

identified a species of Campylobacter. Intensive culture-directed intravenous antibiotics led to resolution of pain and improvement in cranial neuropathies.

Inflammatory Disorders

Cholesterol granulomas are cystic foreign-body reactions characterized by cholesterol crystals surrounded by an inflammatory pseudocapsule. The classically described etiology entails a poorly ventilated air cell space leading to transmucosal hemorrhage followed by blood breakdown and resulting cholesterol crystals. The crystals then would lead to a foreign body response which would become incompletely resolved, walled off and left to expand. Jackler and Cho (Jackler RK et al. 2003) took note of the paradox that cholesterol granulomas typically occur in well pneumatized mastoids. These mastoids are the least likely to suffer from poor ventilation. They postulated that the etiology of these cholesterol granulomas lies in the exposure of marrow into air cells which lead to hemorrhage into mucosal-lined spaces thus leading to the formation of cholesterol and foreign body reaction. In either case, the potential for expansion and compression of surrounding structures leads to the development of hearing loss, tinnitus, headache, vestibular symptoms, facial paresis and diplopia. Because of its lack of a true epithelial lining, the treatment of cholesterol granulomas includes drainage and marsupialization that results in relief of symptoms. Several different approaches to the petrous apex are described but apicotomy approaches such as the infracochlear or infralabyrinthine ones are the most typically used. If the cyst wall is in proximity to the sphenoid sinus without internal carotid intervening, an endoscopic endonasal transsphenoidal approach may be performed for drainage (Zanation AM et al. 2009). For recalcitrant disease, a middle fossa approach may be used to ventilate or exenterate the diseased air cells (Brackmann DE et al. 2002).

Figures 20.8 to 20.10 show the CT scan and pre-contrast T1 and T2 MRI scans of a middle-aged male with a large cholesterol granuloma. The patient underwent endoscopic transsphenoidal drainage with a significant decrease in size of the cyst. If the patient's symptoms recur and/or the cyst should begin to enlarge, the patient will likely undergo repeated drainage through an otologic approach.

NEOPLASTIC DISORDERS

Schwannomas

Vestibular Schwannomas

Vestibular schwannomas are benign tumors arising from the vestibular branch of the 8th nerve. They are relatively common tumors seen by neurotologists and

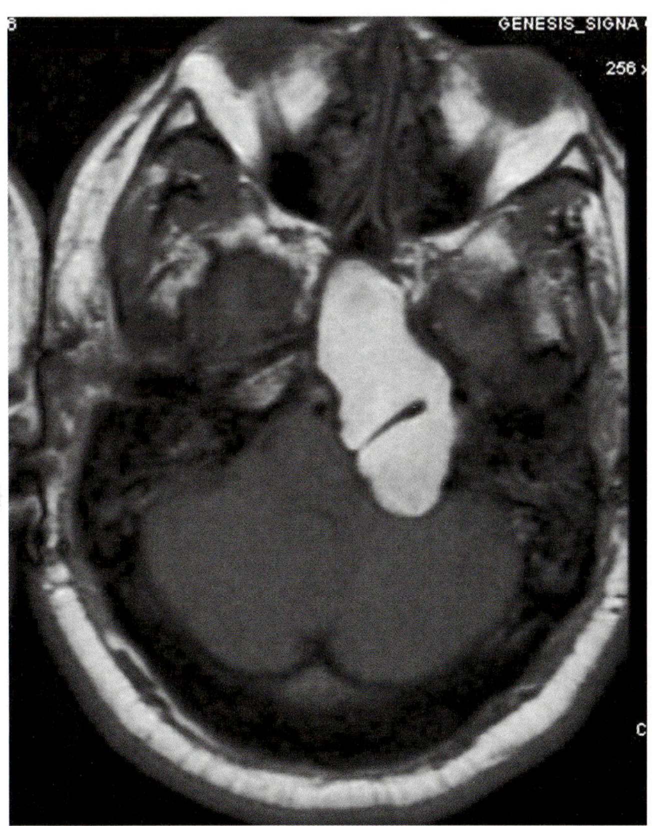

Fig. 20.8: Cholesterol granuloma. This is a T1-weighted non-contrasted axial MRI of a young adult male with a large cholesterol granuloma of the left petrous apex. The lesion is hyperintense on precontrast T1 and T2 with little contrast enhancement due to its cystic nature

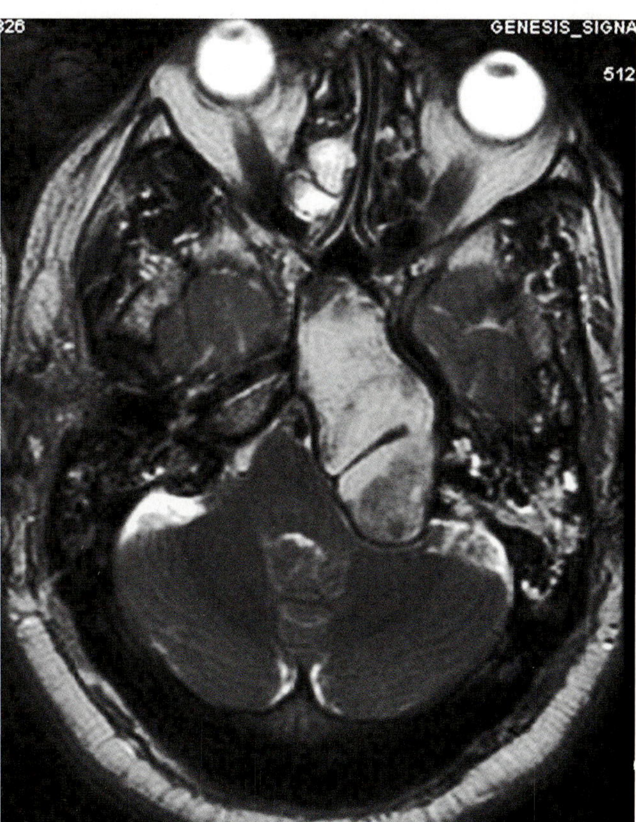

Fig. 20.9: Cholesterol granuloma. This is a T2-weighted non-contrasted axial MRI of the patient from Figure 20.8. Note the fluid signal within the left mastoid which is likely is a result of acquired eustachian tube dysfunction from mass effect. Also note the lateral displacement of the petrous internal carotid artery

the most common tumor occurring in the cerebellopontine angle. As they are benign entities, their treatment algorithm is very complex and depends on the size of the tumor, the patient's life expectancy and hearing status. They may be observed, irradiated and/or surgically removed. Patient survival with little disability is the expectant course of treatment with modern microsurgical techniques; therefore, facial nerve function has become the fundamental outcome measure because of its intimate involvement with these tumors. A more detailed discussion on the management of vestibular schwannomas is beyond the scope of this chapter.

Facial Nerve Schwannomas

As their name suggests, these facial nerve schwannomas are benign lesions that arise directly

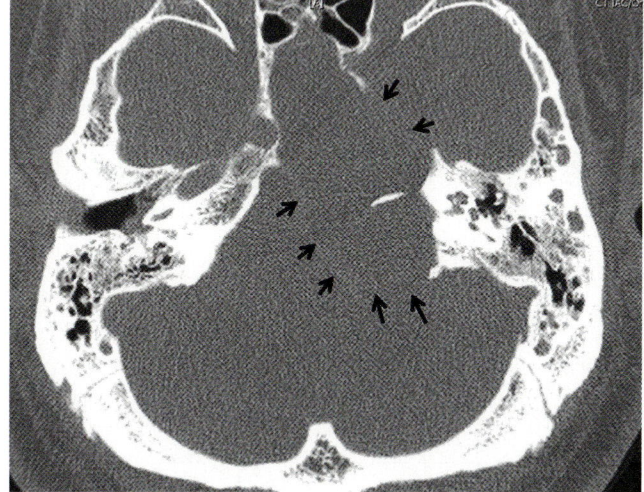

Fig. 20.10: Cholesterol granuloma. This is a non-contrasted temporal bone CT of the patient from Figures 20.8 and 20.9. Note the cystic erosion of the left petrous apex and the slight

from the facial nerve. They are the most common neoplastic lesion of the facial nerve (Thompson AL, et al. 2009) and may occur anywhere along its length. The geniculate ganglion is the most common segment involved. In addition to the symptomatology of vestibular schwannomas, there is a higher rate of facial nerve symptoms such as weakness, twitching and synkinesis as the initial presentation. The management options are similar to those of vestibular schwannomas. However, one must consider that surgical resection of a facial schwannomas has a high risk of facial nerve paresis. A prudent approach is to not perform surgical resection until the patient suffers from compressive effects of the tumor and/or facial nerve function has declined to the point where surgical resection and repair might lead to similar long term postoperative functional results (House-Brackmann grade 3 or 4). At least one author has described a technique for separation of the bulk of tumor away from the facial nerve (Perez R et al. 2005). A more modern option is decompression of the bony encasement of the nerve without resection to prolong and/or stabilize facial function once symptoms of its compromise begin. Radiosurgery raises a theoretical concern that post-radiation edema might lead to further compromise of facial nerve function given its bony confines, but at least two studies demonstrate little progression of weakness after radiation (Kida Y et al. 2007; Madhok R et al. 2009). However, in most cases, facial nerve schwannomas when diagnosed radiologically prior to surgical exploration are treated much more conservatively that vestibular schwannomas. Figures 20.11 and 20.12 demonstrate a CT scan and intraoperative picture of a left sided facial schwannoma in the mastoid sigment of the facial "canal".

Meningiomas

Meningiomas are common intracranial tumors that arise from arachnoid cap cells (Tumors of the Ear and Temporal Bone, 2000). Meningiomas that occur along the petrous apex fall into the category of petroclival meningiomas. These are traditionally difficult tumors to access given their centralized location. The spatial relationship of petroclival tumors to surrounding cranial nerves predisposes the patient to significant morbidity after surgical removal. A full discussion of petroclival meningiomas are out of the scope of this chapter, but their symptomatology varies largely with their size and involvement of adjacent cranial nerves. Treatment options are similar to those of vestibular schwannomas. However, the best surgical approach to such tumors is debated among surgeons (Bambakidis NC et al. 2007). (Fig. 20.13) depicts a large left petroclival meningioma that underwent stereotactic radiosurgery.

Geniculate Hemangiomas

Geniculate ganglion hemangiomas are vascular

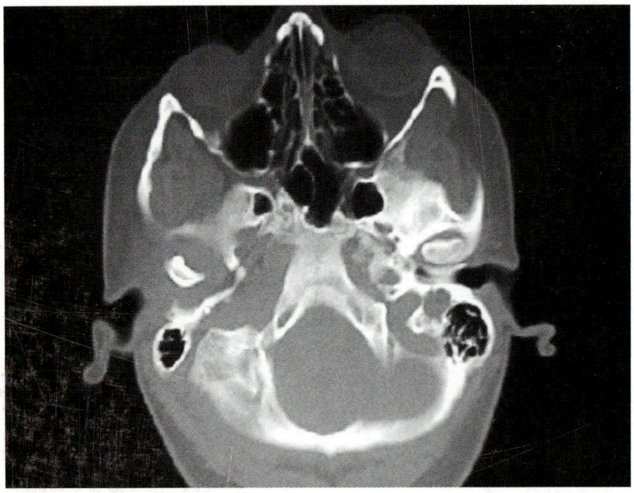

Fig. 20.11: Facial schwannoma. This is a axial non-contrasted CT scan of the temporal bone demonstrating a widened left fallopian canal due to facial schwannoma

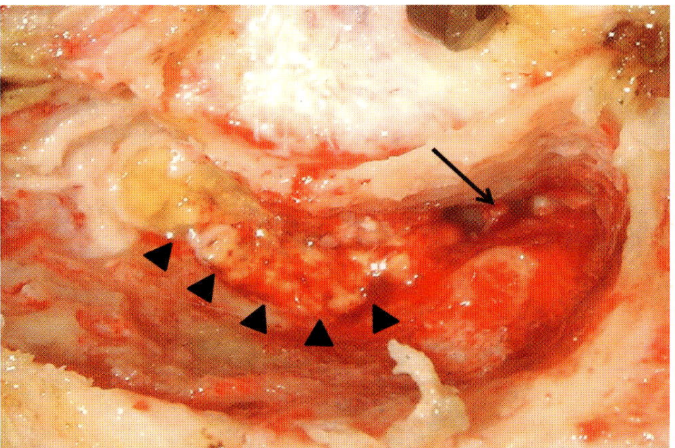

Fig. 20.12: Facial schwannoma. This is the intraoperative view of the left facial schwannoma through a transmastoid approach. The incus has been removed and the arrow points to the stapes capitulum while the arrowheads line the posterior border of the schwannoma within the fallopian canal

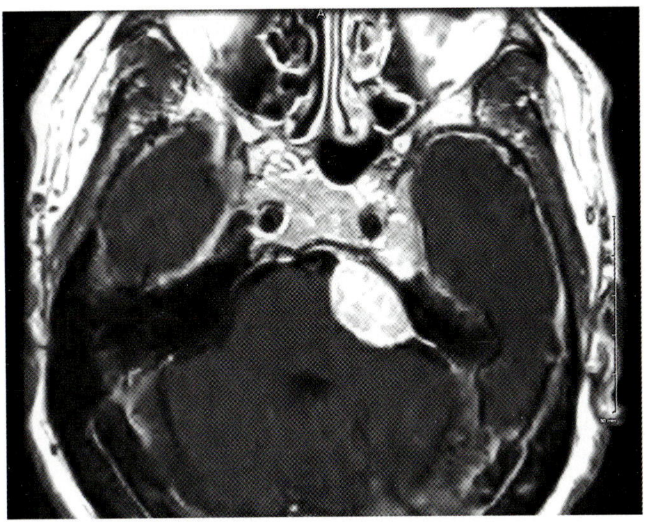

Fig. 20.13: Petroclival meningioma. This is a T1-weighted contrasted MRI of a patient with presumed left petroclival meningioma. Note the brainstem compression

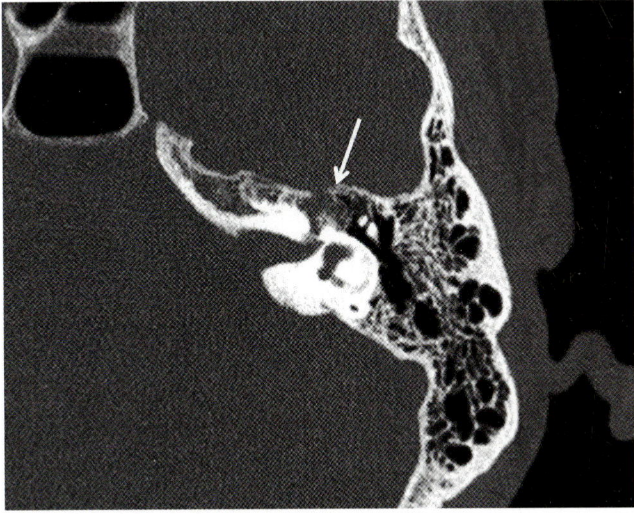

Fig. 20.14: Geniculate hemangioma. This non-contrast temporal bone CT demonstrates the spiculated appearance of bone surrounding this left geniculate hemangioma. CT *courtesy* of William Slattery of the House Clinic

malformations that likely arise from the capillary network along the geniculate ganglion and are not true endothelial neoplasms (Semaan MT et al. 2010). Facial nerve compromise may occur early with these lesions and hearing loss may occur from otic capsule erosion. Their diagnosis can be made with complementary MRI and CT imaging. These tumors may appear as hyperintense lesions on T1 and T2-weighted images and enhance with gadolinium, but they also may be difficult to distinguish from facial schwannomas by MRI alone (Friedman O et al. 2002). CT scanning may helpful in that hemangiomas have a higher tendency to display irregular bony changes ("Honeycomb" appearance) rather than smooth expansion typical of schwannomas. Observation and surgical removal of geniculate hemangiomas are the mainstays of treatment. Surgical removal often involves resection and grafting of the facial nerve. Extraneural dissection and removal of these malformations has been described (Seeman MT et al. 2010). The surgical philosophy on resection of the facial nerve with repair versus extraneural dissection of the tumor with facial nerve preservation varies by institution and surgeon preference. Figures 20.14 and 20.15 demonstrate the typical CT scan appearance of a geniculate hemangioma as well as an intraoperative transmastoid view, respectively.

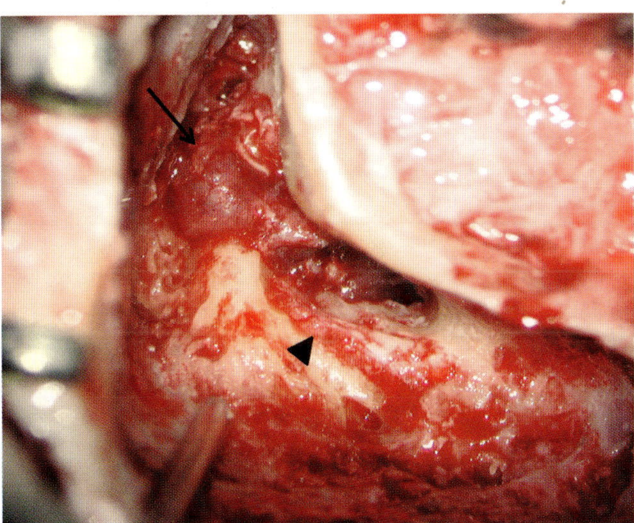

Fig. 20.15: Geniculate hemangioma. Intraoperative transmastoid view of a right facial hemangioma. The arrow points to the geniculate component while the arrowhead points to the descending facial nerve. Photo *courtesy* of William H Slattery of the House Clinic

Chondrosarcoma

Chondrosarcomas are rare malignant lesions of the skull base that arise from sphenopetroclival junction that tend to be of a low-grade histologic type. Their location predisposes affected patients to ocular cranial neuropathies, but other symptoms of lower cranial neuropathy, brainstem compression and hydrocephalus may develop with tumor enlargement. The tentative diagnosis may be indicated by MRI (hypointense or isointense on T1, heterogeneously hyperintense on T2 with variable gadolinium uptake) (Tzortzidis F et al. 2006). High resolution thin-cut CT scans of chondrosarcoma reveal an irregular expansile borders and occasional intratumoral calcification.

Historically, skull base chondrosarcomas have been grouped with the similar-appearing chordomas. Whereas the two have been difficult to distinguish from each other in the past both radiographically and histologically; immunohistochemical stains including cytokeratin and epithelial membrane antigen (EMA) has allowed each entity to be diagnosed with greater clarity. These two stains should be present primarily in chordomas rather than chondrosarcomas. As detailed below, the prognostic difference between the two entities is marked.

Figures 20.16 to 20.19 demonstrate a large chondrosarcoma centered at the right sphenopetroclival junction in a middle-aged female with a 25-year history of diploplia, increasing unsteadiness, and lancinating facial pain. Her facial nerve function and hearing was symmetric and normal as were her remaining cranial nerve function. She underwent transnasal endoscopic biopsy and debulking followed by subtotal resection via a subtemporal approach.

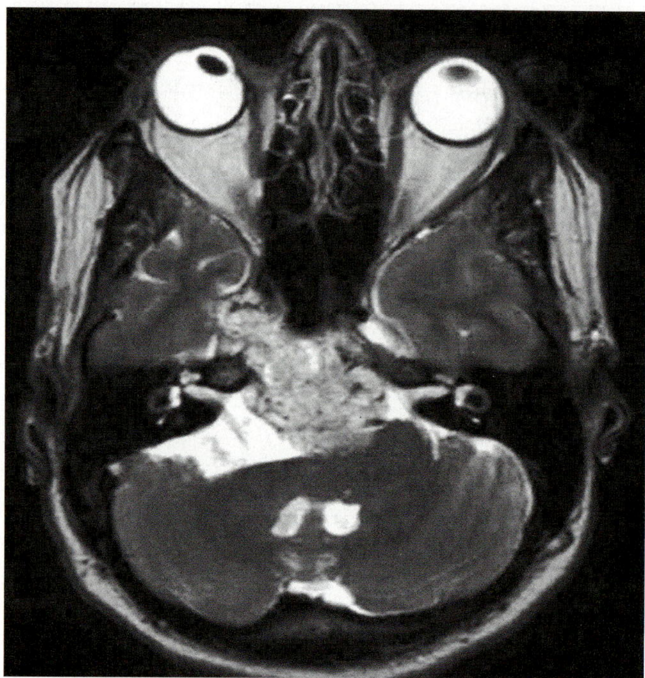

Fig. 20.17: Chondrosarcoma. This is the T2 axial image of the same patient from Figure 20.12. Note the heterogeneous signal on T2 and the obvious displacement of the brainstem. Also detectable on this image is the ipsilateral abducens palsy.

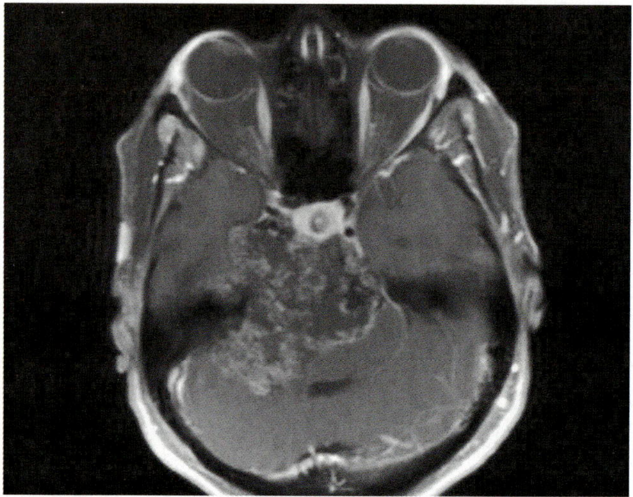

Fig. 20.16: Chondrosarcoma. This Axial T1 MRI performed with gadolinium depicts a large chondrosarcoma with heterogeneous enhancement

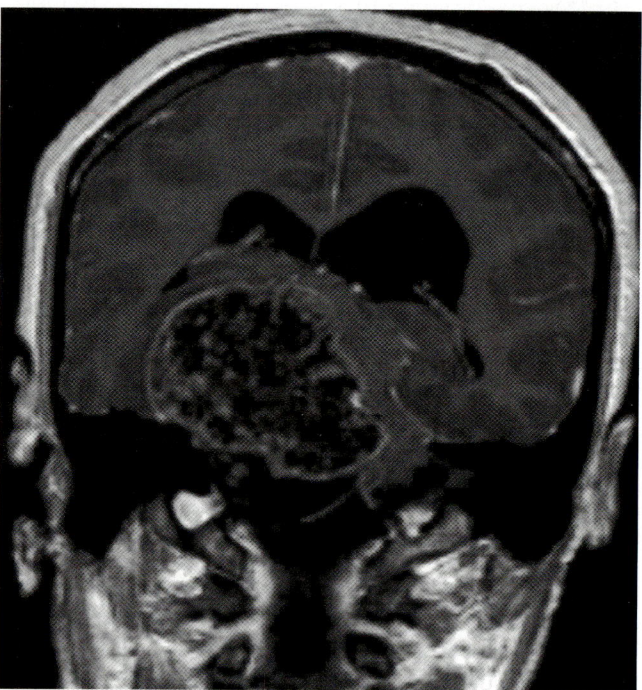

Fig. 20.18: Chondrosarcoma. Coronal contrasted T1 MRI of the patient from Figures 20.12 and 20.13. Note compression along the ventricles by the tumor

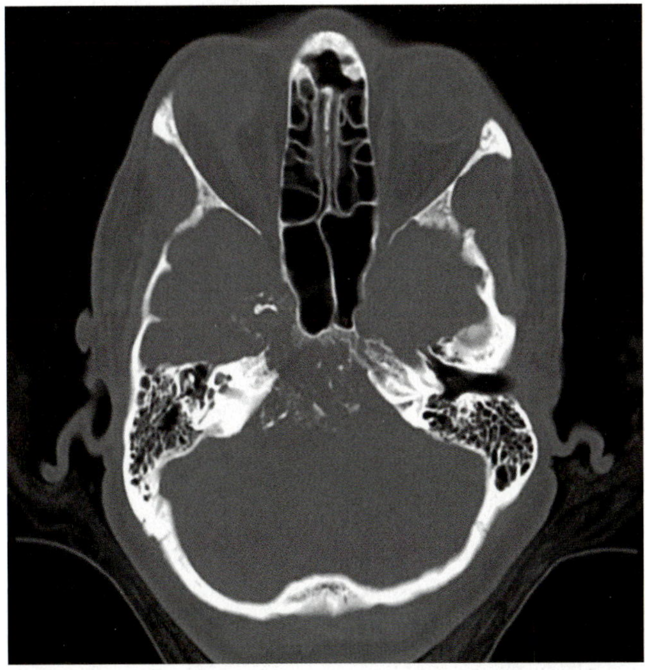

Fig. 20.19: Chondrosarcoma. Axial CT scan of the skull base. This image hints that the lesion is a chondrosarcoma rather than chordoma because it appears to be centered along the right sphenopetroclival junction. The latter tends to originate more centrally. This patient underwent transnasal biopsy and debulking confirming chondrosarcoma and then later subtemporal partial resection

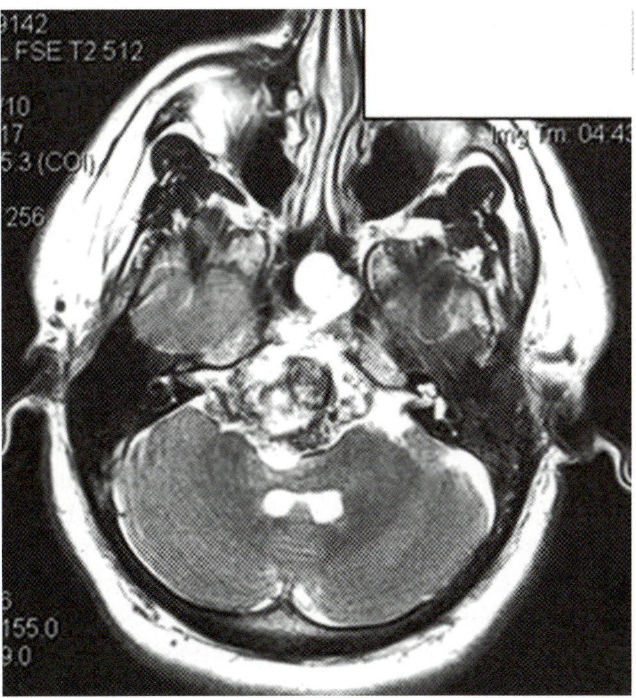

Fig. 20.20: Clival chordoma. This is an axial T2-weighted image of a young adult male with a clival chordoma. Compared to the patient from Figures 20.12 to 20.15, this lesion appears more centralized. Note its heterogeneity and the brainstem compression. The centralized nature of chordomas and chondrosarcomas makes them difficult lesions to access.

Treatment of chondrosarcomas is typically radical surgical resection with or without postoperative radiation therapy. The best surgical approach depends on the extent of the tumor and the experience and comfort level of the operative team involved. Many centers would advise postoperative radiation therapy, but in the case of total resection of a low grade tumor, the utility of radiation therapy has been brought into question (Tzortzidis F et al. 2006). A large body of literature is dedicated to the specific types of radiation therapies found to be efficacious for the treatment of skull base chondrosarcoma and chordomas. A detailed review of these studies is beyond the scope of this chapter.

Chordoma

Chordomas are tumors derived from the embryonic remnants of the primitive notochord. They tend to be more centrally located at the clivus. As aforementioned, they are differentiated from the chondrosarcoma with some level of probability by their more central location along the skull base and with certainty by immunochemical staining for cytokeratin and EMA. Figure 20.20 shows the T2-weighted MRI of a young male with a clival chordoma. The patient underwent a combined petrosal approach (middle and posterior fossa approach) to the lesion and postoperative proton beam therapy.

The surgical approaches to chordomas like chondrosarcomas depend on the extent of disease. Either lesion may be approached from anteriorly through a transnasal/transfacial open or endoscopic approach, laterally through an orbitozygomatic or preauricular subtemporal and infratemporal fossa approach, or posteriorly via a transtemporal or even retrosigmoid approach, or a combination of the above approaches. Patients will often require multiple surgical interventions via different approaches to resect extensive disease.

In a review by Al-Mefty et al. 89 chordomas and 20 chondrosarcomas were studied. All the patients underwent surgery and a majority received postoperative radiation therapy. There were no instances of recurrence or death from disease in the chondrosarcoma group while the chordoma group had a 19% mortality rate from disease and a 41.5% recurrence rate. Average follow-up from both groups was 48 months (Al-Mefty K et al. 2007).

CONGENITAL LESIONS OF THE INTERNAL AUDITORY CANAL

Lipomas (Lipochoristomas)

Lipochoristomas are very rare lesions of the internal auditory canal that can initially be confused with vestibular schwannomas. Clinically, they tend to intimately involve nerve fibers of the nerves within the internal auditory canal, possibly because they may arise from within the 8th nerve itself (Wu SS et al. 2003). Diagnosis can be made preoperatively by MRI characteristics consistent with fat. These lesions are hyperintense on precontrast and postcontrast T1 weighted images with a decrease in intensity on fat suppression sequences. Because of nerve fiber involvement and likely indolent clinical progression, conservative treatment of these lesions is the rule.

APPROACHES TO THE PETROUS APEX

Infracochlear Approach

The infracochlear approach can only be used to ventilate the petrous apex and not to perform a comprehensive exenteration of disease. With that in mind, it is ideal for drainage of cholesterol granulomas where the cyst wall need not be removed. It is intended to preserve hearing. Preoperative CT imaging is helpful to determine the size window and access available for drainage.

Technique: A standard postauricular incision is made. The bony ear canal is identified and the cartilaginous ear canal is transected. A superiorly-based tympanomeatal flap is elevated and left tethered on the umbo. The inferior 270° of ear canal skin is elevated with the flap. The inferior tympanic ring is lowered with a drill down to the level of the hypotympanic floor. Care is taken posteriorly as the facial nerve may run lateral to the level of the annulus inferiorly placing it at risk of damage. An inverted triangle is delineated with the cochlea at the superior base, the internal carotid genu anteriorly and the jugular bulb posteriorly. Within these confines, drilling proceeds medially until the cyst wall is encountered as opened. In patients with large, laterally-expanding cholesterol cysts, the drilling time is shorter. Once the cyst is opened, evacuated and irrigated, a stent or drainage tube is placed through the infracochlear triangle and a pressure equalization tube is placed through the eardrum. The tympanomeatal flap is replaced, the ear canal is packed with care not to obstruct the ventilator mechanism and the postauricular incision is closed in standard fashion (Brackmann DE et al. 2002).

Infralabyrinthine Approach

The infralabyrinthine approach is another drainage-only approach to the petrous apex and also serves to preserve inner ear hearing if good technique is used. Its main limitation is that a high-riding jugular bulb prohibits its use. This limiting factor can be determined on preoperative CT scan.

Technique: Through a standard postauricular incision, a wide cortical mastoidectomy is performed and the sigmoid sinus, incus and lateral semicircular canal are identified. With the lateral semicircular canal as a landmark, the descending facial nerve and posterior semicircular canal are skeletonized. The bone inferior to the posterior semicircular canal, anterior to the sigmoid sinus and posterior to the facial nerve is widened to identify the jugular bulb. Drilling is continued superior to the level of the jugular bulb medially until the cyst wall is encountered and opened. As with the infracochlear approach, a stent or tube is placed to maintain patency of the drainage route (Brackmann DE et al, 2002).

Subtemporal or Middle Fossa Approaches

These approaches may be used with drainage or intent to exenterate disease. As the inner ear and internal auditory canal can be navigated surgically, these approaches can be used in an effort to preserve hearing. There is an enormous variety in the technique of these approaches at every level from skin incision to the amount of bone removed from above. The reader should note that the variations and details of these surgical approaches are beyond the scope of this chapter. A standard subtemporal approach is described.

Technique: A temporal incision is made to expose

the temporalis muscle taking care not to damage the frontal branch of the facial nerve. The temporalis muscle may be either split vertically, cut in an inverted horseshoe fashion, or cut along the superior temporal line leaving a cuff of fascia for re-approximation at the end of surgery. Bare temporal squama is exposed and a temporal bone flap is elevated; this bone flap should be about 5 × 5 cm for exenterative purposes. The temporal lobe dura is elevated from the middle fossa floor beginning posteriorly to identify the true petrous ridge and extended anteriorly. Through elevation, the arcuate eminence, GSPN, middle meningeal artery, foramen ovale and margin of Meckel's cave should be identified. Occasionally, the geniculate ganglion and the internal carotid artery may be dehiscent into the middle fossa. With temporal lobe retractor in place, bony removal typically begins medially depending on the extent of disease (Sennaroglu L et al. 2003). If a drainage procedure alone is performed, a drainage catheter can be placed into the cholesterol granuloma, along the floor of the middle fossa and into the mastoid from above.

The middle fossa approach is used as a hearing preservation approach for removal of small intracanalicular tumors. The internal auditory canal can be skeletonized and decompressed from above and medial to the otic capsule for removal of such lesions.

Infratemporal Approaches

Like the middle fossa approaches, there is great variety in the techniques of infratemporal fossa approaches. The basic concept behind infratemporal fossa approaches is the detachment and inferior displacement of the zygomatic arch and temporalis muscle to expose the inferior preauricular skull base. The mandibular condyle is displaced inferiorly or resected. After identification of structures along the skull base including the lateral pterygoid plate, middle meningeal artery, V3 and internal carotid artery; the bone of the skull base is removed using a drill to approach the petrous apex. Along the way, the Eustachian tube may be identified and the petrous carotid needs to be identified and avoided. The middle meningeal artery and V3 may require transection to improve exposure of the anterior petrous apex. One is more likely to use an infratemporal approach to exenterate disease as opposed to ventilate owing to its invasiveness and lack of accessible ventilated mucosal space as a target air-filled reservoir.

Translabyrinthine Approach

The translabyrinthine approach can be used to ventilate or exenterate disease. As its name suggests, hearing is sacrificed through this approach. It is the most direct route to the petrous apex and usually requires little brain retraction.

Technique: A standard mastoidectomy is performed with skeletonization of the sigmoid sinus, middle, and posterior fossa dura. The incus, lateral semicircular canal, and descending facial nerve are identified. A labyrinthectomy is performed and the bone medial to the labyrinth is removed from middle fossa dura superiorly to jugular bulb inferiorly following the posterior fossa dura medially. In doing so, a posterior petrous apicectomy is performed and the internal auditory canal is subsequently identified. Drilling troughs superior and inferior to the internal auditory canal allows access to the anterior petrous apex. If CSF is encountered, then an abdominal fat graft may be required to obliterate the defect after the affected petrous apex has been resected. If the disease is infectious, a vascularized flap may be a better choice to obliterate the defect.

Transcochlear and Transotic Approaches

Both of these approaches are similar to the translabyrinthine approach; the major difference between the two is that the formal transcochlear approach involves more bone removal along the dura and posterior displacement of the facial nerve (Otologic Surgery, 2010).

Technique: In both approaches, a translabyrinthine craniotomy is performed with exposure of the petrous apex around the internal auditory canal. The ear canal is transected and oversewn in at least two layers to prevent cerebrospinal fluid leakage through the lateral ear canal. The bony external auditory canal is lowered to the level of the facial nerve and the cochlea is drilled away leaving tympanic facial nerve as the superior margin and the carotid artery and jugular bulb as the inferior margin of bone removal. This exposure allows more anterior exposure of the petrous apex as well as clivus.

The transcochlear approach also involves cutting the GSPN and removal of the lateral wall of the fallopian canal to allow posterior displacement of the facial nerve from brainstem to stylomastoid foramen. Such a maneuver provides a continuous view of lesions in the cerebellopontine angle but will cause a temporary facial paresis due to surgical trauma and devascularization of the facial nerve.

Combined Petrosal Approaches

Combined petrosal approaches involve combining both a posterior fossa and a middle fossa approach to access the petrous apex. The posterior fossa approaches used are typically retrolabyrinthine, translabyrinthine, and transotic/transcochlear while the middle fossa approach may also involve a petrosectomy from above. The only approach not previously described in the chapter is the retrolabyrinthine approach which involves a mastoidectomy, decompression of the posterior and middle fossa dura, and skeletonization of the labyrinth. Bony removal posterior to the sigmoid sinus is of great importance as this allows posterior displacement of the cerebellum and sigmoid sinus for greater anterior access.

The posterior fossa approach is then combined with a middle fossa approach via a temporal craniotomy followed by division of the tentorium, superior petrosal sinus, and posterior fossa dura to allow a view of the petrous apex continuously both above and below the tentorium. Division of the tentorium medially places the 4th cranial nerve at risk as it lies along the medial edge of the tentorium (Oghalai JS et al. 2003).

Transnasal Endoscopic Approaches

Endoscopic skull base surgery is a rapidly developing field. Lesions of the petrous apex may be drained or even fully resected transnasally without any external incisions. Zanation AM et al. describe their experience of 20 cases of petrous apex lesion including cholesterol granuloma, petrous apicitis and solid tumors (most commonly chondrosarcomas) managed via an endonasal endoscopic approach. The authors concluded that for selected patients this was a safe approach that avoided facial nerve damage and allowed hearing preservation in the hands of an experienced surgeon (Zanation AM et al, 2009).

BIBLIOGRAPHY

1. Almefty K, Pravdenkova S, Colli BO, et al. Chordoma and chondrosarcoma: similar, but quite different, skull base tumors. Cancer. 2007;110(11):2457-67.
2. Bambakidis NC, Kakarla UK, Kim LJ, et al. Evolution of surgical approaches in the treatment of petroclival meningiomas: a retrospective review. Neurosurgery. 2007;61(5 Suppl 2):202-9;discussion 209-11.
3. Brackmann DE, Toh EH. Surgical management of petrous apex cholesterol granulomas. Otol Neurotol. 2002;23(4):529-33.
4. Friedman O, Neff BA, Willcox TO, et al. Temporal bone hemangiomas involving the facial nerve. Otol Neurotol. 2002;23(5):760-6.
5. Isaacson B, Vrabec JT. The radiographic prevalence of geniculate ganglion dehiscence in normal and congenitally thin temporal bones. Otol Neurotol. 2007;28(1):107-110.
6. Jackler RK, Cho M. A new theory to explain the genesis of petrous apex cholesterol granuloma. Otol Neurotol. 2003;24(1):96-106; discussion 106.
7. Kefalidis G, Riga M, Argyropoulou P, et al. Is the width of the labyrinthine portion of the fallopian tube implicated in the pathophysiology of Bell's palsy?: a prospective clinical study using computed tomography. Laryngoscope. 2010;120(6):1203-7.
8. Kida Y, Yoshimoto M, Hasegawa T. Radiosurgery for facial schwannoma. J Neurosurg. 2007;106(1):24-29.
9. Madhok R, Kondziolka D, Flickinger JC, et al. Gamma knife radiosurgery for facial schwannomas. Neurosurgery. 2009;64(6):1102-5; discussion 1105.
10. Oghalai JS, Jackler RK. Anatomy of the combined retrolabyrinthine-middle fossa craniotomy. Neurosurg Focus. 2003;14(6):e8.
11. Otologic Surgery. 3rd edn. Philadelphia, PA: Elsevier; 2010.
12. Perez R, Chen JM, Nedzelski JM. Intratemporal facial nerve schwannoma: a management dilemma. Otol Neurotol. 2005;26(1):121-6.
13. Semaan MT, Slattery WH, Brackmann DE. Geniculate ganglion hemangiomas: clinical results and long-term follow-up. Otol Neurotol. 2010;31(4):665-70.
14. Sennaroglu L, Slattery WH. Petrous anatomy for middle fossa approach. Laryngoscope. 2003;113(2):332-42.
15. Thompson AL, Aviv RI, Chen JM, et al. Magnetic resonance imaging of facial nerve schwannoma. Laryngoscope. 2009;119(12):2428-36.
16. Tumors of the Ear and Temporal Bone: Lippincott Williams & Wilkins; 2000.
17. Tzortzidis F, Elahi F, Wright DC, et al. Patient outcome at long-term follow-up after aggressive microsurgical resection of cranial base chondrosarcomas. Neurosurgery. 2006;58(6):1090-8; discussion 1090-8.
18. Visosky AM, Isaacson B, Oghalai JS. Circumferential

21

Anesthesia for Otologic Surgery

CM Despande, Aditi N Modi

INTRODUCTION

The important role of an anesthesiologist in any surgery is not only to give pain relief to the patient; but also to provide an excellent operative field, as hemorrhage is a problem for both the surgeon and the anesthesiologist. In microsurgery of the ear, a near bloodless field is essential. The magnification offered by the operating microscope makes even minimal bleeding appear excessive, thus making surgery very difficult. Since 1917, intentionally reducing arterial blood pressure to moderately hypotensive levels during surgery has been used to provide a good surgical field. When such a deliberate hypotension is combined with the proper positioning of the patient such that the operative site is above the heart level, permitting gravitational venous drainage away from the wound to the dependent portions of the body, the technique has been named Controlled Hypotension or Induced Hypotension.

ANESTHETIC AIMS FOR MIDDLE EAR SURGERIES

- Thorough preoperative preparation which includes:
  - Anxiolysis
  - Control and optimization of systemic medical diseases
  - Treatment of active infection of the surgical site
- Maintenance of an adequate depth of anesthesia, ventilation and deliberate hypotensive measures
- Providing anesthetic conditions to facilitate intraoperative facial nerve monitoring
- Smooth calm awakening and extubation
- Prevention of postoperative nausea and vomiting
- Adequate postoperative analgesia.

Thorough Preoperative Preparation

Anxiolysis

To ensure a calm and relaxed patient in the preoperative period. This can be achieved by:
- Establishment of good rapport with the patient
- Drugs:
  - *Benzodiazepines*: These cause sedation and anxiolysis.
- For example; oral diazepam 0.2 mg/kg on the night prior to the surgery or

- Intravenous midazolam 0.03-0.07 mg/kg as premedication
  - *Antihistaminics*: These are beneficial in view of their sedative, anti-tussive and antiemetic properties. For example, intravenous promethazine 0.5 mg/kg as premedication.
  - *α 2-adrenergic agonists*: For example, oral clonidine 3-4 mcg/kg as premedication.
  - *β-blockers*: For example, intravenous metoprolol 0.1 mg/kg as premedication.

Optimization of Systemic Medical Diseases

Optimization of systemic medical diseases like hypertension and uncontrolled diabetes is important so that hemodynamic instabilities and fluctuations do not lead to troublesome oozing of blood in the surgical field and interfere with wound healing.

Treatment of Active Infection

Eliminating an active infection is very important.

Induced Hypotension

It is known that a patient who is awake and conscious bleeds less than a patient who is under general anesthesia. However, all patients do not allow surgery under local anesthetic infiltration and any movement of the patient during surgery may hamper success of the operative procedure.

The anesthetist's skill lies in providing conditions that give the surgeon:
- The best operative field to operate with precision
- To permit accurate delineation of lesions without trauma to the surrounding delicate structures
- To indirectly help improve viability of grafts and diminish hematoma formation
- Reducing overall sepsis and fibrosis.

Blood loss during surgery depends on bleeding from the cut vessels. It may be divided into arterial, capillary or venous.

Arterial bleeding: It is related to the mean arterial pressure and heart rate. It can be decreased by a reduction in mean arterial pressure or the heart rate.

Capillary bleeding: It is dependent upon the local blood flow and can be reduced by local vasoconstriction achieved by infiltration of vasopressors like adrenaline.

Venous bleeding: It is related to venous return and venous tone and thus can be dependent on posture. It can be reduced by the use of vasodilators like sodium nitroprusside and nitroglycerine and proper positioning of the patient to promote venous drainage.

Methods of Achieving Induced Hypotension (Simpson et al. 1992).

Physical Methods

Posture: A 2.5 centimeter elevation (i.e. a 10°-15° elevation) of surgical site reduces blood pressure by 2 mm Hg by:
- Improving the venous drainage
- Producing relative regional ischemia if the operative site is above the level of the heart.

  Augmenting the effect of agents like sympathetic ganglion blocking drugs.

Thus, for surgery in the head and neck region such as the middle ear surgery, a little head elevation is very effective in reducing hemorrhage at the operative site.

Physiological Methods

Effect of intermittent positive pressure ventilation (IPPV) and controlled ventilation: Under normal circumstances venous return to heart occurs during inspiration when the negative intrathoracic pressure enhances blood flow to the heart. During IPPV, inspiration is associated with positive intrathoracic pressure leading to reduction in venous return which will in turn reduce the mean arterial pressure.

Thus, IPPV is a useful adjunct to any hypotensive technique as it:
- Augments any pharmacological method to decrease the arterial pressure.

  Applies positive end expiratory pressure (PEEP) to airways thus limiting venous return and assisting in reduction of arterial blood pressure.

Moderate hypocapnea: Carbon dioxide is a vasodilator. Thus, reduction in carbon dioxide ($PaCO_2$) to 30 mm Hg leads to vasoconstriction. Hypocapnea can be achieved by moderate hyperventilation.

Pharmacological Methods

Mean arterial pressure (MAP) is the most important factor determining the extent of intraoperative bleeding. MAP is directly related to cardiac output

(CO) and systemic vascular resistance (SVR).

$$MAP = CO \times SVR$$

Cardiac output is in turn dependent upon myocardial contractility determining stroke volume (SV) and heart rate (HR).

$$CO = SV \times HR$$

Peripheral vasodilatation is controlled by sympathetic activity. Thus, sympathetic blockade leads to vasodilatation leading to decreased venous return and decrease in cardiac output and hence mean arterial pressure.

- *Local*: Local infiltration using sympathomimetic amines.

  Adrenaline is used frequently to induce local vasoconstriction. Concentration should be sufficient to induce vasoconstriction without causing intense or persistent vasospasm. Concentration commonly used is 1:200000-1:400000; total dose should not exceed 10 mg/kg.

- *Systemic*:
  - *Propofol*: It is a non-barbiturate induction agent. It has a rapid onset of action which is within one arm-brain circulation time and clinical recovery occurs within 10-15 minutes even after prolonged infusion
- Propofol causes fall in systemic vascular resistance leading to hypotension that is greater than one seen with thiopentone
- It causes mild bradycardia probably due to central vagal activity
- It attenuates pressor response to laryngoscopy and intubation
- It is an antiemetic
- It depresses pharyngeal and laryngeal reflexes thus laryngospasm and bronchospasm is uncommon with use of propofol
- It also reduces the intracranial pressure.

  Clinical uses of propofol are as an induction and maintenance agent, hypotensive agent and for its cerebroprotective action.

  Dose of propofol in adults is 2-2.5 mg/kg intravenously for induction of anesthesia and 4-12 mg/kg/hr intravenously for maintenance of anesthesia.

- *Remifentanil*: Remifentanil is a synthetic opioid analgesic. It is a phenylpiperidine derivative of fentanyl (a pure mu opioid agonist), with a similar potency. It is the ideal agent for intravenous administration as an infusion in combination with an intravenous anesthetic agent like propofol used for maintenance of anesthesia and provision of deliberate hypotension. It is available as a powder to be constituted and diluted before use with 5% dextrose or 0.9% saline. The usual dose range is 0.03-3.00 mcg/kg/min. Opioid induced bradycardia and hypotension along with respiratory depression which obviates the need for administering repeated doses of muscle relaxants; make ideal anesthetic and operating conditions for facial nerve surgery.

The combination of propofol and remifentanil as a total intravenous anesthesia regime (TIVA), provide ideal perioperative conditions for middle ear surgery.

- *Volatile anesthetic agents*: Halogenated inhalational anesthetic agents such as halothane, enflurane, isoflurane and the newer sevoflurane are the most commonly used agents which maintain intra-operative anesthesia and help in reduction of mean arterial blood pressure (Eltringham et al. 1982).
- *Halothane*: It causes moderate degree of peripheral vasodilatation, thus reducing the total peripheral vascular resistance. It also has a direct effect on the myocardium leading to bradycardia and decrease in cardiac output in small concentrations. In higher concentrations, it leads to increased intracranial tension and severe myocardial depression. It can also sensitize the myocardium to catecholamines giving rise to dangerous ventricular arrhythmias, thus should be used with caution in conjunction with adrenaline infiltration. Hence, it is best avoided in otoneurosurgery.
- *Enflurane*: The mechanism of action is the same as halothane. The myocardial depression and vagal stimulation is more significant if excessive dose is used. It is also known to be epiletogenic, hence best avoided in otoneurosurgery.
- *Isoflurane*: It has minimal effect on myocardium at low inspired concentration. It causes peripheral vasodilatation that can be controlled by altering the inspired concentration. It is non-arrhythmogenic, as unlike halothane it does not sensitize the myocardium to endogenous and exogenous catecholamines. It is a good agent to use in otoneurosurgery.
- *Sevoflurane*: Actions are similar to isoflurane. Because of rapid induction, better hemodynamic profile and rapid recovery it is preferred.

- *Desflurane*: Actions are similar to isoflurane and sevoflurane. But as compared with all the above volatile anesthetic agents, desflurane has the fastest onset and recovery profile with minimal organ dependent metabolism. It requires a special electrical vaporizer because of its low boiling point (23°C), which can make using desflurane slightly more expensive if not used appropriately with very low-flow anesthetic techniques.
    - *Muscle relaxants*: Various depolarizing and non-depolarizing agents are used in anesthesia practice. Non-depolarizing muscle relaxants like pancuronium, vecuronium, rocuronium and atracurium are most commonly used in the intraoperative period to achieve muscle relaxation.
- *Vecuronium*: This intermediate acting non-depolarizing muscle relaxant is advantageous in view of its cardiostable properties. It attenuates rise in blood pressure and heart rate, thus maintaining a near normal, in fact, lower pulse rate; aiding the deliberate hypotensive technique.
- Rocuronium is essentially, a rapid onset acting vecuronium, which can be easily and specifically reversed by suggammadex.
    - *Hypotensive agents*
- *α-adrenergic blockers*: These drugs include phentolamine and phenoxybenzamine. The main clinical use of these drugs is for pheochromocytoma and certain hypertensive emergencies.
- *β-adrenergic blockers*: These drugs bind selectively to β-adrenergic receptors and interfere with ability of catecholamines or other sympathomimetics to provoke the beta response. The main advantages of β-blockers are the reduction of heart rate and cardiac output by reducing myocardial contractility. Maintenance of a slow heart rate without any additional hypotension controllably reduces bleeding. They can also be used to counteract the tachycardia caused by the ganglion blocking agents or the direct acting vasodilators. Common β-blockers are propranolol, esmolol, metoprolol and labetelol.

Metoprolol, is a selective β-1 adrenergic receptor antagonist. It prevents inotropic and chronotropic response while conserving the bronchodilator, vasodilator and metabolic effects of β-2 receptors intact. Its duration of action is 3-4 hours. It is given in the dose of 0.1 mg/kg intravenously at the time of induction of anesthesia to reduce hypertensive response to intubation and surgical stimulus as well as to reduce intraoperative bleeding (Benfield et al. 1986).

- *Vasodilators*:
    a. *Sodium nitroprusside*: It is an arterial dilator. It allows the rapid reduction in arterial blood pressure and equally rapid restoration to normal value. It is the only drug capable of producing 'Dial a pressure' hypotension over short periods. As a vasodilator it causes an increase in intracranial tension, and so should not be used during neurosurgery before the skull is opened in a patient with increased intracranial tension. A major side effect is cyanide poisoning when used in high doses and over prolonged period. It is used in the dose of 0.3-10 µg/kg/min intravenously to produce controlled hypotension during surgery and anesthesia and for treatment of hypertensive emergencies. An invasive blood pressure monitor is essential while using this drug.
    b. *Nitroglycerin*: It is predominantly a venodilator. It produces a steady and less dramatic reduction in arterial blood pressure with greater effect on systolic blood pressure than diastolic blood pressure and therefore, can be used without invasive arterial pressure monitoring. It maintains the blood flow to vital organs and improves coronary blood supply. It is used in the dose of 0.5-5 µg/kg/min.
- *α 2-adrenergic agonists*: The perioperative use of α 2- adrenergic agonists is finally coming of age. Since a decade now, clonidine has been registered for clinical use and dexmedetomidine has been approved for use in anesthesia in recent times. The clinical responses to α 2-agonists are predictable based on the physiology of α 2-adrenergic receptors (Takahiko et al. 2000).

α 2-Adrenoceptor agonists have several beneficial actions during the perioperative period. They decrease sympathetic tone, attenuate the neuroendocrine and hemodynamic responses to laryngoscopy, intubation, anesthesia and surgery, reduce anesthetic and opioid requirements and cause sedation and analgesia. They decrease intraoperative lability of blood pressure thus maintains stable hemodynamics. They allow psychomotoric function to be preserved. They prevent postoperative shivering.

Clonidine is a selective partial agonist for α 2-adrenoreceptors that decreases sympathetic nervous system output from central nervous system (CNS). It is rapidly and completely absorbed after oral administration and reaches a peak plasma level within 60-90 minutes by this route; elimination half-life being between 8-12 hours. Sedation, anxiolysis and anti-sialogogue action are all attractive attributes of clonidine making it a preferred premedication agent.

Preoperative clonidine in doses of 3-5 μg/kg is known to decrease postoperative pain and analgesic requirements.

Use of clonidine in middle ear surgeries is preferred for the following reasons:
- Calm sedated patient preoperatively
- Smooth induction with attenuated intubation response
- Stable hemodynamics in the intraoperative period with mild bradycardia and hypotension enabling maintenance of a clear surgical field
- Reduction of anesthetic requirement of nitrous oxide and other anesthetic agents for maintenance of anesthesia
- Sedated but arousable and responsive patient in the postoperative period facilitating smooth extubation
- Reduction of postoperative nausea and vomiting
- Reduction of postoperative analgesic requirement.

Dose: 3-5 μg/kg oral tablets in young (18-55 years of age) normal patients about 60 minutes prior to surgery give best results.

Dexmedetomidine is a much more selective α 2-adrenoreceptor agonist compared to clonidine. Dexmedetomidine is shorter-acting drug than clonidine and has a reversal drug for its sedative effect, atipamezole. These properties render dexmedetomidine suitable for sedation and analgesia during the whole perioperative period: as premedication, as an anesthetic adjunct for general and regional anesthesia, and as postoperative sedative and analgesic. The mechanism of action is unique and differs from those of currently used sedative agents, including clonidine. Activation of the receptors in the brain and spinal cord inhibits neuronal firing, causing hypotension, bradycardia, sedation and analgesia. It also leads to decreased salivation, decreased secretion, decreased bowel motility, contraction of vascular and other

smooth muscle, inhibition of renin release, increased glomerular filtration and increased secretion of sodium and water in the kidney, decreased intraocular pressure and decreased insulin release from the pancreas. Dexmedetomidine combines all these effects, thus avoiding some of the side effects of multiagent therapies.

A bolus of dexmedetomidine, 50 mcg/kg/min diluted to 10 ml in normal saline intravenous given over 20 mins, 30 mins before induction of anesthesia and 7 mcg/kg/min (10 ml/min) thereafter until the end of surgery.

Some studies have shown that dexmedetomidine anesthesia raises the tympanometric parameters, however they never exceeded the limits of normal.

- *Magnesium Sulfate*: This drug has recently found a widespread increase in use because of its varied actions. It causes vasodilatation, helping to lower blood pressure which is pertinent to its potential role in middle ear surgery. It also acts peripherally at the neuromuscular junction, decreasing acetylcholine release and may in higher doses and continuous use prolong the duration of action of muscle relaxants; but this is insignificant for a single intraoperative dose. Dose is 0.5-2 gm (2-8 mmol) slowly intravenously.

Use of nitrous oxide: Nitrous oxide is a highly diffusible gas known to enter all body cavities causing them to distend. It diffuses into the middle ear cavity, raising its intracavitary pressure and distending it. This can have detrimental effects; so ideally, nitrous oxide must be discontinued from the anesthetic mixture about 30 minutes before temporalis fascia graft placement and can be restarted after the same.

Prevention of Postoperative Nausea and Vomiting

Postoperative nausea and vomiting (PONV) was known to be one of the common sequel of general anesthesia and surgery. However, in this era of modern day-case anesthesia and surgery, the incidence of PONV has decreased considerably owing to:
- Advances in surgical techniques associated with a reduction in surgical and hence anesthesia time
- Use of anesthetic agents with inherent antiemetic properties
- Use of micromotor drills minimizing vestibular stimulation.

Drugs commonly used for prophylactic antiemesis are:

- Intravenous metochlorpromide: 0.2 mg/kg as a premedicant or after induction
- Intravenous dexamethasone: 0.25 mg/kg at induction
- Intravenous ondansetron: 0.1 mg/kg before reversal
- Intravenous promethazine: 0.5 mg/kg as a premedicant
- Intravenous propofol: As a maintenance anesthetic agent as it has significant antiemetic properties by virtue of its potential antagonist action at D2 dopamine receptor
- Use of oral clonidine as a premedication.

Smooth Calm Awakening and Extubation

It is essential to have a sedated, yet arousable patient postoperatively to avoid a stormy recovery.

Analgesia

Pre-emptive analgesia, i.e. obtaining an adequate state of analgesia without waiting for the patient to complain of pain and then supplementing analgesic medications is the sine-qua-non of modern balanced anesthesia.

Intraoperative Facial Nerve Monitoring

The probability of iatrogenic injury to the facial nerve during microsurgery of the ear can be reduced by facial nerve monitoring. (Herbert Silverstein, 1991). Anesthesia per se' may interfere with routine facial nerve monitoring and the factors are:

- *Level of anesthesia*: Light levels of anesthesia have been shown to cause spontaneous muscle contraction artifacts that may be detected by an EMG monitoring system. If the patient awakens, the EMG may get activated. Therefore, it is a must to have an adequate depth of anesthesia around the time that this sort of monitoring is required.
- *Drugs*: Muscle relaxants may inhibit muscle contractions and electrical activity. Sometimes the effects of these drugs linger and reduce the sensitivity of the facial nerve to stimulation. Stimulation of peripheral nerves by a stimulator can demonstrate whether the effect of the relaxant is still present; thus using a peripheral nerve stimulator becomes empirical in all cases where facial nerve monitoring is essential. Moreover, the use of a remifentanil infusion may reduce the need of administering muscle relaxants too frequently.

- *Electrical interference*: Noise from electrocautery units, video equipment, and other monitoring equipment can cause false muscle contraction artifacts in the EMG monitoring system. Hence as far as possible, the volumes of all monitors inside the operation theater should be kept to a minimum audible tone.

SUMMARY

Both local anesthesia and general anesthesia have their own applications in otologic surgeries. However, general anesthesia has the advantage of better control over the hemodynamic status and muscle relaxation, which is most important in advanced otologic surgeries. A wider spectrum of surgeries can be done under general anesthesia such as facial nerve decompressions, acoustic neuroma and vestibular nerve sections. Thus, general anesthesia has a definite place in the further advancement of otologic microsurgery.

BIBLIOGRAPHY

1. Benfield Paul, Clissold Stephen P. Metoprolol Drugs. 1986;31:376-429.
2. Celil Uslu, Guldem Turan, Emine Dincer, et al. Comparison of Dexmedetomidine, Remifentanil and Esmolol in Controlled Hypotensive Anaesthesia, Internet J Anesthesiol. 2008.
3. Durmus M, But AK, Dogan Z, et al. Effect of dexmedetomidine on bleeding during tympanoplasty or septorhinoplasty. Euro J Anesthesiol. 2007;24(5):447-53.
4. Eltringham RJ. Hypotensive anesthesia for microsurgery of the ear, a comparison between Halothane and Enflurane. Anesthesia. 1982;37:1028-32.
5. Farah Nasreen, Shahjahan Bano, Rashid Manzoor Khan, et al. Dexmedetomidine used to provide hypotensive anesthesia during middle ear surgery. Indian J Otolaryngol Head & Neck Sur. 2009;61(3):205-7.
6. Herbert Silverstein, Seth Rosenberg. Intraoperative Facial Nerve Monitoring, Otolaryngol Clinics N Am. 1991;24(3):709-14.
7. JH Ryu, IS Sohn SH Do. Controlled hypotension for middle ear surgery: a comparison between remifentanil and magnesium sulphate. Br J Anaesth. 2009; 103(4):490-5.
8. Simpson P. Perioperative blood loss and its reduction-the role of the anesthetist. Br J Anes. 1992;69:498-507.
9. Takahiko Kamibayashi, Katsumi Harasawa, Mervyn Maze. Alpha 2 Adrenergic Agonists: Recent Advances in Anesthesia Analgesia. 2000;21:1-7.

Index

Page numbers followed by *f* refer to figure and *t* refer to table